WEST SLOPE COMMUNITY

WASHINGTON

D0016142

The Autoimmune Solution

The Autoimmune Solution

Prevent and Reverse the
Full Spectrum of Inflammatory
Symptoms and Diseases

Amy Myers, M.D.

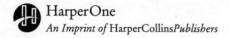

HarperOne
An Imprint of HarperCollins*Publishers*

HarperOne

This book contains advice and information relating to health care. It should be used to supplement rather than replace the advice of your doctor or another trained health professional. If you know or suspect you have a health problem, it is recommended that you seek your physician's advice before embarking on any medical program or treatment. All efforts have been made to assure the accuracy of the information contained in this book as of the date of publication. This publisher and the author disclaim liability for any medical outcomes that may occur as a result of applying the methods suggested in this book.

THE AUTOIMMUNE SOLUTION: *Prevent and Reverse the Full Spectrum of Inflammatory Symptoms and Diseases.* Copyright © 2015 by Amy Myers, M.D. All rights reserved. Printed in the United States of America. No part of this book may be used or reproduced in any manner whatsoever without written permission except in the case of brief quotations embodied in critical articles and reviews. For information, address HarperCollins Publishers, 195 Broadway, New York, NY 10007.

HarperCollins books may be purchased for educational, business, or sales promotional use. For information, please e-mail the Special Markets Department at SPsales@harpercollins.com.

HarperCollins website: www.harpercollins.com

HarperCollins®, 📖®, and HarperOne™ are trademarks of HarperCollins Publishers.

FIRST EDITION

Designed by Terry McGrath
Interior illustrations by Ali Fine

Library of Congress Cataloging-in-Publication Data
Myers, Amy
The autoimmune solution : prevent and reverse the full spectrum of inflammatory symptoms and diseases / Amy Myers, MD.
    pages cm
ISBN 978-0-06-234747-3
1. Autoimmune diseases—Popular works. I. Title.
RC600.M94 2015
616.97'8—dc23   2014017620

15 16 17 18 19   RRD(H)   10 9 8 7 6 5 4

To DAD
and
those with autoimmune conditions.
May you find another way and
a solution in this book.

Contents

Part One

The Autoimmune Epidemic

CHAPTER 1

My Autoimmune Journey— and Yours

ABOUT TEN YEARS AGO I developed an autoimmune condition—and conventional medicine failed me. I don't want it to fail you too.

If you're one of the fifty million Americans suffering from an autoimmune disease, this book is for you. If you're one of the hundreds of millions of people struggling with an inflammatory condition that puts you at risk for developing an autoimmune disease—disorders like arthritis, asthma, eczema, or cardiovascular disease—this book is for you. And if you're one of the millions of people whose parent, spouse, sibling, friend, or child is currently coping with an autoimmune condition, this book is for you too. Whether you want to reverse your autoimmune disorder, keep from getting an autoimmune disorder, or support someone who has an autoimmune disorder, this book can change your life.

I'm an M.D. myself, so I don't like to criticize other doctors, let alone their standard protocols, but the truth must be told: When it comes to the treatment of autoimmune conditions, conventional medicine has failed miserably. The typical weapons of choice are medications that might or might not ease your symptoms; that might disrupt your life with harsh side effects; that often keep you permanently anxious about the possibility of developing an infection; and that might stop working after a few years, causing you to take even more powerful medications. The accepted philosophy is that autoimmune disorders are inevitable, that they can be managed but neither prevented nor reversed. The result is that patients are reduced to complete dependence on their doctors and their prescribed medications, unable to live their lives without constant fear and often without pain.

In these pages, I'll show you how to use a healthy diet, lifestyle, and high-quality supplements to eliminate symptoms, get off your medications, and enjoy the kind of vibrant, total health you've always wanted. I'll show you why changing your diet and healing your gut can make a world of difference, along with freeing your body of its toxic burden, healing your infections, and reducing your load of stress. I'll help you take charge of your health, making the choices that support your body and keep you glowing, fit, and full of energy.

Why do I sound so confident? Because over the years I've treated thousands of patients with this approach—and I've also treated myself. Like I said, conventional medicine failed me, so I had to develop an autoimmune solution, one that would help me overcome the staggering side effects of conventional treatments and enable me to live a busy, healthy life.

If you give me just thirty days, I can help you take back your life too. If you suffer from autoimmunity, I can show you how to reverse your disorder, eliminate your symptoms, and even get off your medications. If you suffer from an inflammatory condition, I can help you heal that condition and keep it from turning into a full-blown autoimmune disorder. If you know someone who is struggling with autoimmunity, I can teach you how to offer your loved one the kind of support and guidance that could make a life-changing difference.

Sound good? Then let's get started. I can't wait for you to find your own autoimmune solution.

THE FAILURE OF CONVENTIONAL MEDICINE

Before we look at the much-needed alternative, let's take a quick tour of what most of you or your loved ones are dealing with, or of what you might be dealing with if your inflammatory condition turns into autoimmunity. You might start out bouncing from doctor to doctor because nobody can figure out what's wrong with you. There are more than one hundred recognized autoimmune conditions and many are not well understood by conventional medicine.

As a result, most doctors and care providers are at a loss if you come in with a collection of autoimmune-like symptoms that don't quite match a diagnosis they recognize. This problem is compounded by the way conventional medicine has been fractured into so many discrete specialties. If you are diagnosed with an autoimmune condition, you don't go see an "immune specialist" (unless you come to see me!). You are more likely shuttled off to a specialist who focuses on the system that is being attacked: a rheumatologist for rheumatoid arthritis; a gastroenterologist for celiac disease, Crohn's disease, and ulcerative colitis; an endocrinologist for Graves' disease, Hashimoto's thyroiditis, and diabetes; and so on. And if you have two autoimmune conditions, as many people do, you are likely to see two separate specialists; for three conditions, three specialists; and so on.

This fragmentation suggests that your problem is a disease of a particular organ, but in fact, it is a disease of the immune system as a whole. All these diseases—despite affecting different organ systems—stem from the same common cause: an immune system gone rogue. My approach is based on getting to the root of the problem: removing the elements that derailed your immune system in the first place and strengthening your immune system rather than suppressing it. That's why using this approach enables you to reverse and prevent many different autoimmune conditions at once.

Because there is a genetic component to autoimmune disorders, your doctor might be especially concerned if you have a family history of autoimmunity that includes at least one parent, sibling, aunt, uncle, or grandparent. You might have begun searching for answers when you realized that one or more people in your family had a condition like rheumatoid arthritis, Crohn's disease, lupus, or Hashimoto's thyroiditis.

Whether or not you have a family history, you are likely to hear that your genes hold the key to whether or not you will develop autoimmunity, that there is nothing you can do to prevent it and no way to reverse it once it strikes. This can make the search for a diagnosis rather ominous, since at the end of the road is not a promise of health but only the prospect of an ever-worsening disease.

How an Autoimmune Disease Progresses

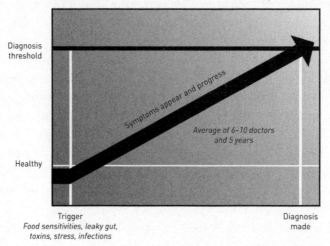

In most cases, your primary care doctor will send you to a special-ist, either with or without a diagnosis—perhaps a rheumatologist, endo-crinologist, gastroenterologist, or neurologist. If you have been diagnosed with a painful, debilitating condition such as rheumatoid arthritis—an inflammation of the joints—the specialist will likely tell you that this disorder, like all autoimmune diseases, is irreversible. The joint pain that sent you to the doctor in the first place? Well, that was just the beginning. Eventually it will become so severe, so disabling, that you'll be in more or less constant pain, and you'll find it very difficult to move. Forget about enjoying a romantic walk along the beach or taking your grandkids to the amusement park. You'll be lucky if you can climb a flight of stairs or take a quick drive to the mall.

The specialist will offer you an array of powerful medications to combat your symptoms and ease your pain.

"What about side effects?" you ask.

"Well, yes, these drugs have significant side effects," she replies. "They are something you are going to have to learn to live with."

Or perhaps your diagnosis is a milder one, such as Hashimoto's thyroiditis, a condition in which your immune system attacks your thyroid and keeps it from producing enough thyroid hormone. Now your specialist has far more cheerful news to share: You just have to take a thyroid hormone supplement every day for the rest of your life. But the medication is inexpensive, you won't notice any side effects, and even though your dosage will probably keep increasing, life will basically go on as before.

You don't really like the idea of your thyroid slowly, steadily being destroyed by your own body. Still, the doctor's suggestions don't sound so bad—until you go home and do your own research. You soon discover a fact that most doctors don't share with their patients: Having even one autoimmune condition makes you three times more likely to develop another. What if the next one is some-

WARNING SIGNS

An autoimmune condition is one in which a disordered immune system begins attacking the body's own tissue. The following symptoms and/ or diagnoses could signal either a full-blown autoimmune disease or an inflamed immune system that is at risk of becoming autoimmune:

- acid reflux
- acne
- ADD/ADHD
- allergies
- Alzheimer's
- anxiety
- arthritis
- asthma
- B12 deficiency
- blood clots
- brain fog (difficulty focusing or just not feeling "sharp")
- cardiovascular disease
- depression
- digestive issues (gas, bloating, indigestion, constipation, diarrhea, reflux/heartburn)
- dry eyes
- eczema
- fatigue
- fibrocystic breasts
- gallstones
- hair loss
- headaches
- infertility
- joint pain
- muscle pain
- obesity or excess weight, especially around the middle
- pancreatitis
- sleep problems (trouble falling or staying asleep)
- swollen, reddened, or painful joints
- uterine fibroids

thing really debilitating, like lupus or multiple sclerosis?

You ask your doctor about this frightening prospect at your next visit, and she confirms that your research was correct: Having one autoimmune condition triples your risk of developing others. But she also tells you there's nothing you can do to prevent that from happening. As far as conventional medicine is concerned, your genes are in charge of your sickness, and your doctor is in charge of your health.

Whatever your condition, appointments with a specialist are likely to be brief. Insurance reimburses doctors for fifteen-minute appointments, so that's usually all they can afford to give you. You have a whole list of questions you'd like to ask, but in most cases, you'll have just enough time to hear the specialist confirm that there is very little you can do to slow the progression of an autoimmune condition, let alone reverse it. You simply have to take the drugs required by the conventional "standard of care" and hope that they make some difference without causing too many side effects. If you're one of the lucky ones, the medications will eliminate all your symptoms. Often, though, you can expect only limited relief. Even if your symptoms disappear completely, the autoimmune storm is still raging inside your body, and you have no idea what its next effects might be.

Then you learn that even if your doctor can find a drug that works,

YOU CAN BENEFIT FROM THIS BOOK IF . . .

- you have an autoimmune disorder;

- you suffer from autism, chronic fatigue syndrome, fibromyalgia, or any other condition that is closely related to an autoimmune disorder; or

- you are on what I call the "autoimmune spectrum"—a path where diet, lifestyle, and/or genetics put you at risk for developing autoimmunity.

Although each of these conditions has different symptoms, they all result from digestive and immune imbalances. By healing your gut and supporting your immune system, The Myers Way is effective in treating all autoimmune and related conditions. It is also an effective way to prevent autoimmune disorders.

IS AUTISM AN AUTOIMMUNE DISORDER?

Recent research suggests that there might be an autoimmune component to autism. Indeed, I have treated children on the autism spectrum in
my clinic, and all have benefited greatly from following The Myers Way. If
your child is on the autism spectrum, following the program in this book
will certainly be helpful.

it might eventually *stop* working. Best-case scenario: Your doctor finds
you another medication, and that too works for a while. Second-best:
The new medication saddles you with some disruptive side effects,
maybe even painful ones. Worst-case: You embark on an endless
journey of frustration, pain, and despair, trying out one powerful
drug after another, while your condition grows ever more painful and
restrictive, and your life seems to be grinding to a halt.

As your treatment progresses, you learn that the worst side effects
aren't always the medical ones: There is also the personal price you
pay for the disease. Perhaps you can't play with your grandchildren
because your joints hurt too much or because the immunosuppressant
you're taking makes you far too vulnerable to a potential cold or flu.
Maybe you can't take that second honeymoon or family vacation
you've been looking forward to because your muscles ache, you feel
exhausted, or you simply feel too weak. You might find yourself taking extra sick days at work or cutting back on your hours. Perhaps
you even risk being fired or laid off.

Or maybe it's your social life that takes the hit. After all, so much
of the time you feel exhausted, cranky, and "not like yourself." Your
friends call, suggesting a dinner, a concert, a hike, or even just a long,
cozy chat on the phone. But too often you just don't have the energy.
Maybe you feel too despondent to join in the fun. Or you fear you
will become such bad company that your friends, family, and loved
ones will eventually grow tired of being with you.

Worst of all, you discover, is the disempowerment. You feel that
your body, your health, and your life itself are essentially out of your
control. You ask your doctor if there's anything you can do to make
things better—maybe alter your diet? You saw someone on a talk

show who said that gluten contributes to autoimmune conditions. Maybe you should give up bread and pasta or try to go gluten-free? Recently a friend sent you the link to an article about a condition known as "leaky gut." Should you be finding out more about that?

Again, conventional medicine is very clear. Autoimmune conditions concern the immune system, says your doctor, not the digestive system! Diet makes little or no difference. Demonizing gluten? That's just a fad. True, some people do suffer from a gluten-related autoimmune condition known as celiac disease, but we've already tested you for that and you don't have it, so gluten is nothing for you to worry about.

Your physician tells you the best you can do is accept your condition, learn to live with your side effects, and hope that your medications continue to work.

Fortunately, there is another way.

THE MYERS WAY: A SOLUTION

Conventional medicine seeks a diagnosis and medicates symptoms. The Myers Way, by contrast, is based in functional medicine, a medical approach that looks at how all the body's systems interact and seeks to get them all functioning optimally. Diet, lifestyle, environmental factors, and stress are all seen as playing a huge role in either making you sick or keeping you well.

No approach, not even The Myers Way, can cure autoimmune conditions. In medical science, "cure" means that a disease has been definitely ended, as opposed to "remission," when a disease is temporarily ended, or "reversal," when a disease remains within your body but shows no symptoms.

Because no one has yet learned how to cure autoimmune conditions, The Myers Way offers you the next best thing: reversal and prevention. The Myers Way relieves your symptoms, helps you get off your medications, and enables you to live a vital, energetic, and pain-free life. It's not about learning to live with a disease. It's about creating a lifelong condition of health.

This approach rests on four pillars, each of which has been tested through experimental research and has seen amazing results over my own years of practice as a physician:

❶ **Heal your gut.** After all, 80 percent of your immune system is in your gut. The gut is the gateway to your health, so if your gut isn't healthy, your immune system won't be either.

❷ **Get rid of gluten, grains, legumes, and other foods that cause chronic inflammation.** Inflammation is a system-wide immune response that, in small doses, can actually help you heal. But when inflammation becomes chronic, it stresses your entire body, especially your immune system. If you suffer from an autoimmune condition, inflammation provokes your symptoms and makes your condition worse. If you are on the autoimmune spectrum, increased inflammation can push you over the edge into a full-blown autoimmune disorder.

Gluten—a protein found in wheat, rye, barley, and many other grains—stresses your digestive system, putting you at risk for a disorder known as leaky gut, which further burdens your immune system. Many other foods, including gluten-free grains and legumes, also trigger inflammation. That's why on The Myers Way you will cut out gluten and clean up your diet, thereby healing your gut, soothing your inflammation, and reversing autoimmunity.

❸ **Tame the toxins.** Every day we are assaulted by thousands of toxins—at home, at work, and outdoors—and our immune systems feel the burden. If you have an autoimmune condition, or if you're anywhere on the autoimmune spectrum, the degree of your toxic burden can make the difference between health and sickness.

❹ **Heal your infections and relieve your stress.** Certain infections can also trigger an autoimmune condition, as can physical, mental, or emotional stress. In a vicious cycle, stress can also trigger or retrigger an infection, while infections add to your body's burden of stress. So when you lighten those burdens on your immune system, you go a long way toward reversing your symptoms.

The Myers Way is based in the latest cutting-edge research published in the most respected scientific journals. In fact, I just finished conducting interviews for my Autoimmune Summit (www.auto immunesummit.com) with forty researchers, scientists, physicians, and teachers from around the country, all of whom agreed with the validity of this four-pillar approach. It is also based on my personal experience as both patient and physician. Unlike conventional medicine, The Myers Way is an empowering and optimistic treatment that offers you the chance to live a vibrant, energized, and pain-free life.

Yes, you can play with your grandchildren again. Yes, you can slow, stop, and even reverse the progression of your disease, eliminating your symptoms, freeing yourself from pain, and reducing or even eliminating your medications. Yes, you can become the vital, energetic person you used to be—or, if you've been suffering from your condition since adolescence, you can become the confident, healthy person you've always wanted to be. And, yes, you can manage your condition yourself.

After you have completed thirty days on The Myers Way, you will feel significantly better, and within a few months, you should be symptom-free. Some of you might need the help of a functional medicine practitioner to achieve full recovery, but in most cases, this book is all you need.

I've used this approach with thousands of my patients, and I have seen it work. In fact, people come to me from across the country— often at considerable effort and expense—because they are so eager to find another, better way of treating autoimmune disorders. They are not happy with the conventional care their own physicians have offered them; they want an autoimmune *solution*. The Myers Way is that solution: an effective, long-term approach to reversing and preventing autoimmune disorders.

I've also used The Myers Way on myself. For years I struggled with an autoimmune condition that launched me into my own painful search for a better type of treatment. In the end, I had to invent my own solution.

MY AUTOIMMUNE JOURNEY

I couldn't believe this was happening to me.

I was lying in bed, clutched in the grip of a panic attack. I wanted desperately to continue with my second year of medical school. But I was struggling with the nightmarish symptoms of Graves' disease, an autoimmune condition in which the thyroid gland attacks itself and overproduces its own hormone. Awful as the symptoms were, the helplessness was worse—the feeling that my life was no longer my own.

The first signs had shown up early into my second year of medical school at Louisiana State University Health Sciences Center in New Orleans. As happens with most autoimmune disorders, I had no idea what was going on. For the first time in my life I was seized by panic attacks. Despite barely exercising and consuming massive quantities of pizza and oatmeal cookies, I was shedding weight like a marathon runner. I went from a size 4 to a size 0 within a few months. Yeah, that sounds like the ideal weight-loss plan, but in fact, it was terrifying to suddenly drop so much weight for no apparent reason. I was always in a mild sweat. My heart never stopped racing. My mind was racing too, partly from the disease and partly because I was just so scared. I never knew when a panic attack might strike. My legs were so weak, they shook every time I went down a flight of stairs. When I picked up a pen to take notes in class, my hand shook with a tremor I could barely control.

Then the insomnia kicked in. I tossed and turned, night after night. If you've ever had insomnia of your own, you know what a torment it can be to lie awake for hours at a time, crazed with exhaustion and yet unable to fall asleep. Soon, the prospect of facing another sleepless night becomes almost as bad as the insomnia itself. I felt as though I were living in a prison of anxiety, dizziness, and fatigue. "There *has* to be a solution," I told myself as I stared miserably at my peacefully sleeping dog, Bella. But this was my life now, and I couldn't help wondering whether this would always be my life.

Finally, my tremor got so bad that my friends noticed it. They were alarmed and convinced me to go see a doctor—who quickly brushed aside my concerns.

"I think this is just stress," she said briskly. "You're a second-year medical student, and it's very common to think you have every disease you're currently learning about. I wouldn't worry about it."

Painful as her response was, it provided a valuable lesson. Today, when a patient comes to me in tears, insisting that there's a part of her story that her physician has overlooked, I am always ready to hear her out. "You know your own body better than I do," I tell my patients, wishing that first doctor had said something similar to me.

At least I knew enough to trust my own instincts. After all, I'd been through plenty of stressful times in my life, and I'd never responded like this. Like the feisty Louisiana woman I had been raised to be, I demanded a full workup and lab testing.

It turned out my instincts were right on the money. I wasn't just panicking over courses and exams. I wasn't mysteriously going insane. I had an actual, diagnosable condition: Graves' disease. Finally, my misery had a name.

Graves' disease is a condition in which the thyroid overperforms. It enlarges to up to twice its normal size, producing all the symptoms I had been suffering from: racing heart, tremors, muscle weakness, disturbed sleep, excessive weight loss. Learning the name of my condition was just about the last comfort I got, however, because the conventional medical treatments for Graves' were pretty terrifying. There were three choices on the menu, and none of them seemed like the route to a happy life.

The first and least invasive choice was to take a drug known as propylthiouracil (PTU). The PTU was supposed to stop my thyroid from working so hard and keep it from overproducing the hormone.

That sounds good, right? Then I looked at the side effects. Here's just a partial list: rash, itching, hives, abnormal hair loss, changes in skin pigmentation, swelling, nausea, vomiting, heartburn, loss of taste, joint or muscle aches, numbness, and headaches. A less common but still possible side effect related to the therapy is a condition known as agranulocytosis, which is a decrease of white blood cells, bringing with it infectious lesions of the throat, the gastrointestinal tract, and the skin, along with an overall feeling of illness and fever.

Okay. What were my other options?

Well, basically they were two different ways of destroying my thyroid gland. I could have it removed surgically. Or I could have a procedure known as thyroid ablation, which involves swallowing a radioactive pill to kill the gland.

Despite my enrollment in a conventional medical school, I believed there were other roads to health besides medications and surgery. For example, nutrition was clearly instrumental in short-term and long-term health.

When I was a kid, my mom made much of our food from scratch: whole-wheat bread, plain organic yogurt, granola and oatmeal cookies, and peppers and tomatoes that she grew right in our own garden. We didn't go in for packaged, processed foods; we barely had any canned foods in our cupboards. We always ate our meals together, as a family—mostly 1970s health food, like brown rice, tofu, sprouts, and vegetables. We rarely got sick, and I was proud of the healthy diet that kept us well. At age fourteen, I even became a vegetarian.

Then my mom got cancer.

She was only fifty-nine at the time, and I was only twenty-nine. I had just spent two exciting years as a Peace Corps volunteer in rural Paraguay and was back in the States, completing my prerequisites for medical school. When I got the news about my mom, I simply couldn't believe it. My mother had always been the vision of health. She looked ten or fifteen years younger than her actual age, jogged three miles each day, and even taught yoga. But out of the blue she had been diagnosed with pancreatic cancer, a disease for which conventional medicine has no cure.

That was a real wake-up call for me. I discovered that you can be doing all the right things—or what you believe to be the right things—and still get terribly ill.

To some extent this is because most serious illnesses are multifactorial. Genetics plays a role. So does our toxic environment. We don't have perfect control over the conditions that create our disorders.

I also discovered—although not for several more years—that our "healthy" family diet had actually been poisoning us all. The whole-wheat bread, grains, and legumes that formed the basis of our family meals were full of inflammatory chemicals that might well have triggered my mom's cancer, worsened my father's autoimmune disease (a condition known as polymyositis, marked by joint pain and muscle weakness), and set me up for my own health problems.

Meanwhile, Mom's illness made it crystal clear how completely resistant most conventional doctors are to any unconventional approach, especially when it concerns nutrition, supplements, or something natural. When I asked Mom's doctor about some new healing foods I had learned of, her doctor simply scoffed, mocking the very idea that nutrition could play a major role. "Your mom could put a watermelon in her ear and jump up and down on one foot, and that might help too, but it probably won't," he told me. As I prepared for medical school, I understood that this response would be typical of the mind-set I would encounter. My plan from the start had been to become an integrative physician who viewed the body as a whole and used diet and natural approaches as much as possible. Mom's experience simply confirmed just how difficult it would be to integrate these two approaches.

Meanwhile, conventional medicine could offer my mother nothing except chemotherapy, which they didn't even expect to provide a cure, only to delay the inevitable. My mother died less than five months after she was diagnosed. I entered medical school the following year—and one year later I was suffering from Graves'.

I now know that besides diet, stress is a big factor in the development of autoimmunity. The stress of my mother's death had clearly helped to trigger my Graves' disease. But there were other factors involved as well:

Diet. As a vegetarian, my diet was based on lots of gluten, grains, and legumes, as well as dairy products, nuts, and seeds. These seemingly healthy foods had actually inflamed my system, setting me up for problems with my immune system. If, like many people, I had a genetic predisposition to autoimmunity, this diet would virtually ensure that my predisposition would turn into a full-blown disease.

Leaky gut. My carb-heavy diet set me up for a condition known as "small intestine bacterial overgrowth (SIBO)," which in turn created leaky gut, in which my intestinal walls became permeable, with dangerous consequences for my digestive and immune systems. (You'll learn more about leaky gut in chapters 4 and 5.)

Toxins. Heavy metals are another factor in triggering autoimmune conditions, and I had had a *lot* of exposure to mercury: through the weekly vaccinations I got in the Peace Corps, in all the canned tuna I loved to eat, and on an extended stay in China, where the air pollution is loaded with heavy metals. Had I reduced my exposure to mercury, I could have lightened my toxic burden and perhaps my immune system would not have gone out of whack.

Infections. Certain types of infections are another risk factor for autoimmunity. And guess what. I had had one of them: the Epstein–Barr virus (EBV), which had given me a bad case of mononucleosis when I was in high school. The EBV is also implicated in chronic fatigue syndrome, which is why people who suffer from that condition are also at risk for autoimmune disorders.

If I had known then what I know now, I would have understood how many risk factors I had—and I would have known how to use diet, gut healing, detox, and stress relief to prevent my condition. Had I still succumbed to an autoimmune disorder, I would at least have been able to treat myself, easing my symptoms, regaining my health, and avoiding the horrific options offered by conventional medicine.

But this was back in the year 2000, and functional medical approaches were in their infancy. My conventional doctors gave me the three unpleasant options, and as far as I knew, those were the only choices I had.

Hoping for a better way, I went to a traditional Chinese doctor and started taking lots of herbs in the form of terrible-tasting brown powder. They didn't seem to do much good, plus I was concerned that if I ever needed emergency treatment, the ER docs would have no idea about potential cross-reactions—they wouldn't even know what I had been taking. Despite my growing lack of faith in conventional medicine, I did not want to abandon it entirely.

So, reluctantly, I opted for the PTU. I got my first lesson in the potentially disastrous side effects when I developed toxic hepatitis a few months later as the prescription drug started destroying my liver. The condition was so severe, I was sent for extended bed rest and nearly had to drop out of medical school.

My choices were now surgery or ablation—remove my thyroid or destroy it. Meanwhile, I was still eating my "healthy" grain-based diet, which was still causing my immune system to attack my thyroid.

I chose ablation and said good-bye to my thyroid, a choice I regret to this day. If only I had known about functional medicine, I might still have my thyroid today, living symptom-free and healthy with my body intact.

At the time, though, I knew no other way. I just have to tell myself that I did the best I could with the knowledge I had.

Yet even then I intuitively knew that there *was* a better way—an approach to health that worked *with* the body's natural healing ability instead of attacking the body with harsh drugs and invasive surgery. I had always known that some other type of medicine existed, even though I didn't know what it was called or how to find it. I had entered medical school committed to finding this other type of healing, and I sought out every possible place where I might learn more about integrative and alternative medicine. I was even president of my medical school's complementary and alternative medicine interest group. But no approach I found seemed to get to the root of the problem.

So when I graduated from medical school, I decided to go into emergency medicine. With that specialty, I could always work in international health, which had been my love in the Peace Corps. And since ER doctors don't have an established practice, I would be free to pursue that other type of medicine—as soon as I knew what it was.

I moved to Austin, Texas, where my time was split between the main trauma center at Brackenridge Hospital and the pediatric trauma center at Dell Children's Medical Center. As an emergency room physician, I had the opportunity to treat people in the most extreme conditions, and I was proud of the lives I helped to save. Bringing a child back from the verge of death, and knowing that I had helped not just him but his entire family, made me remember all over again how powerful the right treatment can be.

Yet the vast majority of the people I saw were not coming in for trauma but because of something related to a chronic disease. This was truly heartbreaking, because conventional medicine could do so little to help them. Not only had conventional medicine failed me, now it—and I too—were failing them.

Meanwhile, my own health problems continued. The ablation had released large amounts of thyroid hormone into my bloodstream, which meant that for months I suffered from severe mood swings. Because my system was still inflamed, I developed irritable bowel syndrome (IBS). Even when the worst of my symptoms abated, I never felt really healthy. The best I could feel was "not sick."

Then, finally, I found what I had been looking for. I discovered functional medicine.

FUNCTIONAL MEDICINE: RESTORING YOUR BODY'S BALANCE

These days, functional medicine is fairly well known. The work of such pioneers as Jeffrey Bland, Mark Hyman, David Perlmutter, Alejandro Junger, and Frank Lipman has helped to popularize this powerful approach to health. Instead of carving the body up into separate specialties, as conventional medicine does—the immune system, the digestive system, the adrenals, the thyroid—functional medicine views

AUTOIMMUNITY IN AMERICA

Following are the estimated figures on the incidence of autoimmune disorders in the United States. Some of these conditions are considered autoimmune disorders and some merely resemble autoimmunity. For all these disorders, however, The Myers Way is an effective protocol to reverse the progression of the disease, ease its symptoms, and restore you to a healthy, vigorous life.

Graves' disease—10 million

Psoriasis—7.5 million

Fibromyalgia—5 million

Lupus—3.5 million

Celiac disease—3 million

Hashimoto's thyroiditis—
  3 million

Rheumatoid arthritis—
  1.3 million

Chronic fatigue syndrome—
  1 million

Crohn's disease—700,000

Ulcerative colitis—700,000

Multiple sclerosis—250,000 to
  350,000

Scleroderma—300,000

Diabetes type 1—25,000 to
  50,000

the entire body as one integrated system. In this view, health is achieved not by medicating individual symptoms or even individual diseases. Instead, you treat the entire body, mindful of how all your body's systems are constantly affecting one another.

For example, 80 percent of your immune system is in your intestinal tract. So a functional medicine perspective—and maybe also common sense—would indicate that in order to heal your immune system, you first have to heal your gut.

Functional medicine also relies on nutrition in the form of real food and supplements. "You didn't get Graves' because of a deficiency in PTU or radiation," a functional M.D. might say. "You got Graves' because your body needed some kind of nourishment or protection that it wasn't getting." The role of functional medicine, then, is to give the body what it needs.

Sometimes, of course, that includes prescription drugs. Even so, the goal is always to restore all the body's system to full health, using as natural and noninvasive an approach as possible.

I know this now; in fact, I practice it now. But back in 2009 I hadn't even heard of functional medicine. Luckily, I chose to attend the Integrative Healthcare Symposium, where I heard functional medicine pioneer Dr. Mark Hyman give a talk explaining that inflammation, toxins, leaky gut, and food sensitivities were the root causes of most chronic illnesses. I also learned that there was a connection between gluten and autoimmune disease—especially thyroid conditions.

I was hooked. Completely. I plunged into training at the Institute for Functional Medicine, which confirmed that this was what I had been looking for all those years. This was the approach that I had intuitively known was out there, the approach I'd never been able to name. This was a way of treating patients that made sense to me, focusing not on using medications to cure disease but on using the body's own resources to create health. Finally I could become the physician I had always dreamed of being. So, with immense relief and gratitude, I set up my own practice.

I was also eager to see if this new approach could help *me*. In my first steps toward developing The Myers Way, I cut several inflamma-tory foods out of my diet and waited eagerly for my results. Sure enough, in thirty days I felt better.

I continued to keep these foods out of my diet. I also treated the infections in my gut, optimized my ability to rid my body of toxins, and learned how to better deal with stress.

After so many years of feeling sick, this new diet seemed like a medical miracle. No more anxiety. No more panic attacks. No more irritable bowel. Suddenly I had tons of energy, and I finally felt well. I had found my autoimmune solution. As I saw what it took to reverse my symptoms and bring me to true health, I discovered the basis of The Myers Way.

THE AUTOIMMUNE SPECTRUM

Once you view the body from a functional medicine perspective, you see that there is not one discrete category called "autoimmunity." Instead, there is what I call the "autoimmune spectrum."

At the high end of the spectrum are the people with full-blown autoimmune conditions. Suppose you have, say, multiple sclerosis. If you follow The Myers Way, you might live a long and healthy life, virtually symptom-free. Once your immune system is no longer attacking your spinal cord—the defining feature of MS—your muscles might become strong and healthy. But your immune system is still poised to attack your body's own tissue, and the moment your inflammation levels rise—whether because of poor diet, toxic burden, stress, or some other factor—your former symptoms will return.

In the middle of the spectrum are those of you with full-blown inflammatory conditions and/or symptoms that have not yet turned into autoimmune disorders: asthma, allergies, joint pain, muscle pain, fatigue, and digestive issues. Obesity is also in this category, since excess body fat—especially around the middle—creates inflammation. (Inflammation also makes it harder to lose weight. Talk about your vicious cycles!) These significant signs of inflammation indicate that even if you don't yet have an autoimmune condition, you are at significant risk to develop one.

None	Some	Mild	Moderate	Severe	Diagnosis of autoimmune disease
No inflammation	1 symptom* 1-2 times per month	1-2 symptoms* 1-2 times per week	2-3 symptoms* most days	>3 symptoms* every day	

*Symptoms defined on The Myers Way Symptom Tracker

Finally, at the low end of the spectrum are those of you who are only moderately inflamed. Maybe you're eating a poor diet, but for the time being you can still tolerate it. You have some problems with your gut, which might manifest in digestive problems, such as acid reflux or constipation, or show up as seemingly unrelated symptoms, such as acne, fatigue, or depression. (See the list of symptoms on page 7.) Perhaps you're exposed to a lot of toxins, through the mold in your basement or the mercury in your fillings, but you haven't yet shown signs of illness. Maybe you're leading a super-stressful life, but so far it feels like you can handle it.

At this low end of the spectrum, you might already have minor symptoms of inflammation, such as acne, IBS, excess weight, or a mild case of asthma—something that shows up only occasionally but never completely goes away. However, if your inflammation continues to increase, you will find yourself continuing up the spectrum. Your symptoms are likely to get worse, and you might even develop an autoimmune condition.

Another factor in assessing your place on the spectrum is your family history. The more relatives you have with an autoimmune condition, the higher your risk for developing one too—and your risk increases when they are first-degree relatives (either a parent or sibling). So even if you have relatively few symptoms, having one or more relatives with an autoimmune condition can push you further up the spectrum.

Are you wondering where on the spectrum *you* are? Fill out The Myers Way Symptom Tracker below and then answer the subsequent questions to find out.

THE MYERS WAY SYMPTOM TRACKER

Rate the following symptoms over the past seven days on a scale of 0 to 4 based on severity. 0 = None, 1 = Some, 2 = Mild, 3 = Moderate, 4 = Severe

HEAD

____headaches

____migraines

____faintness

____trouble sleeping

Total ____

MIND

____brain fog

____poor memory

____impaired coordination

____difficulty deciding

____slurred/stuttered
speech

____learning/attention
deficit

Total ____

EYES

____swollen, red eyelids

____dark circles

____puffy eyes

____poor vision

____watery, itchy eyes

Total ____

NOSE

____nasal congestion

____excessive mucus

____stuffy/runny nose

____sinus problems

____frequent sneezing

Total ____

EARS

____itchy ears

____earaches, infections

____drainage from ear

____ringing ears, hearing loss

Total ____

MOUTH, THROAT

____chronic cough

____frequent throat clearing

____sore throat

____swollen lips

____canker sores

Total ____

HEART

____irregular heartbeat

____rapid heartbeat

____chest pain

Total ____

LUNGS

____chest congestion

____asthma, bronchitis

____shortness of breath

____difficulty breathing

Total ____

SKIN

____acne

____hives, eczema, dry skin

____hair loss

____hot flashes

____excessive sweating

Total ____

WEIGHT

____inability to lose weight

____food cravings

____excess weight

____insufficient weight

____compulsive eating

____water retention, swelling

Total____

DIGESTION

____nausea, vomiting

____diarrhea

____constipation

____bloating

____belching, passing gas

____heartburn, indigestion

____intestinal/stomach pain
  or cramps

Total ____

EMOTIONS

____anxiety

____depression

____mood swings

____nervousness

____irritability

Total ____

ENERGY, ACTIVITY

____fatigue

____lethargy

____hyperactivity

____restlessness

Total ____

JOINTS, MUSCLES

____joint pain/aches
____arthritis
____muscle stiffness
____muscle pain/aches
____weakness, tiredness
Total ____

OTHER

____frequent illness/
      infections
____frequent/urgent urination
____genital itch, discharge
____anal itch
Total ____

Preliminary total _____

Now answer the following questions and add the points to the preliminary total to get your overall total:

❶ Do you have an autoimmune disease? If yes, add 80 points. _____

❷ Do you have more than one autoimmune disease? If yes, add 100 points. _____

❸ Do you have elevated inflammatory markers, such as ESR (erythrocyte sedimentation rate), CRP (C-reactive protein), or homocysteine? If yes, add 10 points. _____

❹ Do you have any diagnosis ending with "itis," such as arthritis, colitis, pancreatitis, sinusitis, or diverticulitis? If yes, add 10 points. _____

❺ Do you have a first-degree relative (a parent or sibling) with an autoimmune disease? If yes, add 10 points for the first relative and add 2 points for each additional first-degree relative. _____

❻ Do you have a second-degree relative (a grandparent, aunt, or uncle) with an autoimmune disease? If yes, add 5 points. _____

❼ Are you female?[a] If yes, add 5 points. _____

Overall total _____

YOUR PLACE ON THE AUTOIMMUNE SPECTRUM

<5	5–9	10–19	20–39	40–79	>80
No risk	Some risk	Mild risk	Moderate risk		Severe risk

Take your overall total from The Myers Way Symptom Tracker.

If your overall total is less than 5, congratulations! Your inflammation is very low, and at this point you are unlikely to develop an autoimmune condition. For lifelong protection, follow The Myers Way to keep your inflammation at this healthy level.

If your overall total is from 5 to 9, you are at the low end of the autoimmune spectrum—but you *are* on the spectrum. You have a few risk factors for autoimmunity, raising the possibility that you might develop an autoimmune condition. To reduce your risk and lower your inflammation, follow The Myers Way.

If your overall total is from 10 to 30, you are in the middle of the autoimmune spectrum, with significant symptoms that reveal considerable inflammation and mild to moderate risk of developing autoimmunity. You can reverse your condition, heal your symptoms, and avoid the risk of an autoimmune condition by following The Myers Way.

If your overall total is over 30, you are at moderate risk either because you have one or more close family members with the condition or because you already have progressed quite far along the autoimmune spectrum. You may already have been diagnosed with an autoimmune condition, or you may have a condition that has not yet been diagnosed. If you do not currently have an autoimmune disorder, your family history and/or high levels of inflammation put you at risk for one. To reverse course and restore optimal health, follow The Myers Way.

GOING FORWARD

I've included a copy of this test and symptom tracker in appendix G. Make five photocopies, then fill one out on the first day you begin The Myers Way and another every week thereafter, on the same day of the week. You will be able to track your progress as you watch your symptoms resolve. If you still have some symptoms at the end of thirty days, make a few more copies and fill the symptom tracker out once a month. If you're not satisfied with your progress, look for a functional medicine practitioner (www.functionalmedicine.org) to help you explore some of the issues that will be discussed in chapters 6 and 7.

THE AUTOIMMUNE EPIDEMIC

If you are familiar with conventional medicine, you will know that the standard belief is that autoimmunity is a genetic condition. In this view, autoimmunity is a given, something your genes simply command your body to do. When, where, and how is up to your genes, not you. So you might be wondering how I can claim that there is an autoimmune epidemic. Since human genetics evolves very slowly, the incidence of autoimmune conditions should remain more or less constant, especially over a few generations.

However, in the past fifty years the incidence of autoimmunity in the United States has tripled. Just as allergies and asthma have taken on epidemic proportions in recent years, so have autoimmune disorders. Since the human gene pool cannot possibly have changed so rapidly, there must be something in the environment that is triggering autoimmune disorders (as well as those other epidemics). And rates are developing so rapidly that autoimmune conditions are now the third leading chronic illness in the United States, right behind cardiovascular disease and cancer.

INFLAMMATORY CONDITIONS ALONG THE AUTOIMMUNE SPECTRUM

Following are the estimated figures on the incidence of inflammatory conditions in the United States:

Acne—85 percent of all Americans at some point in their lives

Obesity—90 million

Excess weight—88 million

Cardiovascular disease— 80 million

Allergies—50 million

Arthritis—50 million

Asthma—25 million

Eczema—7.5 million

Irritable bowel syndrome— 1.4 million

Furthermore, we know of many documented cases of people who have developed autoimmune conditions with no known family history. The reverse is also true: In my years of treating thousands of patients with autoimmune disorders, I have come to believe that most—perhaps all—could have been prevented had my patients only known about The Myers Way and followed it *before* their immune systems went so severely out of balance.

What is triggering this alarming increase in autoimmune disorders? There are four key factors:

Gluten-saturated diets. Gluten today is *everywhere*, dominating our diets in a way that our grandparents could not even have imagined. Moreover, the type of gluten to which we are exposed is not the same protein our ancestors knew but rather a new substance that is far more dangerous to our health. (For a fuller explanation of these issues, see chapter 5.)

Leaky gut. Diet, toxins, stress, and medications all contribute to leaky gut, a condition in which your intestinal walls become too permeable. As a result, partially digested food leaks through, ramping up the stress on your immune system in many different ways and causing all sorts of other health hazards besides. You'll learn more about leaky gut in chapters 4 and 5, where you'll discover that it is an essential precondition for developing an autoimmune disorder. So leaky gut is a key player in our new autoimmune epidemic—and healing leaky gut is a key element in The Myers Way.

The toxic burden. As you will see in chapter 6, we are exposed to a toxic burden that, again, far outweighs anything our grandparents ever had to contend with. The overwhelming amount of chemicals in our air, water, and food—toxins that we're exposed to virtually nonstop at home, at work, and in our environment— has stressed our immune systems to an unprecedented extent.

Our stressful lives. It's hard to compare stress levels across the generations, because our experience of stress is so subjective. But since levels of stress-related illnesses are on the rise, and since stress has been shown to trigger and intensify autoimmune disorders, I'm going to say that this too is a key factor in the current epidemic. (For more on stress and autoimmunity, see chapter 7.)

THE HYGIENE HYPOTHESIS

There is another key theory about why rates of autoimmunity are skyrocketing: the "hygiene hypothesis." While we usually think of bacteria as harmful, most bacteria are either neutral or friendly—and some are absolutely crucial to our health. According to the hygiene hypothesis, these bacteria are being depleted, and as a result, our immune systems are taking a tremendous hit.

As you shall see in chapter 4, caesarean sections and bottle-feeding deprive infants of crucial friendly bacteria picked up in the mother's birth canal and from breast milk, thereby depleting the immune system. (Bottle-feeding also deprives children of immune factors received through breast milk.)

Antibiotics—frequently given to children at the least provocation—kill off and deplete friendly bacteria, weakening the immune system. And because children are given vaccinations, their immune systems are insulated from immune challenges, leaving them with fewer resources to fight off infections.

But the immune-weakening process doesn't stop there. Children are less likely to play in the dirt these days and less likely to have contact with farm animals, both of which further deprive their immune systems of opportunities to repel bacteria. Antibacterial soaps and hand sanitizers kill off still more friendly bacteria, while refined flour, unhealthy fats, too much sugar, and GMOs support the bad bacteria and destroy the good.

Modern sanitation, antibiotics, and vaccinations have undoubtedly saved many lives, but they are also costing many of us healthy immune systems. I suggest we look for a middle ground. Let your kids play in the dirt, stay away from the antibacterial soaps, and take the probiotics I recommend on page 197. And before you allow your doctor to prescribe antibiotics for your children, make sure the treatment is really necessary. Their immune systems will thank you for it.

FINDING HOPE

Almost invariably, when conventional practitioners address autoimmune disorders, they offer to "manage" your condition rather than "solve" it. The reason for that is simple: They do not believe that autoimmune disorders *can* be solved.

That's where we differ, because I *do* believe we can resolve autoimmune disorders. While there is not yet a cure that will permanently allow you to ignore your condition, there *is* a treatment that can resolve your symptoms, get you off your medications, restore you to vitality, and free you to lead a fulfilling life.

I call my program The Myers Way because it is not simply a treatment plan but a way of life. Often a single family member comes into my office seeking answers for a particular health problem. Slowly but surely that person's quest for answers goes on to transform the entire family, as everyone begins to avoid toxic foods and seek out healing ones. I've often noticed that poor health has a momentum of its own, but so, happily, does good health. The Myers Way has proven on many occasions to be the inspiration to get that momentum going.

It can be challenging to navigate the medical maze, negotiate dietary restrictions, and simply bear up under the prospect of living with an autoimmune disorder. But I know how to help you because I've guided thousands of patients through this experience, and I live it myself, every day. So think of me as your big sister, your mentor, and your role model as well as your physician, your researcher, and your science teacher. In this book, I will be all those things. And by the time you've finished reading, you will know everything one book can teach you about healing your immune system, healing your symptoms, and getting any additional help you might need.

Whether you have a full-blown autoimmune condition or are somewhere along the spectrum, I am excited to welcome you to The Myers Way. This approach can make an immediate and long-lasting improvement in your health, bringing you relief from symptoms, increased vitality, and the energy you need to live the life you want. The sense of empowerment you can gain from taking charge of your own health is extraordinary. And the sense of hope in knowing that you will no longer be defined by your disease is perhaps the greatest benefit of all.

As you will see in chapter 12, the patients who commit to following The Myers Way achieve tremendous results. They find relief from their symptoms. They feel energized and vibrant. They are able to get off their medications and lead rich, full lives, no longer shadowed by pain, fear, and an endless parade of doctor visits. Sooner than they would have believed possible, "feeling good" becomes their new normal. That can be your story too.

CHAPTER 2

Myths and Facts About Autoimmunity

IT's SAD BUT TRUE: When it comes to treating autoimmune conditions, conventional medicine just doesn't work. I've treated thousands of patients whose physicians gave them powerful medications, putting them at risk for disruptive side effects and leaving them with a quality of life that was challenging at best and pitiable at worst. These patients were told that they had no choice but to accept their fate: a dire, incurable disorder that could not be stopped and could barely be slowed.

Yet I have seen these same patients after thirty days on The Myers Way glowing with health, full of vitality, their pain forgotten, and their lives restored. So why won't conventional medicine recognize that there *is* an autoimmune solution?

As I've pondered this question over the years, I keep thinking about Ignaz Semmelweis. You might not have heard that name before, but everyone who graduates from medical school knows the story of this pioneering Hungarian physician.

Semmelweis worked in an obstetrical clinic in Vienna in the mid-nineteenth century, an era when thousands of women died in childbirth from a disease known as puerperal fever. In those days doctors treated one woman after another on the maternity wards without even washing their hands between patients. As a result, "childbed fever" took at least one woman in ten.

At this point in medical history Louis Pasteur had not yet discovered germ theory. Somehow Semmelweis intuited that doctors' lack of proper hygiene was helping to spread disease. He suggested that if doctors were to wash their hands between each delivery, fewer women would get sick.

Now, of course, we know that Semmelweis was absolutely right. He even had the evidence to prove it: When he required his interns to cleanse their hands with a chlorinated lime solution, mortality rates from puerperal fever dropped dramatically, falling to less than 2 percent.

You would expect his colleagues to be astounded at Semmelweis's success and to quickly adopt his methods. Yet doctors resented the notion that they were somehow unclean, and they refused to start this newfangled business of washing their hands. Semmelweis's theories would not become common medical practice for another fifty years.

Why couldn't those doctors see what seems so obvious to us today? I picture them with their dirty hands, delivering babies in the same blood-spattered suits they had been wearing all day, pooh-poohing our modern notions of well-scrubbed hands and a sterile surgical field. Then I think of today's conventional physicians who refuse to accept the key role of diet, gut health, toxins, infections, and stress in treating autoimmunity—and, indeed, in all types of disease. I believe that within the next decade these doctors will seem just as quaint, just as wrongheaded—and just as dangerous—as their nineteenth-century colleagues.

A conventional doctor will tell you that diet doesn't matter. It does—and I have seen countless patients reverse their conditions and get off their medications through the power of diet alone. A conventional doctor will tell you that medications are your only option. They aren't—and, again, I have the patient stories to prove it. I don't want to sound contentious. But sometimes black is black and white is white; and, yeah, sometimes the emperor of conventional medicine really is just sitting there buck naked, and it takes us functional medical practitioners to point that out.

I realize that this might be a fairly big leap for you to make. You're sitting at home watching TV, and in the course of a one-hour show, you might see as many as three commercials for various autoimmune medications, each one with pretty music and flowers and smiling

EIGHT MAJOR MYTHS ABOUT AUTOIMMUNE CONDITIONS

Myth One: Autoimmune disorders cannot be reversed.

Myth Two: Your symptoms won't disappear without harsh medications.

Myth Three: When you treat an autoimmune disorder with medication, the side effects are no big deal.

Myth Four: Improving digestion and gut health have no effect on the progression of an autoimmune disorder.

Myth Five: Going gluten-free won't make any difference to your autoimmune disorder.

Myth Six: Having an autoimmune disorder dooms you to a poor quality of life.

Myth Seven: When it comes to autoimmune disorders, only your genes matter; environmental factors do not matter.

Myth Eight: Your immune system is what it is; there is nothing you can do to support it.

people and that seductive voice-over at the end: "Ask your doctor about . . ." So you ask your doctor, or maybe you've been put on that medication already and you feel pleased that you've already done what the commercial is asking you to do. You're in sync. You're in step. You're following that powerful message that begins with "Everybody knows . . ."

Yet if you ask your doctor about giving up gluten, let alone passing on the rice, quinoa, and legumes, you're likely to be given a pitying look and a sad shake of the head. Maybe your doctor will warn you to stay away from "quack theories" or refuse to even discuss an alternative approach. Several of my patients have actually been fired by their specialists because they dared to request a protocol for working their way off prescription drugs. In all three cases the doctors insisted that the medications they had prescribed were "standard of care," a term for what the medical community agrees is the best possible treatment. Then those doctors refused to treat their "rebellious" patients any longer.

"If you can't trust me, we can't work together" was the exact phrase from a doctor to a young woman who later became my patient. This woman lived in a tiny town in rural Texas where there was only one specialist equipped to handle her condition. But because she dared to question conventional medical wisdom, she was left without any treatment at all. I don't want anyone to have to be in this position again.

I've seen the science, I've reviewed the research, and I've treated thousands of patients. As both physician and patient, I'm confident that The Myers Way works, and I want you to be confident too. So let's take on conventional wisdom, myth by myth, dismantling each misconception and replacing it with the truth.

MYTH ONE: AUTOIMMUNE DISORDERS CANNOT BE REVERSED

If you're like most autoimmune patients—and remember, I've spent years on the patient side myself—this is what you're likely to hear when you sit down in the doctor's office:

> I'm so sorry. You have an autoimmune disease. Once the genes that produce this condition have been turned on, they can't be turned off. We can't cure the disease. The only thing we can do now is to manage your symptoms—and the only way to do that is with drugs.

Like many aspects of conventional medicine, there is a great deal of truth in those remarks. But they are also very much misguided. Yes, there is a genetic component in autoimmune disorders. However, twin studies have shown that autoimmunity is only 25 percent heritable, which means that the environment is a far more significant part of the picture: 75 percent, to be exact.

Moreover, as we have learned from the brand-new field of epigenetics, genetic expression can be modified. Certainly you cannot change your genes. You can, however, turn some genes on while turning others off, thereby changing your genetic expression—the extent to which your genetic qualities are actually expressed.

Yes, there is a genetic component to your illness. But those genes are not the whole story. For you to develop an autoimmune disorder, something in your environment, diet, or personal circumstances has to *turn on* the group of your genes that causes autoimmune disorders. Once those genes are turned on, you can work to turn them off, or at least to turn them down. Through diet, intestinal healing, and reducing your toxic burden, you can instruct your problematic genes to turn off

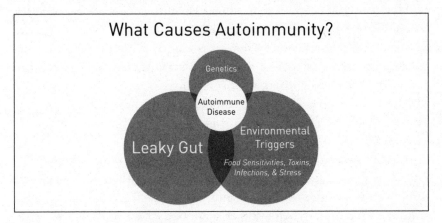

What Causes Autoimmunity?

Genetics

Autoimmune Disease

Leaky Gut

Environmental Triggers

Food Sensitivities, Toxins, Infections, & Stress

again, thereby restoring your beleaguered immune system to health. And if you are on the autoimmune spectrum, you can often *prevent* autoimmune disorders by the diet and lifestyle choices you make.

MYTH TWO: YOUR SYMPTOMS WON'T DISAPPEAR WITHOUT HARSH MEDICATIONS

It's sad to say, but most conventional practitioners dismiss the importance of nutrition as a major factor in our health. Most are also unaware of the power of gluten to disrupt our digestion, torpedo our immune systems, and trigger autoimmune responses. Conventional medical practice also tends to dismiss the harmful power of the toxins that lurk not only in our food, air, and water but also in our shampoos, deodorants, cosmetics, and home cleaning products, not to mention in our furniture, carpeting, mattresses, TVs, and computers. The very concept of a toxic burden is foreign to most health-care professionals, let alone the power of removing that burden from those who suffer from autoimmune disorders.

As a result, when it comes to fighting autoimmune conditions, conventional medicine really has only one weapon in its arsenal: drugs.

One especially dangerous class of drug used to treat autoimmunity is known as "immunosuppressants"—medications that suppress your immune system. The reasoning is that if an overactive immune system causes the problem, then suppressing your immune system offers a solution.

However, you need your immune system to cope with the bacteria, viruses, toxins, and other threats that surround you every day. And you can't disable a major system in the body without expecting significant repercussions. As a result, this type of treatment is painful, risky, and frequently disrupts normal life.

However, people with more severe disorders are routinely told by conventional practitioners that drugs, along with their potential side effects, are the only possible treatment.

Instead of using medicine to suppress the immune system, The Myers Way uses food and supplements to strengthen and support it while you make sure to heal the gut. Easing the toxic burden on your immune system also helps to get your body back in balance, as do healing infections and reducing stress. Medications are *not* your only option in treating autoimmune disorders.

MYTH THREE: WHEN YOU TREAT AN AUTOIMMUNE DISORDER WITH MEDICATION, THE SIDE EFFECTS ARE NO BIG DEAL

I wish this myth were true—but it isn't. Conventional practitioners, trying to bring aid and comfort to their patients, are likely to reassure you that your medications won't cause side effects and that the side effects they do cause are minor. As a former "conventional medicine patient," I know this all too well.

In fact, the side effects of the drugs most often used to treat autoimmune disorders are common, frequent, and disruptive. There are some exceptions, such as Hashimoto's thyroiditis, Sjögren's, vitiligo, and psoriasis, which usually require more gentle treatments. Most people with autoimmune conditions, however, are not so lucky. Take a look at the following chart—and then be thankful that there is another way, one whose only side effects are increased energy, better mood, improved brain function, and better health.

SIDE EFFECTS FROM COMMONLY PRESCRIBED MEDICATIONS FOR AUTOIMMUNE CONDITIONS

There are three main classes of autoimmune medications:

First line of treatment: **Steroids,** which suppress your immune system, and **nonsteroidal anti-inflammatory drugs (NSAIDs),** which suppress inflammation.

Second line of treatment: **Disease-modifying antirheumatic drugs (DMARDs),** which interfere with DNA and cell replication.

Third line of treatment: **Biologics,** which interfere with how your immune cells communicate with one another.

STEROIDS

Prednisone[b], used to treat arthritis, skin problems, eye problems, and immune disorders:

- nausea
- vomiting
- loss of appetite
- heartburn
- sleep problems
- sweating
- acne
- muscle pain or cramps
- irregular heartbeat
- weight gain
- fever
- depression, mood swings, agitation
- increased blood sugar
- possible allergic reaction

NONSTEROIDAL ANTI-INFLAMMATORY DRUGS (NSAIDs[b])

Advil, Aleve, Motrin (ibuprofen), used to treat all types of pain and inflammation, including joint and muscle pain, and headaches:

- stomach pain
- constipation
- diarrhea
- gas
- heartburn
- nausea
- vomiting
- dizziness

DISEASE-MODIFYING ANTIRHEUMATIC DRUGS (DMARDs)

CellCept (mycophenolic acid), used to treat autoimmune conditions:

- infection
- symptoms of infection, such as fever and headaches
- risk of serious infection
- decreased red and white blood cell counts
- easy bruising or bleeding
- fatigue
- dizziness or fainting
- diarrhea
- abdominal pain
- swelling of ankles and feet
- high blood pressure
- lymphoma
- skin cancer

Enbrel (etanercept), used to treat rheumatoid arthritis and other autoimmune conditions:

- tuberculosis and other infections
- hepatitis B
- nervous system problems, including multiple sclerosis, seizures, inflammation of the nerves or eyes
- blood problems
- heart failure
- psoriasis
- lupus-like syndrome

Imuran (azathioprine), used to treat rheumatoid arthritis:

- risk of skin cancer, lymphoma, other cancers
- anemia
- swollen glands
- swollen or painful abdomen
- night sweats
- itching
- fever
- sore throat
- easy bruising or bleeding
- fatigue

Trexall (methotrexate), used to treat rheumatoid arthritis and psoriasis:

- infection
- fever or chills
- fatigue
- flu-like symptoms
- easy bleeding or bruising
- possible damage to liver, lungs, and kidneys
- severe abdominal pain
- nausea, loss of appetite
- painful, widespread mouth sores
- cough with yellow sputum
- shortness of breath
- difficulty urinating, increased frequency of urination, burning during urination
- blood in the urine
- hair loss
- diarrhea
- birth defects
- severe sore throat
- sinus pain with yellow mucus
- shingles
- irreversible liver or lung damage

Plaquenil (hydroxychloroquine), used to treat lupus and rheumatoid arthritis:

- nausea
- cramps
- loss of appetite
- diarrhea
- dizziness
- headaches
- anxiety, depression

BIOLOGICS

Humira (adalimumab), prescribed for rheumatoid arthritis and Crohn's disease:

- tuberculosis
- hepatitis B
- infections caused by bacteria, fungi, or viruses that spread throughout the body
- cancer
- heart failure
- immune reactions, such as pain, joint pain, shortness of breath
- allergic reactions, such as trouble breathing; hives; swollen face, eyes, lips, or mouth
- nervous system problems, such as numbness, tingling, vision problems, weakness in the extremities, dizziness
- blood problems, such as persistent fever, tendency to bruise or bleed
- liver problems, such as fatigue, poor appetite, vomiting, abdominal pain
- psoriasis
- sinus infections
- upper respiratory (chest) infections
- nausea
- headaches

Kineret (anakinra), used to treat rheumatoid arthritis:

- lowered ability to fight infection, including neutropenia (which is the loss of infection-fighting white blood cells known as neutrophils)
- increased risk of lymphoma
- severe rash
- swollen face
- difficulty breathing
- injection site reaction, including swelling, bruising, itching, stinging
- upper respiratory and sinus infections
- joint pain
- headaches
- nausea
- diarrhea
- abdominal pain
- flu-like symptoms
- worsening of rheumatoid arthritis

MYTH FOUR: IMPROVING DIGESTION AND GUT HEALTH HAVE NO EFFECT ON THE PROGRESSION OF AN AUTOIMMUNE DISORDER

I heard it from my doctors when I was a patient, and I hear it from my colleagues now that I'm a functional medicine physician: The immune system and the digestive system are two different aspects of the body, and never the twain shall meet.

But, in fact, you have *one* body, all your systems "talk" to each other, and the vast majority of your immune system is located in your gut. So how can digestion and immunity be unrelated?

If you go to a conventional practitioner with an autoimmune disorder and ask about digestive issues, you are likely to be referred to a gastroenterologist. It's sad to say, but most gastroenterologists would order an endoscopy or a colonoscopy before they'd ever ask about your diet.

Here's the problem with ignoring the gut: Since the majority of your immune system is located there, it is essential to focus on the digestive system and heal your leaky gut if you want to reverse your autoimmune symptoms. In order to be healthy, you must have a healthy gut. And I can show you thousands of patients who have seen immune-system results—almost immediately—from digestive-system healing.

MYTH FIVE: GOING GLUTEN-FREE WON'T MAKE ANY DIFFERENCE TO YOUR AUTOIMMUNE DISORDER

"Gluten-free? That's just some crazy fad people are trying to cash in on. We've been eating wheat for thousands of years, so why all of a sudden would it turn out not to be healthy?"

That's what many people believe about the role of gluten in our health, and most conventional practitioners are no different. Tell your doctor that you are concerned about gluten, and most likely he or she will say two things: "We can run a blood test and see if you have celiac disease" and "Do you have any digestive issues? No? Then you don't have to worry about gluten."

In chapter 5, I provide a full explanation of just why gluten is bad for your autoimmune condition; how celiac disease, which is rare, differs from gluten sensitivity, which is common; and how you might be suffering from gluten sensitivity without showing any digestive symptoms at all. I explain why, even if you don't have celiac disease, you still might be gluten-sensitive, and I talk you through exactly how gluten is making your autoimmune disorder worse.

The idea that gluten doesn't make any real difference to your condition is one of the most dangerous myths about autoimmune disorders. Taking apart that myth might be the single greatest service I can do for you.

MYTH SIX: HAVING AN AUTOIMMUNE DISORDER DOOMS YOU TO A POOR QUALITY OF LIFE

"My doctor said that, over time, I could expect to get weaker and weaker."

"I've had to tell my son not to bring the grandkids over—I can't take a chance on getting sick."

"Sometimes the pain gets so bad, I can't even take a walk with my husband."

These are the kinds of problems that someone with an autoimmune disorder can frequently expect—but they are by no means inevitable. Although conventional medicine would counsel you to accept a poor quality of life as the likely outcome of your condition, I'm here to tell you that it is not at all inevitable. If you follow The Myers Way, you can expect to be symptom-free, pain-free, and vigorous. Getting your autoimmune condition under control takes some people longer than others, and you might need support beyond what I can provide in this book (although I will point you to all the resources you need). Ultimately, if you clean up your diet; eliminate gluten, grains, and legumes; fix your leaky gut; lighten your toxic burden; heal your infections; and ease your stress load, you can look forward to an excellent quality of life.

MYTH SEVEN: WHEN IT COMES TO AUTOIMMUNE DISORDERS, ONLY YOUR GENES MATTER; ENVIRONMENTAL FACTORS DO NOT MATTER

Well, genetics does account for about 25 percent of the chance that you will develop an autoimmune disorder. But that means the remaining 75 percent of the picture is environmental—and therefore up to you. I find that an incredibly empowering statistic.

Avoiding gluten, grains, and legumes; healing your gut; taming your toxins; and relieving your burden of stress all play an enormous role in determining whether a genetic predisposition will be activated or remain dormant. Healing and preventing infections can also make a significant difference. Even after an autoimmune condition has been triggered, diet, toxins, infections, and stress can either make the condition worse or help to reverse it.

So don't become a prisoner of your genetics. Whatever genes you were born with, you have the power to manage your body's response to autoimmunity—and the power to create a happy, healthy life.

MYTH EIGHT: YOUR IMMUNE SYSTEM IS WHAT IT IS; THERE IS NOTHING YOU CAN DO TO SUPPORT IT

This myth might be the one that speaks most eloquently to the difference between conventional approaches and The Myers Way. Conventional practitioners treat autoimmune conditions by medicating the symptoms and suppressing the immune system. The Myers Way treats autoimmune conditions by strengthening the immune system, which includes cleansing and supporting the gut.

This divergence in approach is related to the differences between conventional medicine and functional medicine. Conventional medicine often goes for the quick fix: an acid-blocking medication rather than a change in diet to overcome acid reflux; immunosuppressants rather than a diet and lifestyle that promote health. Conventional approaches to autoimmune conditions frequently produce more side effects, which require more medications, which produce still more side effects—a vicious cycle that often seems to get worse and worse.

By contrast, The Myers Way creates a "virtuous cycle." By sup-porting your immune system through diet and detoxification, you create more vitality and health. Your mood, mental function, and overall energy level improve. As your inflammation subsides, your skin glows and even your hair gets healthier. You look better, feel better, and function better. Now you are creating positive side effects, rather than negative ones, in an ongoing upward spiral of health.

My approach is fundamentally different. I feel hope every day I go into my office and see the patients whose lives have been changed. I want to share that hope with you, so you can let go of the myths that surround you and embrace the promise of this powerful approach.

I know following The Myers Way can empower you to reverse your symptoms naturally, restoring you to energy, vitality, and health. But you don't have to take my word for it. Just give me thirty days and see the results for yourself.

CHAPTER 3

Your Enemy, Yourself

How Autoimmunity Works

ONE OF THE WORST THINGS about an autoimmune condition is feeling as if some alien presence has taken over your body. Out of nowhere, you are occupied by a mysterious force that makes you tremble, ache, panic, weaken, turn red, fail to sleep, and fail to focus, not to mention overwhelm you with fatigue, brain fog, and muscle weakness.

I have never felt more out of control than when I was struggling with my Graves' disease, and I see that same panicky confusion in so many of my patients when they first come to see me. It's bad enough feeling weak, dizzy, and exhausted. Okay, fine—you feel that when you have the flu, and you know you can get over it and go back to life as you know it. But with an autoimmune condition, if your conventional doctor has given you the conventional perspective, you feel as though the disease has taken all your power—as though it, not you, gets to decide your future. Can you go on vacation with your family? Ask the disease. Can you take on a challenging new assignment at work? Ask the disease. Can you apply for med school or grad school or law school, take off for a "gap year" in Nepal, start a family with your spouse, or train for a triathlon? Ask the disease, because now that you have this mysterious disorder, you no longer get to count on your body—or your energy level, your mental focus, or your emotional well-being. You *might* be fine in a month or two; you might even feel better than you do now. *If* those new medications work the way they're supposed to, *if* you don't develop some unexpected side effects, *if* the stress of traveling or extra work or childbirth doesn't derail your temperamental immune system, *if* you don't pick up yet another infection or stress or challenge abroad, your life might be able to continue in a satisfying way—or it might not. Ask the disease.

Even if you have a milder condition, like psoriasis, Hashimoto's, or Sjögren's, the idea that your body is destroying itself can be disturbing. Your immune system seems to have suddenly gone rogue, attacking your skin, thyroid, mucus membranes, or some other vital part of your anatomy. At least you know you can go on with your life as you have known it, that you can continue to throw yourself into travel or grad school or a demanding new promotion, that you can continue to play with your grandkids or go on a second honeymoon with your spouse. But lurking in the back of your mind is the knowledge that you now have a medical condition—for life—that can never really be reversed, only managed. Something went wrong, and because the conventional view is that it was caused by your genes, you couldn't have prevented it, which means that you can't prevent another disease from striking either, perhaps a worse one next time. Or perhaps this one will get worse at some point, and you won't be able to prevent that either. Even if the symptoms are not so bad, the feeling of disempowerment is.

Those of you on the autoimmune spectrum have an additional issue to combat. Not only do you have to deal with some disturbing symptoms, causing you to feel out of control, you most likely don't have a conventional medical diagnosis to explain what is happening to you. If you don't know what is happening to you, or why, how can you take charge of your health, let alone your life? How can you prevent your symptoms from getting worse, let alone act to make them any better? You ask your conventional doctor, "Are there any medications for my symptoms?" or "How long do I have to keep taking this?" or "What do we do if these medications stop working, the way the last ones did?" and there aren't any good answers. You ask, "Is there anything I can do to make things better?" and there isn't a good answer for that either. Feeling sick is bad enough. Feeling like your mysterious, nameless symptoms have taken all your power is worse.

I want to give that power back to you. In my view, power starts with knowledge. So I'm going to give you a quick science lesson—a highly simplified but still useful explanation of how your immune system works—so you can understand exactly what is going on inside your body. This explanation of the problem also contains the seeds of a solution, because once you understand the material in this chapter, you'll be able to see exactly why following my recommendations will work to reverse your symptoms, prevent them from getting worse, and bring you to a whole new level of health and vitality.

The key is to view your body as a friend and ally rather than as an enemy and saboteur—but how can you do that if you don't understand what your body is doing and why it is responding as it is? Reading this chapter will solve that problem. Knowing your own physiology empowers you to take action to strengthen and support your immune system, end your symptoms, get off your medications, and reclaim your health.

THE IMMUNE SYSTEM, YOUR PROTECTOR

When you think of it, the human body is quite a vulnerable organism. Bacteria, viruses, and parasites land on your skin. They float around you in the air, enticing your lungs to breathe them in. And of course these microscopic dangers crawl over your food and creep into your water, so you unknowingly introduce them into your body by swallowing them. Sometimes it seems remarkable that any of us survive at all.

In the midst of this toxic soup, what keeps you safe? Your heroic immune system, an extraordinarily complex and intricate configuration of biochemicals whose number-one priority is to protect you.

It's amazing to think that your immune system is at work every minute, even though most of the time you're probably not even aware that you *have* an immune system. It's as though you're being protected by some unsung security team, toiling away behind the scenes, sniffing out danger, quietly fending off attackers, calmly neutralizing threats. When your security team does its job properly, it really is one of the great marvels of the human body.

But when your immune system fails to do its job properly, chaos ensues. Conventional medicine responds by using drugs to *control* your immune system: suppressing it, modulating it, and compensating for it, while medicating the symptoms that result from its failures.

For example, a common conventional treatment for many autoimmune conditions is steroids, perhaps in the form of prednisone. Steroids suppress the immune system, so the reasoning is that they will work to calm an overactive immune system and get it down to a normal level so that it will stop attacking your own tissue.

There are two problems with this approach, however. First, prednisone has a number of problematic side effects, as you saw on page 37. Second, when the prednisone suppresses your immune system, it doesn't necessarily get it down to a normal level—it might suppress it down to *below* a normal level, so that you are dangerously vulnerable to threats a healthy immune function would be able to shake off, even such seemingly minor threats as a cold virus or some bacteria clinging to poorly washed food. That's why people on immunosuppressants often have to be unusually careful about contact with children, being in a crowd, flying, and other situations where they might be exposed to illness or infection.

Another common treatment for autoimmune conditions is Trexall (methotrexate), which also interferes with immune function, again in order to get an overactive immune system to function at a normal level so that it stops attacking your own tissue.

We don't know exactly how methotrexate works. It was originally developed as an anticancer drug, because it seems to prevent cells from using folate (a form of vitamin B) to manufacture DNA and RNA, keeping your cells from multiplying. This is good for blocking the spread of cancer cells, but it also interferes with the division of your normal, healthy cells, particularly the fast-growing ones that line your gut and replenish your bone marrow. Again, the danger is that the medication suppresses your immune system below a normal level, to the point where you are vulnerable to illness and infection.

Meanwhile, there is a risk of side effects (page 38), which are even more severe than those associated with prednisone.

Another example of an even more severe immunosuppressant is CellCept (mycophenolic acid), originally developed to suppress immune systems in organ recipients, so that their bodies wouldn't reject the transplanted organ. Later, researchers discovered that it could also be used to suppress an overactive immune system in people with autoimmune conditions. But, again, there's no way to calibrate how far the medication suppresses your immune system, and the danger does always exist that your immune system will be suppressed too far.

Of course there are also potential side effects (page 37), even more disturbing than those for other types of immunosuppressants.

Instead of suppressing your immune system, we're going to take a different approach. We are going to *support* your immune system, removing the obstacles that interfere with its work and making sure that it has all the resources it needs. We're going to feed your immune system the food it needs, as well as nourish it with some high-quality supplements. We're also going to remove the obstacles that keep your immune system from doing its job as we heal your gut, lighten your toxic burden, lower your stress load, and heal your infections. Your immune system will become strong and healthy, your symptoms will disappear, and "I feel great!" will become your new normal.

A BARRIER AGAINST DANGER

Your immune system begins its job at the boundaries between your body and the outside world. When bacteria land on your skin, part of what keeps them from infecting your body is the actual physical structure of your epidermis. But your immune system is also operating on your skin's surface, ready to engage (as you will soon see) in close combat with any invasive organism that seeks to enter through your pores.

Likewise, when you breathe in bacteria or toxins through your nose and lungs, the tiny hairs inside your nose and the hair-like cilia inside your lungs act as a *physical* barrier to prevent the invaders from entering. At the same time, your immune system creates a *chemical* barrier, producing the mucus in your nose and lungs that entrap and neutralize many dangers.

Your immune system's true glory, however, emerges when you swallow, for then it produces a whole slew of killer chemicals ready to destroy any problematic bacteria, viruses, or other potential dangers you might ingest with your food. Since most of the dangers you encounter come in through your mouth, scientists estimate that 80 percent of your immune system is located in your gut.

What that means is that when your gut isn't working properly, your immune system is compromised. As you shall see in chapters 4 and 5, the lining of your gut wall—your epithelium—is only one cell thick. A great deal of your immune system is just on the other side of that wall. So when your gut wall cells are healthy, your immune system can relax and do its job properly. When those cells are compromised, allowing partially digested food to leak through the intestinal wall, your immune system is also compromised. An overactive immune system and, eventually, autoimmune diseases can be the result. *You must have a healthy gut to have a healthy immune system.*

YOUR INNATE IMMUNE SYSTEM: YOUR FIRST LINE OF DEFENSE

Your immune system has two parts: "innate" and "adaptive." Your first, fastest, and most immediate line of defense is the innate system. This is the more primitive part of your immune system, the part you have in common with plants, fungi, insects, and multicelled organisms.

Your innate immune system is set up to act quickly and efficiently. It has no "memory"; it does not confer lasting immunity. Another part of your immune system does have a kind of memory, preventing you from getting certain diseases more than once or keeping you safe from a disease once you have been vaccinated for it. That slower, "smarter" branch of the team is known as your adaptive immune system, and we'll get to that in a minute. However, your innate immune system is both faster and less well informed. It doesn't keep a history of every disease you've ever had; it has to start from scratch every time it encounters a threat, rushing to your defense and fighting off the invaders just as if it had never seen them before. It's like the part of the security team that responds immediately, before it has time to look at the intelligence files or run background checks on a computer.

Your innate immune system frequently works through a mechanism known as "acute inflammation." "Inflammation" is just what it sounds like: a hot, fiery reaction that represents your body's efforts to fight off infection. "Acute" means that the inflammation is a specific, time-limited response to a problem, as opposed to "chronic inflammation," which is an ongoing, persistent response. (Chronic inflammation is the response we worry about and the one I'll be talking about throughout the book.)

Suppose you cut your finger on a rusty gate. That filthy old gate is simply swarming with harmful bacteria, and now that you've cut your finger, you've basically opened the door to those bacteria and thrown them a welcome party. If some form of protection doesn't show up, those harmful bacteria are basically going to infect your finger and maybe take over other parts of your body as well.[c]

The innate immune system to the rescue. It sends a whole team of killer chemicals to the site of the infection, creating the acute inflammation that is its primary weapon. Acute inflammation is actually an attempt to heal the infection, even though that healing can be an uncomfortable, even a painful, process, which by definition involves redness, swelling, heat, and pain:

Redness. Blood cells rush to the infection site, carrying immune chemicals with them. The extra blood cells beneath the surface of your skin cause it to turn red.

Swelling. Fluids also flow to the site. Some bring more killer chemicals. Others are there to carry away the dead cells that will result from this epic battle. These extra fluids cause the "battleground" to swell.

Heat. All that blood is warm, from the heat of your body. Extra blood generates extra heat.

Pain. The by-products of these chemical reactions stimulate your nerve endings, creating the nervous-system reaction known as pain. The pain is useful, because it alerts your body that you have been attacked and that the attack is serious. You didn't just get yelled at or threatened; you actually got cut, hit, or infected. The pain warns you to turn back and get help.

YOUR ADAPTIVE IMMUNE SYSTEM: YOUR SECOND LINE OF DEFENSE

Your innate immune system never really "learns" anything. Think of it as the entry-level portion of your security team, the guys who don't keep records or develop targeted approaches for particular intruders. These guys are great at rushing to the scene the instant there's a threat, but they don't vary their approach all that much. "Intruder equals inflammation" is basically the only formula they know.

Your adaptive immune system, by contrast, takes a little longer to kick into action. In fact, it develops over time, because it gathers and retains tons of information about which intruders have threatened you and how best to attack them. You can only find this portion of the immune system higher up on the evolutionary chain—basically, among vertebrates (animals with backbones).

The adaptive immune system evolved because, as an active, mobile being, you might find yourself encountering multiple environments with a wide variety of potential threats. Your adaptive immune system allows you to recognize some of these threats and develop permanent protection against them.

Every single time you cut your finger, you are vulnerable to infection from harmful bacteria. That's why open wounds are the job of the innate immune system. But once you encounter a disease like, say, measles, you never have to worry about getting that particular disease again. That's because your adaptive immune system takes over. After its first encounter with the measles virus, your adaptive immune system figures out how to give you long-term immunity—a targeted set of weapons that can nip that virus in the bud if it ever tries to invade your body again.

That's how vaccinations work. When you are vaccinated against polio, your body is exposed to a tiny amount of the poliovirus. Your adaptive immune system learns to recognize that virus and develops a long-term strategy against it. Thanks to this long-term strategy, you're protected for the rest of your life against that particular invader.

Of course some adaptive immune responses last a shorter time— weeks, months, or years, rather than a whole lifetime. That's why some vaccinations have to be administered more than once.

ANTIBODIES: YOUR ADAPTIVE IMMUNE SYSTEM'S WEAPONS OF CHOICE

Your adaptive immune system recognizes and targets intruders through an ingenious biological mechanism known as the "antibody."

An antibody is a large, Y-shaped protein produced by a portion of your immune system known as the "B cell," and it's secreted by your white blood cells. Sometimes another type of cell, known as the "T helper cell," is needed to help activate the B cell.

In order for your adaptive immune system to function properly, all these different types of cells need to be healthy. You don't need to remember the name of each type of cell, though. Just remember the antibody.

Antibodies are part of your security team's "special forces." Basically, your adaptive immune system studies a particular threat and then devises a protection strategy designed to target only that one threat. This protection strategy involves mobilizing immune cells to create inflammation that will in turn destroy the intruder—but this reaction is targeted and intruder specific. The inflammation flares up only when the antibody has detected the particular threat it has learned to recognize.

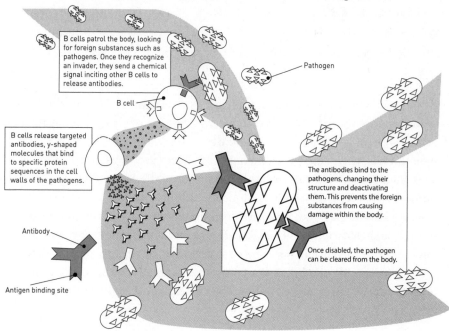

B cells patrol the body, looking for foreign substances such as pathogens. Once they recognize an invader, they send a chemical signal inciting other B cells to release antibodies.

Pathogen

B cell

B cells release targeted antibodies, y-shaped molecules that bind to specific protein sequences in the cell walls of the pathogens.

The antibodies bind to the pathogens, changing their structure and deactivating them. This prevents the foreign substances from causing damage within the body.

Antibody

Once disabled, the pathogen can be cleared from the body.

Antigen binding site

MEET YOUR "SECURITY SQUAD"

Your immune system is a complex system with many different players, but here are the key squad members. You don't need to remember all their names, but it's nice to know they're on the job!

Antibodies identify invaders and incite inflammation to go after them.

Lymphocytes are a type of immune system cell manufactured in the lymphatic system. They include B and T cells.

B cells produce both antibodies and inflammation. They also produce cytokines, "messenger" chemicals that signal other parts of the immune system to generate inflammation, which in turn brings more B cells and T cells to the scene.

Killer T cells are part of your inflammatory response. They attack invaders.

Helper T cells tell the B cells and Killer T cells what to do.

Regulatory T cells help instruct the inflammatory process when to turn on and when to turn off, so that your immune system doesn't remain on permanently high alert and your body doesn't remain permanently inflamed.

That's why we have so many different vaccines. The antibodies you develop against polio won't give you one bit of protection against measles, just as the antibodies you develop against measles won't give you even a tiny defense against polio. Each group of antibodies is designed to attack only one specific target while leaving every other microbe, bacterium, or virus alone.

You can see why an adaptive immune system would be so useful to animals that can move around the planet, encountering many different types of conditions. The vast majority of organisms are either neutral or good for you. If your immune system went into high alert every time it encountered a new organism, you would be in a state of constant inflammation: red, swollen, feverish, and in pain. Because inflammation is such a painful and demanding process, you want to save it for when you really need it—for when a genuine threat is attacking you.

The great paradox of your adaptive immune system is that it makes you both more vulnerable and stronger. So, yes, you can get measles *once* because your immune system doesn't spring into high alert every time it encounters an unfamiliar organism. The first time you meet the measles virus, it gets a free pass. Then, once your adaptive immune system figures out that the measles virus actually is bad for you, it produces targeted antibodies—sort of like posting a photograph of a known threat in the security squad's Command Central. "Watch out for that guy," the antibodies are told. "If you see him again, let us know, and we'll hit him with all the inflammation we have!" Meanwhile, other strange organisms—maybe a new food you've never tried or a new bacterium in a country you've never visited—get that same free pass.

Of course sometimes there is crossover. The antibodies that protect you against one disease occasionally do respond to one or more other diseases. In fact, vaccines themselves were invented when eighteenth-century physician Edward Jenner realized that people who had had cowpox—an unpleasant but not fatal disease—seemed to be immune to smallpox, which often was fatal. Jenner figured out that if he could give his patients a mild case of cowpox, they would then be protected against smallpox.

Jenner didn't understand exactly how this worked, but we do: Once a patient had the cowpox antibodies, those antibodies triggered an inflammatory response that targeted both the cowpox virus and its look-alike, the smallpox virus. It's as though the team in Command Central looked at the smallpox virus and thought, "Hey, that looks an awful lot like the guy in our cowpox photograph. Let's go after him too!" So antibodies go after particular targets—but sometimes they attack look-alikes as well.

This is how the flu vaccine works, by the way. The actual vaccine infects your body with three strains of the flu virus, but if another strain begins to spread that year, the vaccine should help protect you against that one too.

Let's recap this whole process:

Your adaptive immune system learns to recognize particular threats and develops antibodies in response. When an antibody detects a threat, it instructs your immune system to destroy the threat with a flood of inflammatory chemicals. Although each antibody is targeted to a particular threat, antibodies can get "confused" and target new threats that are simply look-alikes.

HOW DIFFERENT TYPES OF ANTIBODIES CREATE ALLERGIES AND SENSITIVITIES

All antibodies are not created equal. Each type works in a different way and at a different speed, giving you more flexibility against different types of threats.

The following are some of the main types of antibodies involved with autoimmunity and gut health. As you can see, each antibody is named "Ig," which is short for "immunoglobulin," another term for antibody. Each type of immunoglobulin has been randomly assigned a letter: A, E, or G. The letters don't mean anything; they're just the way scientists happened to label them.

IgA. This is the most common type of antibody and it forms the largest part of your immune system. The vast majority of your IgA is found in the mucosal lining of your gut. IgA is also found in your respiratory tract (nose, mouth, and lungs) and your urogenital tract (urinary tract and vagina). These antibodies keep harmful bacteria, viruses, and parasites from colonizing these areas and taking them over. IgA antibodies are also found in your saliva, tears, and breast milk. If you have an overgrowth of yeast in your intestines, then typically there will be a depressed level of IgA on a comprehensive stool test. This is one indicator that your immune system is not functioning optimally and you will have a harder time fighting infections.

IgE. If you have allergies, IgE antibodies are in play. This portion of your immune system jumps into action immediately. As soon as it detects an intruder, it mobilizes your innate immune system to release a whole flood of protective inflammatory chemicals. Unfortunately, the effects of that inflammation can often be worse than the invader. If you have a peanut allergy, for example, a single bite of peanut can trigger a swift and powerful inflammatory reaction. As a side effect of the inflammation, your lungs might swell so much that you become unable to breathe. It isn't the peanut the closes your airways; it's your body's inflammatory response to the peanut.

IgG. This type of antibody triggers an inflammatory response that is far slower and less intense than an IgE response—a response known as a "sensitivity" rather than an allergy. An IgG antibody creates more subtle reactions, which might be delayed for up to seventy-two hours, making it very hard to pinpoint exactly what triggered the symptoms. As a result, your entire system can become inflamed from frequent encounters with various threats, but because your IgG reactions are so delayed, it can be difficult to figure out what the threats are and how to avoid them. Gluten and dairy sensitivities are common results of this type of antibody, and you're going to learn a lot more about this type of reaction in chapters 4 and 5, since preventing IgG reactions is such a key aspect of The Myers Way.

NO INFLAMMATION: A HEALTHY, STRONG IMMUNE SYSTEM

The goal that we are working toward—the goal that The Myers Way is designed to help you reach—is a state of *no inflammation*.

When you have no inflammation in your body, that means your immune system is at rest. It is calm, strong, responsive, and ready to do—but not overdo—its job.

Suppose you are taking a short domestic flight, and the person next to you has the flu. She coughs, and some of the flu virus floats into the air around your face. You breathe in molecules of the flu virus through your nostrils—but you don't catch the flu. That's because your innate immune system, in the form of "macrophage" molecules lining your lungs and nasal passages, is on the alert. The

POSSIBLE RESPONSES TO AN IGG DEFENSE

The following signs of an inflammatory response can be delayed for hours or even days after your IgG antibodies detect a threat:

Brain issues (headaches, anxiety, depression, mood swings, seizures, ADD/ADHD, brain fog, lack of focus, memory problems, sleep problems, sleepiness, fatigue)

Digestive issues (gas, bloating, indigestion, nausea, constipation, diarrhea)

Hormonal issues (irregular periods, hormone imbalances, hot flashes)

Metabolic issues (weight gain, difficulty losing weight)

Musculoskeletal issues (joint pain, joint swelling, muscle pain, back pain)

Skin issues (acne, hives, itching, flushing, rashes)

Ironically, these symptoms are not caused by the actual threat to your body. Instead, they are the side effects of inflammation: your immune system's attempts to protect you.

macrophages (literally "big eaters") surround and absorb the virus molecules, keeping you safe and healthy.

Everything works so well, you're not even aware of the terrific job your security squad is doing for you. By contrast, the passenger in the seat in front of you has a weakened immune system, and even on this two-hour flight, he *does* pick up the flu. The next day, he's lying miserably in bed, his body aching, his fever raging—but thanks to your strong immune system, you haven't missed a beat.

Or suppose you go to the store and buy some broccoli, which you don't wash very well. Broccoli is picked from the ground, and this particular piece of ground had some cow manure on it, swarming with unhealthy bacteria. Without even realizing it, you end up consuming a fair amount of this unhealthy bacteria—and yet you don't get sick. That's because your innate immune system was standing by, ready to destroy the bacteria before they could cause diarrhea or an infection. Those are the blessings of a strong immune system, which is why our goal is to keep yours healthy.

ACUTE INFLAMMATION: A QUICK AND TEMPORARY RESPONSE

Sometimes, even when your immune system is strong, a threat is just too much for you. Then your immune system pulls out its first weapon of choice: acute inflammation.

Suppose that instead of a short, domestic flight, you have to take a long, international trip. Once again, you sit beside someone who has the flu. Your exposure on the domestic flight was relatively brief, but this foreign flight gives you several hours more exposure. With all that extra access, the flu virus finally succeeds in burrowing its way inside you, evading the macrophages and threatening you from within. What happens then?

The innate immune system to the rescue again. It quickly mobilizes a wide variety of killer cells and inflammatory chemicals designed to kill off the invader. Your flu symptoms are caused not by the invader but by your immune system's weapon of choice. Inflammation—not the flu itself—is responsible for your red nose (redness), congested nasal passages (swelling), fever (heat), and achiness (pain). Because this is a case of *acute* inflammation, your immune system calms down as soon as the invader is defeated: The inflammation subsides, and life goes happily on.

Likewise, when you cut your finger on that rusty gate, you will probably experience some redness, swelling, heat, and pain as your innate immune system rushes inflammatory chemicals to the site of a potential infection. Those painful or uncomfortable symptoms are evidence that your immune system is trying to protect you, attacking invaders with acute inflammation. Soon enough, the infection is defeated, and the inflammation subsides.

The key thing to remember is that acute inflammation is triggered by a particular cause . . . and it goes away when the problem is solved. Acute inflammation can be painful or uncomfortable, as anyone who's been up all night with the flu can attest. But once the episode is over, it's over, and in most cases you bounce back to good health.

CHRONIC INFLAMMATION: YOUR IMMUNE SYSTEM ON NEVER-ENDING ALERT

Unlike acute inflammation, *chronic* inflammation sticks around for a long time, maybe even permanently. That is very bad news because chronic inflammation is one of the greatest health risks we face today. It is the underlying cause of nearly every type of disease, from acne to cardiovascular disease, and perhaps even of cancer. And, as you saw in chapter 1 (see "The Autoimmune Spectrum," page 20), chronic inflammation plays a huge role in autoimmune conditions: setting them off, keeping them going, and making them worse.

As you just saw, the inflammatory reaction is supposed to flare up in response to a specific threat, eradicate the threat, and then subside, giving your body a chance to get back to normal. However, when your body is exposed to one threat after another, with no time to fully recover, or when a threat—even a low-level threat—never completely

CONDITIONS ASSOCIATED WITH CHRONIC INFLAMMATION

Bone and joint disorders (back pain, muscle pain, arthritis)

Cancers of all types

Cardiovascular diseases (heart disease, atherosclerosis)

Digestive disorders (acid reflux [GERD], irritable bowel syndrome, ulcers, gallstones, fatty liver, diverticulitis, food sensitivities, food allergies)

Emotional and cognitive disorders (anxiety, depression, ADD/ADHD, Alzheimer's, dementia)

Hormonal disorders (fibrocystic breasts, endometriosis, fibroids)

Metabolic disorders (obesity, diabetes)

Respiratory disorders (sinusitis, seasonal allergies, asthma)

Skin conditions (acne, eczema, rosacea)

Of course chronic inflammation is also associated with autoimmune conditions of all types, along with such related conditions as chronic fatigue syndrome.

IMMUNE COMPLEXES: THE HIDDEN CAUSE OF JOINT PAIN

When your immune system is highly inflamed, it creates clusters of anti-inflammatory chemicals known as "immune complexes." These can travel through your bloodstream and settle in your joints, inflaming your joints and producing—you guessed it—redness, swelling, heat, and pain. That's why inflamed joints are a warning sign: You might be at risk for rheumatoid arthritis, or you might already have it.

Either way, you can heal your symptoms by decreasing the overall inflammation in your body. Once again, lowering inflammation by following The Myers Way is your solution for both reversing and preventing autoimmune conditions.

subsides, your immune system remains on permanent alert and inflammation becomes chronic. It's as if a portion of the rusty gate remains buried in your finger: The onslaught of infection never really goes away. Inflammation keeps getting triggered, and your body suffers as a result.

When inflammation becomes chronic, your immune system is like an overworked security squad whose guys have been on the job six straight days without a break. As you can imagine, they are likely to make all sorts of mistakes—with potentially disastrous consequences for your health.

AUTOIMMUNITY: WHEN CHRONIC INFLAMMATION LASTS TOO LONG

In chapters 4 through 7 you'll find out more about what factors can put your immune system on permanent alert, creating chronic inflammation and putting you at risk for autoimmunity. I'll give you a quick preview: These factors include the intestinal problem known as leaky gut (covered in chapter 4); gluten, grains, legumes, and other common foods in your diet (discussed in chapter 5); environmental toxins (explored in chapter 6); certain types of infections; and an overload of stress (both examined in chapter 7). That's why The Myers Way focuses on improving the diet, healing the gut, lightening the toxic burden, treating infections, and relieving stress. Together, these end chronic inflammation, give your immune system a break, and get it running at peak efficiency once again.

If you don't have an autoimmune condition, please keep in mind that chronic inflammation can trigger one. And if you are currently suffering from an autoimmune condition, chronic inflammation will make it worse. That's why our goal with The Myers Way is always to *reduce, eliminate, and prevent chronic inflammation.*

Check out page 7 for a list of symptoms that might occur when you are chronically inflamed. This is the list of warning signs for the autoimmune spectrum, because chronic inflammation is what *puts* you on that spectrum. The more inflamed you are, and the longer your chronic inflammation continues, the greater your risk of an autoimmune condition.

No one knows exactly how chronic inflammation translates into autoimmunity. What we do know is that there is a high correlation between the two conditions. Chronic inflammation stresses your immune system, and when your immune system becomes too stressed, it's likely to go rogue.

Let's go back to our image of the security squad: five or six guys sitting in Command Central, surrounded by hostile invaders. The invaders—infections, toxins, stressors, harmful bacteria, and a host of other elements—keep assaulting the building, ceaselessly, relentlessly. The guys are exhausted—they haven't had a break in days—but they can't afford to leave their post, even for a meal or a good night's sleep, because the attacks just keep on coming. All they can do is load up on coffee and doughnuts and hope that they're up to the job.

What are they likely to do? At first, they might be selective about whom they fire at, choosing their targets with care. As the assaults wear on and they become increasingly exhausted, they begin to spray the entire surrounding area with all the firepower at their command. They just want the attacks to stop, and at this point they aren't thinking too clearly about how to distinguish big threats from little ones, or even how to distinguish real threats from imaginary ones. They're just bringing out the biggest guns they have in a desperate attempt to protect their position.

That's how your immune system responds when it's assaulted

continuously with the wrong types of food, the toxins in your environment, certain dangerous infections, and an overload of stress. Initially, maybe, it could handle one or two challenges. But if the challenges keep on coming, the inflammation ratchets up higher and higher. Eventually, your beleaguered immune system might simply go rogue and start attacking your own tissue. This is the danger zone: the state in which you develop an autoimmune condition. Until you find a way to stop the attacks and bring down the firepower, your own innocent body will be caught in the crossfire, with ever-worsening symptoms and ever-declining health.

As previously mentioned, your conventional doctor might respond by prescribing immunosuppressants—powerful drugs that suppress your immune system. In effect, conventional medicine tries to disarm those guys in Command Central so that they can't shoot at the wrong targets. Unfortunately, those medications also suppress the *entire* security team, even the guys who are well rested and properly regulated. With your entire security team off the job, you are now vulnerable to invasion from a real enemy, which is why when you take immunosuppressants you must be incredibly careful to keep your hands clean, avoid sick people, and maybe even give up time with your grandchildren, just in case you catch a bug.

As a functional medicine physician, I respond differently. I have a lot of sympathy for those guys in Command Central, and I want to make them stronger, not weaker. My goal is not to disarm the security

NO MORE COFFEE AND DOUGHNUTS!

Remember how your security team kept itself going on coffee and doughnuts? Caffeine and sugar often do seem to provide a quick fix when you're tired or stressed—but, in fact, they only make the problem worse, and both items actually *suppress* your immune system. So for your first thirty days on The Myers Way, I'm going to ask you to pass on the caffeine and sugar, just to give your poor, beleaguered security team the support they need. You might be able to add small amounts of these foods back into your diet once your immune system is strong enough, but I personally avoid them except for special occasions and so do many of my patients.

team but, rather, to give them a break, allowing them to come back to the job rested, relaxed, and ready to use good judgment. My strategy is to stop the assaults—to reduce the number of factors your immune system has to deal with by cleaning up your diet, healing your gut, lightening your toxic burden, treating your infections, and reducing your overall load of stress. Once these assaults are reduced, your immune system will calm down, stop attacking you, and save its firepower for the real threats.

TOLERANCE OF SELF

If I tell you that you've got to have "tolerance of self" to be healthy, I'm not talking about a state of psychological self-acceptance (important as that might be!). I'm speaking of the way your immune system has to tolerate the elements of your own body.

Autoimmunity occurs when your immune system loses tolerance of self and begins attacking your tissue. If you have Hashimoto's, your immune system attacks your thyroid. If you have multiple sclerosis, it attacks the myelin sheath surrounding your brain and spinal cord. If you have polymyositis, it attacks your muscles. Once your immune system goes rogue in this way, that's it. You have an autoimmune condition and there is no known cure.

Fortunately, there is an effective treatment. You can put a stop to your chronic inflammation while easing the burden on your immune system in many other ways. When your immune system is not quite so stressed, it regains tolerance of self and stops attacking you. (The full scientific explanation involves your thymus's ability to produce, regulate, and balance your T cells.)

If your inflammation levels rise again, however, your immune system is likely to go out of whack, just as it did before. Your antibodies will once again confuse your own tissue with that of an invader. You will lose your tolerance of self, and your symptoms will return.

This is why, regardless of where you are on the autoimmune spectrum, you must remain on The Myers Way, because keeping your inflammation levels down is the only way you can protect yourself. As you heal your gut, get off your medications, and become symptom-free, you might have leeway with some aspects of The Myers Way:

eggs, nightshades, an occasional alcoholic or caffeinated drink, small amounts of sugar, maybe even a gluten- and dairy-free muffin as a special treat. (After you have completed your first thirty days on The Myers Way, go to my website for a special bonus chapter on how to find out what you can add back in, and when.) However, gluten and dairy are so inflammatory, and gluten causes so many other problems, I want you avoiding these foods 100 percent of the time.

I explained this to a patient recently who was struggling with the idea of letting go of familiar foods. Although she accepted that her health depended on her adopting this new diet, she felt sad and somewhat panicky about all the things she might never be able to eat.

"Look," I told her, "your gut is leaky right now. It's as if a dam broke and we are fixing it brick by brick. If you eat a gluten-free muffin or a scrambled egg at this point, it would knock out the few bricks we just managed to get back into place.

"Pretty soon, though—maybe in a couple of months, maybe a bit longer—you will have healed your leaky gut, resolved all your symptoms, and gotten off all your medications. At that point your gut will be a lot stronger, and if you want to have some quinoa or an omelet or even a gluten-free muffin, sure that will knock out a few bricks, but we can easily repair the leak and put those bricks back without much trouble. Of course even at that point, if you eat some gluten, you'll knock out *all* the bricks and we will have to start over again. But you should be able to tolerate a few more foods at that point than are safe for you now."

It really helped my patient to visualize those bricks. She liked knowing that she would be able to strengthen her gut and withstand a few more challenges, and she understood that her tolerance for those challenges was not unlimited. Meanwhile, she was happy to work on the "repair job" in front of her, knowing that it was part of a process that would continue to carry her forward.

So the good news is that you *can* overcome chronic inflammation—and go on to enjoy boundless good health. And once your gut is healed and your immune system is in balance, you can loosen up on some of the provisions of The Myers Way. Your first step, though, is to follow the diet strictly for thirty days. Only 100 percent compliance is going to give you the exciting results you want and deserve.

Part Two

Get to the Root

CHAPTER 4

Heal Your Gut

MY PATIENT SHENNA WAS EXCITED. We were just beginning our first appointment, and she was hoping to finally resolve her symptoms and get off her medications.

Shenna had been diagnosed with lupus about six years ago. Lupus is a chronic inflammatory condition in which the immune system attacks a wide variety of the body's tissues and organs, which can include joints, kidneys, skin, heart, lungs, brain, and blood cells.

Before she came to see me, Shenna had been working with a conventional medicine doctor, who had prescribed her Plaquenil, one of the usual first-line drugs for her condition. For most of those six years, Shenna had managed to lead a relatively normal life, although she often suffered from headaches, fatigue, and depression. Her doctor told her that all three symptoms were common side effects of lupus—caused either physically by the disease or psychologically by the challenges of living with a serious illness. In response, the doctor gave Shenna a prescription for Lexapro, a common antidepressant.

Shenna wasn't happy about the many problems she faced. Still, like so many people with autoimmune conditions, she didn't think she had any other options.

Then Shenna had a new "flare": the technical term for a lupus episode and also the term used with many autoimmune conditions when the symptoms suddenly get worse. Now she was suddenly also coping with chest pain, shortness of breath, joint pain, and unnerving bouts of memory loss. She couldn't remember the names of people she had met, she forgot several familiar phone numbers, and she began having trouble finding where she had parked her car. In response, her doctor added another, more powerful medication: prednisone, a steroid typically ordered when lupus seems to be progressing.

Shenna was hopeful that prednisone would help bring this flare under control. But after three months, it still hadn't—and now she was facing a whole new set of side effects: weight gain, easy bruising, increased depression, and a blood pressure reading that had her primary care doctor worried.

Between her symptoms and her side effects, Shenna's "normal" life turned into a constant round of missed work, canceled dinner plans, and anxious trips to the doctor. So she began to look for another way. A friend had forwarded her one of my newsletters, and Shenna checked out my website. She was inspired by the message of hope I offered—the prospect of a life without symptoms, medications, or side effects; a life of vibrancy, energy, and health.

So here we were in my office.

"I'm really hoping you can help me," Shenna said softly, "but I'm not sure that anybody can. My grandmother had lupus too, and my mother has rheumatoid arthritis. I know autoimmune conditions are genetic, and I just feel like my genes have doomed me."

She shook her head, looking down. "The worst thing is that I have a twelve-year-old daughter. Given the way things have gone for the women in my family, it's hard not to feel like she's doomed too."

"Shenna," I said firmly, waiting until she looked back up at me, "I'm going to tell you something very important. Yes, you probably have a genetic predisposition to autoimmunity, but that's only 25 percent of the story. The other 75 percent is up to you. Which means that you can turn things around for yourself, and you can likely keep your daughter from ever having to face what you've gone through."

I pointed to the thirty-page intake form that I ask all my patients to fill out, with detailed questions about every aspect of Shenna's life.

"We are going to determine how your autoimmune condition developed," I told her, "and all this information is going to help us figure that out."

"Yeah, there really were a lot of questions. None of my doctors have ever asked me about any of those things," Shenna said. "You even asked me whether I was breast-fed or bottle-fed and if I was born by C-section. I'm so curious. What does that have to do with being autoimmune?"

THE FUNCTIONAL MEDICINE DETECTIVE

One of the best attributes of functional medicine is the way it allows me to personalize my approach. Each patient has their own story, full of valuable information and important clues. That's why one of the first things I ask my patients to do is fill out a detailed intake form covering every possible relevant area. Then I ask them to tell me their story.

After all, the heart of functional medicine is understanding the many ways that seemingly unrelated factors can interact. What you eat, how well you sleep, which toxins you're exposed to, and the degree of stress in your life all play a key role in your health, along with many other factors that sometimes take a bit of digging. As a functional medicine physician, I have to be a kind of detective, looking for clues about how my patients' health issues began and progressed.

As you recall from chapter 1, many people who do not yet have an autoimmune disorder are on the autoimmune spectrum (page 20). When I meet with my autoimmune patients, I try to figure out how they progressed up that spectrum and what factors led to their symptoms progressing. That way we can see how to move them back *down* the spectrum, reducing their inflammation and creating health.

As you saw in chapter 3, 80 percent of the immune system is located in the gut, meaning that if you don't have a healthy gut, you can't have a healthy immune system. That's why gut health is a vital part of what I want to uncover. If I find out where a patient's gut was compromised, I can usually see what made them autoimmune. That's why *Heal your gut* is the first pillar of The Myers Way.

Most of my patients don't come in looking for solutions to gut problems, however. They're focused on the condition that brought them in. Likewise, Shenna thought her story started six years ago, when her lupus was first diagnosed. I asked her to go back further.

"You didn't get lupus overnight," I pointed out. "Your inflammation must have been building up for a long time. In fact, that C-section and that bottle-feeding I asked about might have a lot to do with your health right now."

And so Shenna and I began putting her story together. As always, I focused on two questions:

How had Shenna's gut health been compromised?

How had that created problems for her immune system?

We'll get back to Shenna's story in a minute. But first, in order to truly understand Shenna's story, you need to know a little bit about the gut.

THE GUT: THE GATEWAY TO YOUR HEALTH

People always ask me "Why is the gut so important to you?" Simple, I tell them: The gut is the gateway to your health.

The gut is a complex system that includes every part of your body involved in digestion:

- mouth
- esophagus
- stomach
- small intestine
- large intestine (colon)
- anus
- gallbladder
- liver
- pancreas
- nervous system
- immune system
- the trillions of bacteria that live in your gut and elsewhere throughout your body

If any one of these parts of your digestive system goes out of whack, your whole gut suffers—and symptoms result.

If you have an autoimmune condition or are on the autoimmune spectrum, your poor gut is staggering under the weight of a poor diet (even foods that seem like they *should* be healthy), medications, toxins, infections, and too much stress. We've all been there—but now it's time to make a change.

The good news is that when you do heal your gut—which you can begin to do in thirty days—you'll be well on your way to reversing and preventing autoimmune conditions, not to mention healing many other symptoms you might never have associated with gut health.[d] A lot of the issues I have to explain are complex, but this one really is that simple: Heal your gut and you heal yourself. In fact, most of your other health problems will simply go away, and they might even disappear for good.

SIGNS OF GOOD GUT HEALTH

You feel good after eating.

You have one to three bowel movements per day—solid and well formed.

You do not experience gas, bloating, cramps, or pain after eating.

You do not notice undigested food in your stool.

You have no need for digestive medications.

You do not experience GERD or acid reflux symptoms.

SIGNS OF POOR GUT HEALTH

Acne

ADD/ADHD

Anxiety

Arthritis

Asthma

Autoimmune disease

Belching

Bloating

Blood sugar imbalances

Cancer

Chronic coughing

Chronic fatigue syndrome

Congestion

Constipation (fewer than one bowel movement per day)

Depression

Diarrhea, loose stools

Difficulty concentrating

Dizziness

Fatigue

Fibromyalgia

Frequent illness

Headaches

Heartburn

Hormone imbalance

Infertility

Insomnia

Intestinal spasms

Irregular periods

Joint pain

Low white blood cell count

Mood swings

Nausea or vomiting

Passing gas

Seasonal allergies

Skin rashes, eczema, hives, rosacea

Stomach pain

Stuffy nose

Thyroid imbalance

Weight gain, inability to lose weight

HOW DIGESTION WORKS

You see and smell food, triggering your salivary glands.

Your salivary glands produce saliva.

The enzymes in the saliva break down simple carbohydrates
(found in starchy foods).

You chew your food, breaking it down into smaller fragments.

You swallow your food, which travels down your esophagus
and into your stomach.

Various chemicals break your food down further,
especially hydrochloric acid (HCl).

Food enters your small intestine, where most of your food is digested.

The small intestine also secretes hormones that signal your
pancreas, liver, and gallbladder to initiate their roles in digestion.

Insoluble fiber and water move on to the large intestine for final absorption.

Any leftover waste is eliminated through the anus.

HEALTHY GUT OR LEAKY GUT?

One of the keys to good gut health is your small intestine, because that's where most of your digestion takes place. Your small intestine is truly an amazing organ. It is "small" in name only: Although it fits snugly within your abdomen, it is more than twenty feet long and has the surface area of a tennis court.

Within the small intestine are tiny projections known as "villi." When nutrients flow through the small intestine, they get caught on these projections, which look like hairy fingers. The little hairs on your villi are called "microvilli," and this whole portion of your small intestine is known as the "brush border," because it looks like a giant, hairy brush.

The hairs of the brush—the villi and microvilli—sweep the nutrients in amid the flow of newly digested food. The nutrients are then directed toward "tight junctions," special channels that hold the cells of your epithelial wall tightly together. (These cells are known as enterocytes.) Passing through the tight junctions, the nutrients enter your bloodstream, which carries that nourishment to every part of your body.

When your digestion is working well, your tight junctions keep all but the smallest molecules of food from passing through your intestinal wall. When your gut health is compromised, however, you develop the condition known as leaky gut.

Leaky gut compromises your small intestine's ability to absorb nutrients. Part of why your small intestine is so amazing is because, with all those folds and villi, it has a huge surface area. The greater the surface area, the more nutrients it can absorb. Just think of how much more water a bath towel can absorb than, say, a tiny square of napkin.

However, if your villi and microvilli become damaged, that reduces the surface area of your small intestine—and your ability to absorb nutrients goes way down. Although conventional medicine recognizes this phenomenon only in celiac disease, my clinical experience leads me to believe that there is a spectrum of this type of damage, which includes many people with leaky gut, keeping them from getting the full nutritional benefit of their food.

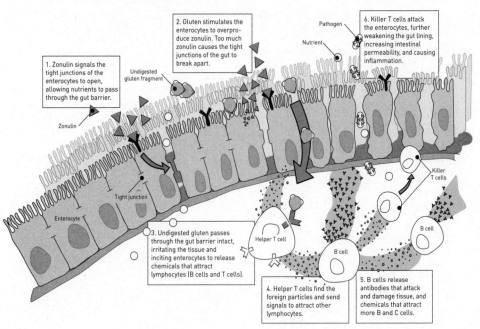

1. Zonulin signals the tight junctions of the enterocytes to open, allowing nutrients to pass through the gut barrier.

2. Gluten stimulates the enterocytes to overproduce zonulin. Too much zonulin causes the tight junctions of the gut to break apart.

6. Killer T cells attack the enterocytes, further weakening the gut lining, increasing intestinal permeability, and causing inflammation.

3. Undigested gluten passes through the gut barrier intact, irritating the tissue and inciting enterocytes to release chemicals that attract lymphocytes (B cells and T cells).

4. Helper T cells find the foreign particles and send signals to attract other lymphocytes.

5. B cells release antibodies that attack and damage tissue, and chemicals that attract more B and C cells.

Undigested gluten fragment

Zonulin

Tight junction

Enterocyte

Helper T cell

B cell

B cell

Pathogen

Nutrient

Killer T cells

Leaky gut not only limits potential nutrient absorption, it also causes the walls of your intestines to leak and your tight junctions to begin to come apart. Then all sorts of forbidden items can slip out of your gut and into your bloodstream, including toxins, unfriendly microbes, and partially digested food. Recent research is also leaning toward the belief that a leaky gut is one of the preconditions for cancer.

What happens when things that belong *in* your gut start leaking *out*?

First, the toxins and unfriendly microbes—elements that would normally have stayed within your gut and passed out during elimination—

HOW DO YOU KNOW IF YOU HAVE LEAKY GUT?

If you have already been diagnosed with an autoimmune condition, then you definitely had leaky gut at some point and still do, unless you have followed or are currently following a protocol similar to the one I recommend in this book.

In fact, whether or not you have an autoimmune condition, just about everybody eating a standard American diet and/or living our typically high-stress lifestyle has some degree of a leaky gut. Some symptoms can clue you in to your own gut health. If you have any of the following symptoms—and especially if the symptom is intense or frequent—you almost certainly have leaky gut and can benefit from the eating plan laid out in chapter 9.

Bones: osteopenia, osteoporosis

Brain: anxiety, depression, brain fog

Digestive system: bloating, constipation, diarrhea, weight loss, fat malabsorption

Hormones: irregular periods, PMS, perimenopausal or menopausal symptoms

Immune system: frequent colds, flu, and infections; joint pain; muscle pain; autoimmune disorders

Infections—gut: parasite, small intestine bacterial overgrowth (SIBO), or yeast overgrowth (candida)

Metabolism: excess weight, obesity, diabetes

Nutrients: iron deficiency/ anemia, omega-3 fatty acid deficiency, vitamin deficiencies

Skin: acne, eczema, rosacea

WHAT CAUSES LEAKY GUT?

Challenging foods and food sensitivities:

- alcohol
- dairy
- eggs
- gluten
- GMOs
- grains and pseudo-grains
- legumes
- nightshade vegetables
- sugar

Chemotherapy

Gut infections and imbalances:

- parasites
- SIBO
- yeast overgrowth

Medications:

- acid-blocking medications
- antibiotics
- birth-control pills
- NSAIDs (aspirin, ibuprofen, and prescription NSAIDs [nonsteroidal anti-inflammatory drugs])
- prednisone

Mycotoxins (toxic mold)

Radiation

Stress:

- physical stress (illness, lack of sleep)
- emotional stress (family, personal, and work pressures)

Surgeries

start to enter your bloodstream, where they definitely do not belong. All of a sudden those guys in Command Central have a lot more toxic invaders to deal with. They start firing off the inflammatory chemicals, and you start suffering from side effects. You get acne or frequent colds or gas or a headache—and your immune system starts feeling strained.

But it gets worse, because along with those bad toxins and microbes, your gut is also leaking partially digested food in forms your body simply doesn't recognize. Instead of the amino acids and glucose molecules your immune system has been trained to expect, much larger and stranger pieces of food make their way into your bloodstream.

Now your immune system really goes crazy. It starts making antibodies for these new invaders—gluten, dairy proteins, egg proteins, and other foods that might otherwise be healthy for you to eat. Every time you eat some of that food, your antibodies alert your immune system, and the guys in Command Central fire off a flood of inflammatory chemicals. You develop chronic inflammation, with all its multiple side effects—and your immune system is now super stressed. You are now firmly on the autoimmune spectrum. If you stay there long enough, you might develop a full-blown autoimmune disease.

Alessio Fasano, M.D., the founder and director of the Center for Celiac Research at Massachusetts General Hospital and a professor at Harvard Medical School, has done the leading research into gluten and leaky gut. He believes that in order to develop an autoimmune condition, you must have leaky gut. This means that if you have leaky gut, you are putting yourself at risk for developing autoimmunity. I can confirm this from my own practice: Leaky gut puts you firmly on the autoimmune spectrum. So if you want to reverse and prevent autoimmune conditions, heal your leaky gut.

SHENNA'S STORY: CHILDHOOD CLUES

When Shenna and I sat down to put her story together, we began at the beginning, with Shenna's birth. Shenna had been born by caesarean section, which meant that she had been taken by the attending doctor right from her mother's womb, rather than passing down the birth canal.

Why was this significant? Well, in order to function properly, your gut relies upon trillions of bacteria that live within your intestines and elsewhere in your body. You actually have ten times more microbial cells than human cells.

You weren't born with these friendly bacteria. Instead, you begin to acquire them from your mother during your passage down the birth canal. Babies who are born by C-section often miss out on some crucial bacteria—bacteria that are vital to good gut health.

I know it might be hard for you to think of bacteria as important for your health. We're used to thinking of them as dangerous invaders, and of course some of them are. But the vast majority of bacteria on this planet are either neutral or helpful.

The friendly bacteria that live in your gut are *incredibly* helpful. They make it possible for you to digest your food, and they maintain the lining of your intestinal walls, the epithelium.

A strong epithelium is crucial for preventing leaky gut. That's why a good population of friendly bacteria is necessary for gut health—and, therefore, to your immune system.

Shenna, though, started out with a deficit of friendly bacteria, so that was our first clue as to what went wrong:

Clue One: Missing Out on Friendly Bacteria in the Birth Canal

Shenna also told me that her mother had difficulty breast-feeding, so she needed to feed Shenna by bottle instead. Breast milk is a second crucial source of friendly bacteria for newborns and infants, along with some key immune factors. By being bottle-fed, Shenna missed out on these two crucial supports . . . and moved a little further up the autoimmune spectrum.

Clue Two: Missing Out on Friendly Bacteria and Immune Factors from Breast-Feeding

These early problems almost certainly affected Shenna's health as a child and likely contributed to her frequent ear infections. Shenna also shared with me that many of her favorite childhood foods were dairy products: yogurt sweetened with fruit for breakfast, a buttery grilled-cheese sandwich for lunch, a sweet bowl of ice cream for a nightly dessert, a glass of warm milk at bedtime.

My inner detective jumped into high gear. Ear infections are frequently a sign of food sensitivity—those delayed IgG reactions you read about in chapter 3—specifically, sensitivity to dairy. If you have food sensitivity, by definition you have a leaky gut, which I inferred had been caused by the lack of friendly bacteria that Shenna was missing as the result of her birth and bottle-feeding.

Let's talk about this. In response, Shenna's immune system might have decided early on that milk was a dangerous toxic invader and created antibodies to target dairy products, with three likely effects:

- Every time Shenna ate any product that contained milk—including baked goods, pancakes, and French toast—her dairy antibodies cued her immune system, which flooded her body with inflammatory chemicals. These chemicals produced a whole slew of side effects—including ear infections.

• Shenna's system was now full of "casomorphins," found in all dairy products. Many people have a gene that causes these substances to enter their morphine receptors, so that dairy products act in a very similar way to morphine: You feel great when the dairy is in your system, and you go through withdrawal when you try to give it up. Shenna seemed to have these receptors, because if she went even a couple of days without eating milk, cheese, yogurt, or ice cream, she began to feel irritable, tired, and "desperate for dairy." So Shenna kept eating dairy—and her inflammation became chronic. (By the way, gluten contains "gluteomorphins," which act in the same manner, which is why so many people crave gluten and have a hard time giving it up.)

• This chronic inflammation further contributed to leaky gut. This stressed Shenna's immune system even more, pushing her further up the autoimmune spectrum.

Clue Three: Frequent Ear Infections = Likely a Dairy Sensitivity

Shenna's ear infections had another important effect: She was treated for them with antibiotics. While antibiotics have many important uses, they also have one very problematic side effect: They kill off your friendly bacteria, which, as you just saw, can lead to leaky gut, chronic inflammation, and more stress for your immune system.

By creating leaky gut, antibiotics can also indirectly affect your brain function. That's because of a relationship most conventional doctors aren't aware of but that is one of the basic premises of functional medicine: the gut–brain connection. When you take antibiotics, you kill off good bacteria in your intestines, which can lead to yeast overgrowth. Yeast likes to spread out in a layer over the inside of your gut. Your gut produces 95 percent of your serotonin, the feel-good chemical your brain uses to combat depression and anxiety, ensure good sleep, keep your moods level, and produce feelings of optimism, calm, and self-confidence. The yeast layer seriously affects the production of neurotransmitters, so continued use of antibiotics goes on to mess with both your immune system and your brain, leaving you vulnerable to brain fog, anxiety, depression, and memory problems.

Clue Four: More Friendly Bacteria Destroyed by Antibiotics

Yeast overgrowth is one of the most common intestinal problems I treat, particularly a type called *Candida* overgrowth. Yeast overgrowth also suppresses your immune system.

When patients come to me, I routinely do a host of blood work and a comprehensive stool analysis, looking for infections and yeast overgrowth. When I see a low white blood cell count, or when the stool test shows low IgA levels, yeast overgrowth is my first thought, whether the rest of my tests indicate it or not. The low intestinal IgA and low white blood cell count are also clear evidence that the patient's immune system is suppressed. It's always satisfying to treat a patient for yeast overgrowth and see their intestinal IgA and white blood cell count bound back up to normal. I love when patients feel better, and I have tests to show them that their immune system is improving too.

As we kept talking, Shenna's current problems came into focus. Perhaps, I suggested, her depression, memory loss, and brain fog were not only side effects of the lupus or the prednisone. Very likely they were also the results of her long-standing yeast overgrowth infection.

CLUES FROM THE TEENAGE YEARS

When Shenna hit puberty, she developed a severe case of acne, a problem that lingered well into her late twenties. Since acne is a common side effect of dairy sensitivities, we had found another clue. (For a list of symptoms that usually indicate chronic inflammation and immune system problems, see page 7.)

To make matters worse, Shenna took antibiotics to help clear up her acne. That destroyed still more friendly bacteria—and made her yeast overgrowth even worse.

Meanwhile, the teenage Shenna was eating a diet high in sweets and starches—lots of sugary baked goods and desserts—which were just the right foods to nourish the unfriendly bacteria lurking in her gut. As a result, she developed a condition known as "small intestine bacterial overgrowth," or SIBO, which gave her gas and bloating.

At this point I'd like you to think of Shenna's gut as a jungle, where the law is survival of the fittest. An epic battle is going on between the friendly bacteria on the one hand and the yeast overgrowth and unfriendly bacteria on the other. Thanks to the many factors we have identified—going all the way back to Shenna's birth and continuing through her childhood and teenage years—the friendly bacteria were losing that battle, while the yeast overgrowth and unfriendly bacteria were taking over the jungle. As a result, Shenna was setting herself up for a whole host of problems, including leaky gut, depression, brain fog, and memory loss.

Clue Five: Acne = Dairy Sensitivity

Clue Six: Antibiotics → More Friendly Bacteria Destroyed → Yeast Overgrowth

Clue Seven: High-Sugar Diet → SIBO

COLLEGE CLUES

In college, Shenna started having problems with acid reflux, especially as a semester would near its end and a stressed-out Shenna felt the pressure of deadlines and exams. Most people—including most conventional medicine doctors—believe that acid reflux results from too much acid. Actually, acid reflux more often results from *not enough* acid, a problem that can result from stress, poor diet, or, again, a lack of friendly bacteria.

When you don't have enough stomach acid, you can't fully digest the proteins you consume. Instead of moving from your stomach into your small intestine, your undigested food sits in your stomach longer than it's supposed to. Sometimes that undigested food backs up into your esophagus, along with small quantities of acid. The acid burns, and you get acid reflux. But if you had had more acid in your stomach in the first place, your food would have kept moving, and you wouldn't have had the reflux.

Your stomach acid is supposed to break down the proteins you digest into much smaller molecules called amino acids, chemicals that your body needs to run virtually every cellular reaction in the body, as well as build muscle, give you energy, and create neurotransmitters, those all-important brain chemicals. So, I told Shenna, her low stomach acid had four troubling effects:

- It gave her acid reflux;
- it kept her from properly digesting her proteins, which deprived her of amino acids, which ultimately contributed to her fatigue and immune issues;
- it kept her from making enough neurotransmitters, which worsened her brain fog, depression, and memory loss; and
- it failed to protect her from any unfriendly bacteria and parasites that might be hitching a ride on her food, setting her up for yeast overgrowth and SIBO.

Clue Eight: Acid Reflux = Low Stomach Acid → Depression, Brain Fog, Fatigue, and Many Other Problems

Like many people, Shenna frequently took acid blockers to fight her reflux. However, acid blockers destroy both stomach acid and key enzymes that your system needs to digest food properly. So Shenna's attempts to solve her acid reflux were actually making that problem worse.

Clue Nine: Acid Blockers = Intensified Digestive Issues, Brain Problems, Yeast Overgrowth, and a Vulnerability to Parasites

Shenna was amazed to learn how far along the autoimmune spectrum she had progressed before she even turned eighteen. But we weren't done yet. Also in college, Shenna told me, she had started taking the birth-control pill, a medication she still relied on. She also told me that she suffered from frequent vaginal yeast infections.

I saw a clear connection between these two seemingly unrelated facts. All those years of being on the pill had raised Shenna's estrogen levels. The estrogen was feeding the yeast overgrowth in her gut, which went on to manifest in the form of vaginal yeast infections. In addition, the systemic yeast overgrowth decreased Shenna's ability to make neurotransmitters (setting her up for depression, brain fog, and memory problems), contributed to her leaky gut, and depressed her immune system.

Meanwhile, in yet another vicious cycle, the excess yeast in Shenna's system craved sugar . . . causing Shenna to crave sugar too . . .

leading her to eat the sweet and starchy foods that created SIBO and fed her yeast . . . which caused her to crave even more sugar. As a result, Shenna gained weight. Her excess body fat was yet another source of inflammation . . . which is often a cause of weight gain . . . leading to yet more inflammation . . . and on the cycle goes, becoming more and more vicious with each passing year.

Clue Ten: Frequent Yeast Infections = Yeast Overgrowth, Probably Caused by Birth-Control Pill

Clue Eleven: Yeast Overgrowth → Sugar Cravings → Weight Gain → More Inflammation, and More Digestive and Immune Problems

The three most common gut infections I see among my patients are SIBO, yeast overgrowth, and parasites. Just based on hearing her story, I thought that Shenna very likely had at least two of the three—and I had not even done any tests yet. These gut infections were contributing to leaky gut even as they pushed Shenna further and further up the autoimmune spectrum, besides creating a whole host of mental and physical symptoms.

Ultimately, for Shenna, the inflammatory burden became too great. Her overstressed immune system went rogue, in the process I described in chapter 3, and she developed lupus.

STOMACH ACID: ONE OF YOUR GUT'S BEST FRIENDS

Your stomach acid

- breaks down *proteins* (from meat, chicken, fish, and other foods) into amino acids, which can later be absorbed in the small intestine;

- provides *amino acids* to support just about every function in your body, including making muscle and bone, keeping your moods even, giving you energy, and supporting your immune system;

- protects you against any *unfriendly bacteria, yeast,* and *parasites* that might hitch a ride on the food you consume; and

- supports proper *digestion* and *absorption,* so you get the full benefit of all the nutrients you consume.

At this point you might be wondering whether *you* have SIBO, yeast overgrowth, or parasites, and if so, what you should do about them. Don't worry. Just check out the tests in chapter 9 to see whether you are suffering from any of these common gut infections. The all-natural supplements you can take to heal these infections are listed on pages 199–200.

SOLVING THE PUZZLE

Now that we had all the clues, it was time to put them together.

- Infancy: missing out on key friendly bacteria
- Childhood: ear infections (dairy sensitivity); killing off friendly bacteria (antibiotics); developing yeast overgrowth (antibiotics)
- Adolescence: acne (dairy sensitivity); killing off more friendly bacteria (antibiotics); developing more yeast overgrowth (antibiotics); SIBO (high-sugar diet)
- College: high estrogen, yeast infections, bacterial overgrowth (birth-control pill); reducing stomach acid and digestive enzymes (acid blockers)

All These Factors → Leaky Gut → Depression, Brain Fog, Autoimmune Spectrum → Lupus

Shenna was amazed to learn about all the different ways her diet, lifestyle, and history had set her up for an autoimmune disorder. "You mean if I had taken care of some of these problems differently, I could have prevented my lupus?" she asked me.

I knew exactly how Shenna felt, because that was my reaction when I discovered functional medicine and realized that my thyroid ablation had been unnecessary. It was exciting to find a new way to treat my Graves' disease, but it was upsetting to think that it all could have been prevented if only I had known.

"Look," I told Shenna, "you might have been able to reverse this journey and get off the autoimmune spectrum *if* you had known about this approach. But I don't want you to blame yourself. You did what your other doctors told you, and until now, you never knew any other

> ## WHEN THE CURE IS WORSE THAN THE DISEASE
>
> Shenna took antibiotics for her ear infections and her acne:
>> Antibiotics destroy friendly bacteria → chronic inflammation → leaky gut and immune issues → yeast overgrowth, SIBO, and/or more acne
>
> Shenna took acid blockers for her acid reflux:
>> Acid blockers destroy stomach acid and digestive enzymes → gut problems, yeast overgrowth, and immune issues → failure to absorb amino acids → fatigue, depression, and/or brain fog

way. All you can do is the best you can with the knowledge that you have at the time."

Shenna nodded slowly, taking this in.

"The good news," I continued, "is that by the time we're done with this appointment, you're going to know exactly how to turn things around. Following The Myers Way gives you the power to reverse your condition and prevent any future autoimmune disorders. It also gives you the knowledge to protect your daughter and to help her prevent getting an autoimmune disease later in life."

THE 4Rs: FOUR STEPS TO GUT HEALING

"Okay, now I see how my gut problems have set me up for lupus," Shenna told me. "But what's the solution?"

Luckily, I told her, functional medicine has developed a very effective protocol to heal and protect your gut: the 4Rs. The name comes from the four key steps: remove, restore, reinoculate, and repair.

Although I break these into four steps to help you picture the process, in fact all four steps are undertaken simultaneously. I explain them here so you can understand what's happening to your body, but you don't need to worry about following them. They're all included in your thirty-day protocol for The Myers Way, so if you just follow the program in chapter 9, you will be doing everything you need to do in order to heal your gut.

Step One: REMOVE the Bad

The first step is to remove anything that disrupts the environment of your GI tract or contributes to your leaky gut. As you'll see in part III, The Myers Way protocol has you remove inflammatory foods, including gluten, grains, legumes, dairy, sugar, nightshade vegetables, and eggs, as well as processed foods, additives, and preservatives. You also remove alcohol, caffeine, and as many medications as possible, because these are likely to stress or irritate your gut. Finally, you'll remove intestinal infections such as yeast, parasites, and small intestine bacterial overgrowth (SIBO), all of which can wreak havoc on your gut as well.

The number-one food to remove, as you shall see in the next chapter, is gluten, a protein found in wheat, rye, and other grains. Gluten appears in pasta, bread, pancakes, waffles, and baked goods. In my opinion, it is the number-one health hazard in America. If you finish this book and decide that you can do only *one* thing to improve your health, removing gluten from your diet is far and away the best thing you can do.

For Shenna, it was also crucial to get rid of dairy, the problem food that had caused her ear infections and probably also her acne. Cutting out gluten and other inflammatory foods would help heal Shenna's gut and reverse her lupus too.

Shenna also needed to clear up the bacterial overgrowth from her SIBO and her yeast infection. Using natural supplements and probiotics—capsules and powders that contain friendly bacteria—I helped Shenna get rid of the unfriendly bacteria and replenish her friendly bacteria. Since the birth-control pills Shenna took had probably contributed to this problem, I worked with Shenna to find another form of birth control.

Step Two: RESTORE the Good

Once the bad is out, it's time to bring back the good. In this step, you restore the essential ingredients for proper digestion and absorption that might have been depleted by diet, medications, disease, or aging.

Adding back in digestive enzymes in supplement form is one key component of this step. Without these enzymes, you don't digest your food properly, which stresses your digestive system and leaves you undernourished. "'You are what you eat' isn't quite accurate," I always tell my patients. "Really, the saying should be 'You are what you digest and absorb.'"

Adding digestive enzymes also restores stomach acid, if needed, since those acids are required for proper digestion. (You can find the exact protocol for how to add in stomach acids on page 198.) Shenna realized that this was a crucial step for her, because it would help heal her acid reflux while lightening the load on her gut. Restoring stomach acid meant that Shenna could properly digest her food, absorb her nutrients, and use those nutrients to make all the neurotransmitters she needed. Proper digestion and absorption would also support Shenna's immune system.

Step Three: REINOCULATE with Healthy Bacteria

As you have seen, your body needs a healthy balance of good intestinal bacteria. These friendly bacteria are frequently depleted by antibiotics, steroids, acid-blocking medications, poor diet, stress, and many other factors.

Because of her delivery by C-section and her lack of breast milk as an infant, Shenna had probably started life with a deficit of friendly bacteria. The antibiotics she got for her frequent ear infections, and later for her acne, likely knocked out most of whatever friendly bacteria she had left.

The solution? Probiotics: capsules and powders that replenish your army of friendly bacteria so it can protect you from the world around you—and from yourself. Even if you had a normal delivery and were breast-fed as a child, you are subject to all the other factors that deplete friendly bacteria, including toxins, poor diet, and stress. So I want you taking probiotics too.

By the way, you might have heard the recommendation that fermented foods—yogurt, kefir (a kind of fermented milk), kimchi (pickled Korean cabbage), sauerkraut, and other fermented vegetables—are a great way to support your healthy bacteria. Indeed, fermented foods are full of healthy bacteria, which makes them natural probiotics. They're also full of the fiber and sugars that feed bacteria, which makes them natural "prebiotics"—elements that feed and support your intestinal bacteria.

This is true, but there is a caveat. If you haven't yet balanced your gut bacteria—if you have an overgrowth of yeast or are suffering from SIBO—fermented foods can actually feed the *bad* bacteria. In that case, rather than supporting your gut health, fermented foods can actually make it worse.

Once your gut is healed, I strongly recommend that you load up on nondairy fermented foods: raw sauerkraut, kimchi, and fermented vegetables. Make sure your gut has been healed, though, or you might be doing more harm than good. You can tell that your gut is healed when you are off your medications and your symptoms have dramatically improved.

Step Four: REPAIR the Gut

Like Shenna, most of us suffer from leaky gut. We need to repair that gut wall lining, which we can do through supplements. One of my favorites is L-glutamine, an amino acid that helps to rejuvenate the gut wall lining. Omega-3 fish oils help decrease your inflammation. In addition, licorice root and aloe vera help soothe your gut and cool your inflammation, allowing your gut to heal more quickly. (See pages 198–99 for the supplements you will be taking on The Myers Way.)

WHY DOES THE MYERS WAY WORK SO QUICKLY?

Shenna was excited to get started on the 4Rs, but she was puzzled about why such seemingly simple steps could work so quickly.

There are two reasons for this, I told her. The first is that many of her symptoms were not caused by her autoimmune condition but by her poor gut health. Healing the gut would enable her to get rid of lots of symptoms quickly, even if reversing the autoimmune condition took somewhat longer.

Second, gut cells are renewed at an incredibly fast rate. Every cell in your body has a specific life, after which it dies and is replaced by a new cell. Gut cells live only a few days at most. On the one hand, this means that you need to constantly support your gut, with healthy foods and especially healthy fats, which your body uses to make new cells. On the other hand, the quick cell turnover means that you can make big changes in a relatively short time, because old unhealthy cells are replaced by newer healthy ones.

Shenna liked thinking about how dynamic her gut was—to envision it as a living system that needed to be nourished and cared for. "If I feel like eating something that isn't on The Myers Way," she told me during our second appointment, "I just picture what it will do to my gut, and that helps me to stay on course."

FROM GUT HEALTH TO TOTAL HEALTH

Once Shenna understood how important her gut health was, she felt highly motivated to follow every aspect of The Myers Way. She was encouraged to see that her symptoms began to decrease within her first week of the new diet. Within a month, she was able to function without medications, her autoimmune markers had begun to normalize, and her health continued to improve.

Shenna was also excited to get her daughter on The Myers Way. She had such success reversing her own condition that she was now confident the same protocol would protect her daughter, even if her daughter had inherited Shenna's genetic predisposition to autoimmune disorders.

"I just wish I had known about all these gut stressors earlier," she told me during her last visit. "But the good thing is now I can help my daughter take the healthy path—and hopefully protect her from ever developing an autoimmune disease!"

CHAPTER 5

Get Rid of Gluten, Grains, and Legumes

MARSHALL WAS A TALL, STOCKY MAN in his midfifties who had been suffering from ulcerative colitis for the past two decades. Ulcerative colitis is a painful condition in which the large intestine, or colon, becomes inflamed and develops raw, open sores.[e] For most of the past few years, Marshall's conventional medicine doctor had been treating his condition with mesalamine, a powerful drug whose side effects include diarrhea, nausea, cramping, and flatulence.

That was bad enough, but when the disease was at its most intense, Marshall's doctor sometimes gave him prednisone, the same steroid that Shenna had been taking for her lupus. Marshall suffered from a different—but no less frustrating—group of side effects than Shenna, including weight gain, anxiety, and feeling as though his thoughts and emotions "just run away with me, like I can't control them at all."

Like Shenna, Marshall had grown tired of fighting what increasingly felt like a losing battle. As he told me about raising two kids, holding down his job as a high school science teacher, and trying to maintain a close relationship with his wife, I could see his jaw clench.

"I'm just so tired of my life being controlled by this disease!" he finally burst out. "The diarrhea, the cramping, the fevers!"

Marshall shook his head. "I'm at the end of my rope," he admitted. "I really hope you can help me, Doctor, because I have seen a grand total of *five* doctors over the past three years when this started getting worse, and they all just loaded me up with drugs. Sometimes the drugs worked and sometimes they didn't, but eventually, they always *stopped* working. And after that last round of steroids, I've put on another twenty pounds."

Abruptly, Marshall stopped talking and looked me straight in the eye. "Can you help me, Dr. Myers?" he said bluntly. "*Am* I going to feel better? Because I'm just so tired of feeling this bad."

I reassured Marshall that hope was indeed at hand. We would work to get him off his medications and into a full remission: no symptoms, no pain, not even any discomfort. His mind and his emotions would feel like his again. He would even be able to lose the unwanted weight.

Marshall breathed an enormous, heartfelt sigh of relief. "Okay, Doc. Thank you. What do I do?"

DIET DELUSIONS

As all my patients do, Marshall had completed a food diary before seeing me. I noticed immediately that there was no meat, chicken, or fish in his diet—just gluten, grains, and legumes, along with some dairy products, eggs, and vegetables.

I asked Marshall if he was a vegetarian and learned that, like me, he had become one at age fourteen. For breakfast, he told me, he had a bowl of low-fat Greek yogurt, sprinkled with some organic granola, and a couple of slices of homemade whole-wheat toast. Sometimes, for variety, he had shredded wheat instead. His lunch was either a veggie stir-fry with tofu (made from soy) and seitan (made from wheat) or a big bowl of miso soup (soy). Dinner was brown rice and black beans or maybe some type of vegetable stew over quinoa or millet. Every so often, Marshall told me, he had eggs or, for a special treat, some whole-wheat mac and cheese.

Marshall was clearly proud of this organic, whole-grain, low-fat diet, which he had gotten his whole family to follow. As he described the way he and his wife made their own yogurt, I recalled making yogurt with my mother. I remembered those wonderful family meals of my childhood—and I also remembered the Graves' disease that had ultimately resulted from them.

GLUTEN, GRAINS, AND LEGUMES: FOODS TO REMOVE

Gluten is a group of proteins found in many grains, including wheat, rye, and barley. Gluten is not found in rice, millet, corn, or quinoa. While oats don't inherently contain gluten, virtually all conventionally farmed oats are cross-contaminated either in processing or in storage, so for all practical purposes, they are not considered gluten-free.

Grains are the seeds of starchy plants cultivated for human or animal food. Examples of grains include wheat, rye, barley, rice, millet, and oats. While corn and quinoa are technically not grains, they contain proteins very similar to grains.

Legumes are plants that grow their edible seeds in long cases. Examples of legumes include lentils, chickpeas (garbanzos), peas, green beans, and other types of beans: red, white, black, and kidney.

But while I respected Marshall's choices, I wanted him to understand the health problems involved. The second pillar of The Myers Way is *Get rid of gluten, grains, and legumes, and other foods that cause chronic inflammation* because these foods are so problematic for people with autoimmune disorders. So, just as I had done with Shenna, I worked with Marshall to identify the clues that had led to his current health problems. I explained how the lectins in grains and legumes had inflamed Marshall's body, triggering his immune system to go onto autoimmune alert and interfering with his gut's ability to absorb nutrients. I also showed him how his symptoms were caused by his diet. I explained that gluten was part of what made him feel so foggy, anxious, and depressed; and I showed him how all those black beans and soy products were triggering his bloating, gas, and diarrhea.

What really hit home for Marshall, though, was when I explained that he—along with the rest of us—was being massively overexposed to gluten, in amounts that would shock our grandparents. Because let's face it, people, gluten is just about everywhere, even in places you wouldn't think to look for it in a thousand years. You might have known that gluten can be found in cereals, breads, and other baked goods. But did you know that it is also in almost every processed food and in such unexpected hideouts as ketchup, canned soup, soy sauce, and cold cuts?

I have an even bigger surprise for you: Gluten can also be found in toothpaste, shampoo, conditioner, and many brands of lotions, moisturizers, and personal-care products. If you're not careful, you might find yourself absorbing gluten—either through your mouth or through your skin—almost every hour you're awake. I guess if you use a nighttime moisturizer, you could keep on absorbing gluten even while you sleep.

Basically, I told Marshall, gluten, grains, and legumes are all highly inflammatory foods. Since inflammation is the biggest risk factor for autoimmunity, cutting out these "hot" foods only makes sense. For each of my patients, I try to find the source of his or her inflammation, and Marshall's diet was clearly fanning the flames.

But Marshall still couldn't wrap his mind around the idea that his "healthy" diet was so deadly dangerous. Maybe many of you out there can't either.

So let's start with the basics. What is gluten, and how exactly does it disrupt your gut, sabotage your immune system, and threaten your health?

WHAT IS GLUTEN?

Gluten is a group of proteins made up of the peptides gliadin and glutenin. It's found in many grains, such as wheat, semolina, spelt, Kamut, rye, and barley. Oats don't naturally contain gluten. However, due to cross-contamination in the processing methods, you should assume that oats do contain gluten unless they are certified gluten-free. (Later in this chapter I'll share with you a number of reasons why even gluten-free grains are likely to cause you problems if you have an autoimmune condition or are anywhere along the spectrum.)

Our English word "gluten" comes from the Latin word for glue. This makes sense, because gluten is what makes dough sticky, giving bread its airy and fluffy texture. Gluten is also considered a "sticky" protein because it holds together the nutrient stores of the plants that contain it. That stickiness is why manufacturers frequently use gluten as a binder and filler.

WHERE'S THE GLUTEN?

Simple Food Sources

Any form of wheat, barley, or rye:

- breads
- cakes
- cereals
- cookies
- crackers
- muffins
- pancakes
- pasta
- pies
- pretzels
- waffles
- ancient wheat grains, such as spelt, Kamut, and triticale
- oats (by cross-contamination)

Some Not-So-Obvious Food Sources

Not all of these always contain gluten, but they do often enough that you're better off avoiding them.

- alcohol
- candy
- cold cuts and luncheon meats
- corn chips
- dry roasted nuts
- gravy cubes
- instant or restaurant mashed potatoes
- meat, chicken, and vegetable stock cubes
- processed crab
- sauces and condiments, such as ketchup, barbecue sauce, and many others
- scrambled eggs in a restaurant (many places mix in a little pancake batter)
- vegan meat substitutes
- vitamins

Additives and Preservatives

- artificial coloring
- baking powder
- caramel coloring/flavoring
- citric acid (can be fermented from wheat, corn, molasses, or beets)
- coloring
- dextrins
- diglycerides
- emulsifiers
- enzymes
- fat replacers
- flavorings
- food starch
- glucose syrup
- glycerides
- maltodextrin
- modified food starch
- natural flavors
- stabilizers
- starch
- wheat starch

Some Sources Outside Your Food

- body and beauty products
- medications, supplements, and herbal formulas
- Play-Doh and paints
- postage stamps and envelopes

(See my website, AmyMyersMD.com, for a more comprehensive list.)

So here's problem number one with gluten: As we discussed, it is found in almost everything. It is such a common additive that our government doesn't even require it be labeled on packages, so it's often hidden under such names as "hydrolyzed vegetable protein," "food starch," "vegetable protein," or even "natural flavors."

If you're going to follow The Myers Way, you need to become a gluten detective, alert to the presence of this dangerous protein everywhere it might be found. To get you started, take a look at the chart on page 95 to see some of the many places where gluten hangs out.

"BUT IF I DON'T HAVE CELIAC DISEASE, WHAT'S THE PROBLEM?"

At this point you might be wondering why you can't have gluten if you don't have celiac disease. So let me lay it out for you.

SCARY GLUTEN FACTS

- More than fifty-five diseases have been linked to gluten.

- An estimated 99 percent of the people who have either celiac disease or gluten sensitivity are never diagnosed.

- Up to 30 percent of people of European descent carry the gene for celiac disease, putting them at higher risk for health problems triggered by gluten.

- A recent study published in the prestigious journal *Gastroenterology* compared ten thousand blood samples from individuals fifty years ago to those taken from ten thousand people today and found that there has been a 400 percent increase in the incidence of celiac disease.

- A study conducted from 1969 to 2008, following thirty thousand patients with diagnosed celiac disease, undiagnosed celiac disease (which was revealed during the study), and gluten sensitivity, found that each of the groups had significantly higher mortality than participants who were not affected by gluten.

As you'll see throughout the rest of this chapter, gluten contributes to leaky gut in a wide variety of ways. If you happen to be perfectly healthy, you can recover relatively quickly—but honestly, why would you put yourself through that? As you'll see in the next two chapters, the world is full of toxins and stressors you can't always avoid, so why subject your body to a challenge you *can* avoid?

In any case, if you have an autoimmune condition or are anywhere on the autoimmune spectrum—if you have any of the symptoms listed on pages 22–24—you can't afford even a tiny push in the direction of leaky gut, let alone the massive assault staged by only small amounts of gluten. I'll put it as bluntly as I know how: Gluten is poisoning you, not just in one way but in several.

Celiac disease is an autoimmune condition—and it is the most serious condition specifically associated with gluten. The gluten triggers your body to attack the cells of your small intestine. This blunts your microvilli, which, as you saw in the previous chapter, help to draw in nutrients from the flow of food while expanding the surface of the small intestine. Without a healthy growth of microvilli, you're unable to absorb the nutrients you consume. You could be eating up a storm—maybe even focusing on healthy foods—and still end up malnourished because your small intestine simply isn't absorbing nutrients and passing them into your bloodstream. Again, what matters is not what you eat but what you *digest* and *absorb*.

Only about 1 person in 133 has celiac disease, however, although that number is rising, both because of the omnipresence of gluten and because, as you'll see in a moment, commercial farms and manufacturers have altered the nature of gluten itself. Meanwhile, though, celiac disease affects less than one percent of the population, and only another half percent have a wheat allergy. So if that isn't you, then what's the problem?

The problem is what I call the "gluten-sensitivity spectrum"—the vast number of people who have a gluten sensitivity. Some statistics put that at a whopping 30 percent of the population, although many experts believe the figure is even higher. Based on my clinical experience, if you have an autoimmune disease, you are somewhere on the gluten-sensitivity spectrum, and therefore you should avoid gluten like the plague.

As you saw in chapter 3, allergies are triggered by the IgE antibod-

ies, which mobilize a swift and sometimes fatal response to a perceived intruder, such as when the intensity of your immune response
inflames your airways, causing them to close. Food sensitivities are
triggered by IgG antibodies, which mobilize a delayed response that
is often less intense in the short run—but incredibly detrimental in
the long run.

Remember, IgG antibodies trigger a response that might not show
up for as long as seventy-two hours. So if you eat some granola or fish
broiled with soy sauce on Monday, you might not realize that your
Wednesday migraine, acne, gas attack, or joint pain was caused by that
seemingly healthy food you no longer even remember consuming.

If you have an autoimmune condition or are on the autoimmune
spectrum, the news is even worse. As you saw in the previous two
chapters, you are engaged in a serious battle with inflammation.
Inflammation will make your symptoms worse if you have an autoimmune disorder, and move you higher on the spectrum, putting you
at greater risk for an autoimmune condition, if you don't have one.
Reducing inflammation is your biggest weapon in reversing and preventing autoimmunity—but gluten inflames your system and keeps
things going in exactly the wrong direction.

Believe it or not, the bad news isn't over yet. In fact, it's about to
get even worse. Two words: "molecular mimicry."

Molecular mimicry is a phenomenon in which your immune system
might actually confuse a part of your own body with a foreign invader.
Remember how the antibodies for cowpox also targeted the smallpox
virus? Well, by the same token the antibodies for gluten can also
target your thyroid tissue, creating a common autoimmune condition
called Hashimoto's thyroiditis. Basically, when gluten molecules leak
through your gut into your bloodstream, your immune system views
them as foreign invaders and makes antibodies to attack them, just
as if they were a dangerous virus or bacterium. Then, if you have
Hashimoto's, those same antibodies get even more confused. Not only
do they treat gluten as a deadly invader, they also treat your own
thyroid tissue as if it were gluten. As a result, your immune system
begins to destroy your thyroid.

This is just one of the reasons why I want you to avoid gluten if
you have an autoimmune condition or are anywhere on the spectrum—I don't want you to trigger a situation where your security

Molecular Mimicry

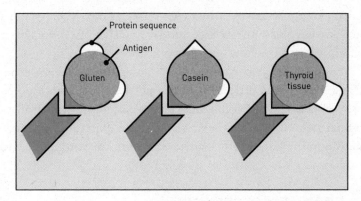

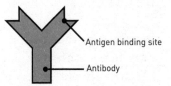

Antigen binding site

Antibody

Antibodies bind to the specific protein sequences of antigens. While gluten, casein, and your own tissues may all be different, they share some of the same protein sequences. A cross-reaction occurs when your immune system cannot distinguish between these molecules.

squad puts a picture of your thyroid up in Command Central next to its picture of the gluten molecule.

Molecular mimicry also occurs in other autoimmune conditions, whereby antibodies that you have developed to gliadin—one of the key proteins found in gluten—confuse other tissue with molecules of gluten. As a result, any time you eat something that contains gluten, your antibodies might cue your immune system to attack your own tissue. Fortunately, as I have seen with countless patients, once we calm the immune system down and support it through the four pillars detailed in this part of the book, molecular mimicry slows down or stops entirely. When you focus on the right diet, heal your gut, and maintain a healthy lifestyle, you can prevent molecular mimicry.

You need to be vigilant, though, because we have recently discovered that if you eat just a small amount of gluten, it can raise those anti-self antibodies for up to three months. So when I tell you to avoid gluten 100 percent, I mean 100 percent, not 99 percent or even 99.5 percent. Even a tiny amount of gluten can set off those antibodies and trigger your immune system to start attacking your own tissue.

It's very counterintuitive, I know. You might be saying, "Hey, I cut back on the gluten—way back! I used to have it several times a day. Now I eat it only four times a year—stuffing at Thanksgiving, chocolate cake for Valentine's Day, pecan pie at our Memorial Day picnic, and sweet rolls with my kids on the first day of school. Four servings of gluten a year—how can that possibly hurt?"

But if you have certain types of gluten-reactive autoimmune conditions, those four little servings might keep your antibodies elevated all year-round. And consuming gluten raises your inflammation levels, which puts you at further risk for developing and/or worsening an autoimmune condition, whichever condition you might have.

A WORD ABOUT TESTING

Many of my patients are confused about gluten because they've been tested and were told they didn't have any problems with it, but I believe that is probably not the case and they actually are suffering from a gluten-related disorder. Let me talk you through the different ways to test for gluten issues and what the limits of those tests are.

First, there is a test for celiac disease. The gold standard for celiac disease testing is an intestinal biopsy, but in some cases blood tests will reveal that certain markers are elevated as well. However, since only 1 person in 133 has celiac disease, this test is not going to reveal more common problems.

Allergists also offer a test for wheat allergy or gluten allergy. This is a test for IgE reactions (page 56). Only about 1 percent of the population has this type of allergy to gluten, so again, this test won't reveal more common problems.

The most common gluten issue is gluten sensitivity—the IgG reaction—and as you've seen, close to one-third of the population suffer from this, possibly more. There are food-sensitivity tests that can look for this, but the problem here is that gluten contains many different gliadins, or proteins, and while you might be fine with several, you could still have a sensitivity to one. And the most common food-sensitivity tests look for only that most common gliadin, known as 33-mer. If you're fine with 33-mer but sensitive to one of the many other proteins in gluten, you might easily get a false negative.

We now have a better test, by Cyrex Laboratories, which checks for a much wider range of gliadins. If you are really concerned to get specification verification for your gluten-sensitivity status, you can ask a functional medicine practitioner to order that test for you.

However, as I always tell my patients, your body knows better than any test. When in doubt, take it out, and see if you feel better. If you do, you can be pretty sure that gluten was the problem, and you should continue to avoid it. Another good clue that gluten is not right for your body is if you've taken gluten out for a few weeks and then feel worse after you start eating it again.

I so frequently see with my rheumatoid arthritis and Hashimoto's patients that they will take gluten out of their diets and begin to feel better within a couple of weeks or even days. The RA patients' joint pain and swelling will disappear. The Hashimoto's patients' antibodies will drop. Their conventional doctor might then say, "Well, maybe gluten *was* your problem. Why don't you start eating it again for a couple of weeks and then we'll test you for celiac disease."

Someday, I'm sure, this will be grounds for malpractice. If you take gluten out of your diet and your health improves, your body is telling you everything you need to know.

GLUTEN AND LEAKY GUT

Now, let me make it perfectly clear why I don't want you eating gluten even if you don't have celiac disease or you aren't allergic or gluten-sensitive: Gluten causes leaky gut. Even if you're doing everything else right to support your immune system—eating healthy foods, detoxing your body, healing your infections, and reducing your stress load—gluten can sabotage those efforts with a single bite.

Our understanding of how gluten affects the intestinal tract is due to the pioneering Dr. Alessio Fasano, whom you first met back in chapter 4. Dr. Fasano discovered that gluten triggers the production of a substance known as "zonulin," which causes the tight junctions of the epithelial cell wall to loosen. In optimal health, the tight junctions soon close up again, and the digestive system continues intact.

But when the body is overexposed to gluten—and, as you just saw, almost all of us are far too exposed to gluten—the zonulin keeps coming and the tight junctions holding your cell walls together remain open.

Now instead of a nice tight epithelial wall, you have a leaky barrier that allows partially digested food to leak through. Your immune system can't recognize these partially digested morsels, so it begins to attack them with all the chemicals it usually reserves for a harmful virus or bacterium. Suddenly, you have an immune system on high alert. Those guys in Command Central are spraying your body with inflammatory fire—and that is the perfect setup for an autoimmune condition.

"BUT WE HAVE ALWAYS EATEN BREAD!"

Many of my patients have a hard time wrapping their minds around the notion that foods as common as bread and pasta are so unhealthy that they can provoke the symptoms of a debilitating and painful disease. "People have eaten these foods for hundreds of years" is a statement I hear frequently. Or "These are the foods my grandmother used to make. How can they be so dangerous?"

Let me tell you exactly why the bread, pasta, and baked goods we buy today are completely different from the ones our grandparents knew.

First, in a quest to create ever lighter, fluffier forms of bread and other baked goods, as well as efforts to create hardier strains of wheat, farmers and corporations have developed new hybrids. Just as food growers have figured out how to create a nectarine by crossing a peach with a plum or how to create hardier tomatoes or new types of roses, they have also developed new strains of wheat.

But many advances come with a price, and the hybridization of wheat and other grains comes with a big one. Hybridization has created new forms of gluten—that is, brand-new proteins that our bodies do not recognize. Interbreeding two different strains of wheat has been known to create several new wheat proteins not found in either of the original strains. Our bodies have not evolved as quickly as the newly developed wheat, and they simply don't know how to respond to these proteins.

Second, scientists have developed a process known as "deamination," which removes one of the amino acids from the proteins that gluten contains. This process enables food companies to load up their goods with gluten, creating supersize cinnamon buns and gigantic fluffy bagels. And because this process makes gluten water-soluble, manufacturers can now use gluten as a preservative and a thickener in all sorts of products in which gluten never used to appear.

Gluten was already in your French toast and spaghetti Bolognese, but deamination means that gluten also shows up in your soy sauce and your sliced deli meats. It means that when you go to an Asian restaurant to feast on stir-fry and rice, when you buy a chef's salad with ham and turkey at a diner, or when you put a little ketchup on your French fries, you are consuming gluten, even though bread, pasta, and baked goods are nowhere in sight. As you have seen, unless you shop very carefully for your personal-care products, you might be consuming gluten when you brush your teeth, shampoo your hair, or smooth lotion onto your body.

In addition, the deamination process itself makes the now omnipresent gluten far more dangerous to your body. First, we're exposed to new types of gluten that our bodies can't handle; then we are massively overexposed to gluten, overloading our guts and our immune systems. In my opinion, the combination of these new proteins and the gluten overload is the double whammy that is a major factor in the skyrocketing autoimmune epidemic.

Another factor that makes gluten more dangerous to us today is the ever-increasing toxic burden each of us carries, thanks to the hundreds of new chemical compounds corporations are pumping into our air, water, and soil. Our immune systems are staggering under their load of industrial toxins, which makes gluten even more problematic. And our guts are leakier than ever. (See the list on page 77 for the factors that cause leaky gut.)

So maybe our grandparents could enjoy their bread and pasta with no ill effects. After all, their gluten was not hybridized and deaminated; it wasn't found in *everything*, and they ate real food, not packaged junk. In all likelihood, their toxic load was lower, they were not on as many medications, and although their lives were hard, they were probably not as stressed by their lives as we are today. As a result, their guts were not as leaky simply because they weren't facing all the other factors that make gluten so deadly for us today—especially those of us who are vulnerable to autoimmune disorders. It's also possible that our grandparents *did* suffer ill effects from their grain-based diets and never made the connection between their migraine headaches, fatigue, or depression and the bread, pasta, and baked goods they consumed.

Regardless of our grandparents' experiences, our own food supply has been transformed so profoundly over the past fifty years that we are literally eating different foods than they were, even when the foods appear similar. Their bread was made from long-known strains of wheat grown in relatively clean soil; ours is made from hybridized, deaminated wheat that has been grown in toxic soil, watered with mercury- or lead-laden water, and doused with pesticides and herbicides. Their legumes were made from natural plants; many of ours are genetically modified and, again, doused with toxins. Even the packaged, processed, and fast foods were safer, cleaner, and healthier fifty years ago.

We don't sprout and soak beans the way our ancestors did; we don't eat slow, communal meals; we don't eat primarily home-cooked foods. And even if you never eat processed food, any time you eat nonorganic meat or chicken, or farm-raised fish, you are getting the genetically modified corn and soy that was in the animals' feed. Virtually all of us are massively overexposed to gluten, corn, and soy— which are used as animal feed, preservatives, flavorings, and fillers—not to mention overexposed to gluten in all the nonfood places we have discussed. So even if our grandparents could digest the gluten, grains, and legumes they relied on, we are not living their lives or eating their foods.

We can't really look to the past to figure out our diets. We have to look at where we are now, what our food supply currently offers us, and what our bodies can handle. Wherever you are on the autoimmune spectrum, cutting out gluten is the right and safest choice.

THE HIGH COST OF "GLUTEN-FREE"

As gluten-free living becomes more popular, many companies are jumping on board to create the next delicious gluten-free waffle, bread, cake, or muffin. These seemingly healthy foods really aren't healthy at all. They're often loaded with sugar, salt, preservatives, additives, and dyes.

Now, if you have a gluten-loving family—especially if that family includes children—gluten-free substitutes might be just the way to help everyone transition to a healthier diet. If your kids live on pizza and mac and cheese, and you get them to eat gluten-free and maybe even dairy-free versions of those foods, awesome. I commend you for making such a healthy change in your family's lives.

But I have to be honest with you: Junk is junk. And just about all the gluten-free foods out there are basically . . . well, junk. Let me tell you why.

First, when wheat is turned into flour, it creates a lot more bulk than other grains or seeds. So if a gluten-free product is made from rice, corn, tapioca, potato, or almond flour, it usually needs something to make up for the bulk and consistency that won't be there without the wheat.

Sugar to the rescue! Sugar adds calories as well as bulk, however, not to mention the way it causes your blood sugar to spike and then crash. Most nonwheat flours are more highly refined than wheat flours, which means that they too will push your blood sugar to spike and crash. As a result, you're putting yourself at risk of weight gain and, potentially, diabetes. And please don't be fooled by products that offer "all natural" sweeteners like refined cane sugar, brown rice syrup, or agave. These are either glucose (the type of sugar found in cane and sugar beets), fructose (the type of sugar found in corn and fruit), or some combination. The fancy names don't make them any healthier.

Even when gluten-free products are labeled "organic" or "all natural," they can be loaded with preservatives. Furthermore, unless the item is specifically marked "non-GMO," it's probably made with corn or soy, and 80 percent of all corn and soy grown in the United States has been genetically modified. (For more on concerns with genetically modified organisms and the foods that are made from them, see "GMOs: A New Kind of Health Challenge," page 114, and appendix A.)

In addition, your immune system might treat even gluten-free grains as though they were gluten, making antibodies and triggering inflammation. To make matters even worse, gluten-free grains (and legumes) contain lectins, inflammatory substances that also inhibit the absorption of minerals and other nutrients.

So ignore the pretty label and the "healthy, organic, gluten-free" logo on the package. There will be no such foods during your thirty days of The Myers Way.

WHEN GLUTEN-FREE IS <u>NOT</u> GLUTEN-FREE

When I told Marshall about the importance of avoiding gluten, he balked at first. Eventually, though, he decided that avoiding gluten was a small price to pay for healing the painful, debilitating condition that had taken over his life.

What he found harder to understand was why I wanted him to give up other grains as well, even supposedly healthy choices like brown rice, oats, and quinoa. (Although quinoa technically is not a grain, it includes grain-like proteins.)

There are several reasons to avoid gluten-free grains. One of the most persuasive is that many such grains are not really gluten-free. A study published in June 2010 in the *Journal of the American Dietetic Association* found that in a sampling of twenty-two grains that were naturally gluten-free, over half of them had evidence of gluten.

How did this happen? Through a process known as cross-contamination. This isn't a biological mystery; it's just simple proximity. Unless a grain is grown on an isolated farm and processed in an entirely gluten-free facility, it's highly likely to come into contact with a gluten-bearing grain. With our highly industrialized food system, there are tons of opportunities for this type of contact, which means that supposedly gluten-free grains are not really gluten-free. Cross-contamination can happen in the fields, in the processing plant, during shipping, or in the bulk bins at your grocer. This is all before these grains even make their way to your home, where there are just as many opportunities for them to come into contact with gluten in your pantry, in your refrigerator, or on your kitchen counters.

Of course you can always make wise food choices and select items that are as minimally processed as possible, but you'll never have complete control over what happens to your food before it reaches the store or your plate. And even a tiny amount of gluten can have a grievous effect on both your gut and your immune system. As you saw earlier in this chapter, if you have an autoimmune condition, molecular mimicry is likely to fool a gluten-sensitive immune system into attacking your body as well as the gluten. Even a few molecules of cross-contaminated gluten can trigger your anti-gluten antibodies to signal your immune system to send out the inflammatory chemicals and, perhaps, to attack your body's tissue.

In addition, as you'll see a bit later in this chapter, even small amounts of gluten can create leaky gut. This can have disastrous consequences on your immune system as well.

Cross-contamination is one powerful reason why I advise my auto-immune patients to avoid all grains. Think of how grievously gluten affects your autoimmune condition or how it could push you up the spectrum into a full-blown disorder, and then follow my motto: When in doubt, go without.

FOODS THAT MIMIC GLUTEN

In chapter 8, you will see lists of foods I'd like you to avoid. Some of them are grains and legumes, but many belong to completely different food groups. Yet all these problem foods have one very important thing in common: They are all foods your body confuses with gluten. As a result, each of them potentially triggers a powerful inflammatory response that ratchets up your level of chronic inflammation. If you have an autoimmune condition, these foods can keep your symptoms going full throttle. If you are on the autoimmune spectrum, these foods might push you over the edge into a full-blown autoimmune disorder.

You saw how this worked in chapter 3, when you watched the guys in Command Central get confused between a potential target and its look-alike. Remember, your adaptive immune system makes antibod-

CROSS-REACTIVITY:
FOODS THAT YOUR BODY MIGHT CONFUSE WITH GLUTEN

Corn	Millet	Rice
Dairy products, including whey protein	Oats	Yeast

ies designed to target particular bad guys—the technical term is "antigens"—that your immune system has decided are likely to do you harm. Once gluten gets tagged as an antigen, your adaptive immune system makes antibodies to seek it out and sound the alarm—but those antibodies can easily get confused and sound the alarm for gluten look-alikes as well.

The scientific name for that process is "cross-reactivity." Basically, your adaptive immune system confuses gluten-free grains with gluten-bearing grains, flooding your body with inflammatory chemicals whether you're confronting wheat, rice, or corn.

In fact, your immune system can confuse other foods with gluten too, including dairy, corn, rice, yeast, and millet. This is why I would like you to avoid all possible substances that might trigger a cross-reaction, especially for the first thirty days of The Myers Way, when you are trying to calm down those guys in Command Central and convince them that they do not have to be on such high alert. Once you've given those poor guys a break, you might be able to introduce some gluten-free foods back into your diet in moderate amounts.

"BUT WE HAVE ALWAYS EATEN BEANS!"

I'm always surprised at the number of people who understand the problem with gluten but stop when it comes to legumes. If right now you are thinking, "But we have always eaten split-pea soup" or bean burritos or any other legume-based dish, I would regretfully respond with a similar explanation. Overexposure to gluten has affected our responses to other grains, creating more cross-reactions. And the toxic burden in our food, water, and air has overwhelmed our digestive and immune systems in ways our grandparents could not even imagine. These sad new elements of modern life mean that the strains placed by lectins upon our systems—once bearable—have now become intolerable, especially for those of us who suffer from autoimmunity.

It's also true that our bean-eating ancestors prepared their legumes differently than we do. Traditionally, these foods are soaked for hours before cooking—a process that helps leach the lectins away and makes legumes safer to eat. Our ancestors didn't eat grocery-store hummus or packaged rice pilaf, so we can't really compare their eating habits to ours. And again, agriculture is only a few thousand years old; our ancestors for a couple million years before that never ate grains or legumes. So I have to tell you what I know will work: Cut these foods out of your diet and watch your symptoms disappear.

Hey, I used to be a vegetarian. Remember? I know how good grains and legumes can taste, how satisfying it can feel when they fill you up, and how nutritious they appear to be. I know how challenging it can be to find substitutes for these foods when you're used to relying on them for most or even part of your diet.

I'm not only a former vegetarian, however; I'm also a person with an autoimmune disorder. I know firsthand just what havoc can be wrought by those tasty bowls of vegetarian chili or those tangy hummus wraps. I'm here to spare you what I went through—and that means changing your diet.

Even most of the people who tell you to avoid gluten don't realize the damage that is also being done by these other types of food. Like I always say, knowledge is power, so let me empower you with some vital information about why you shouldn't eat grains and legumes.

LOOKING AT LECTINS

Lectins are carbohydrate-binding proteins—that is, they are proteins that help keep two carbohydrate molecules together. Lectins are everywhere—in animals, plants, and microorganisms—but the ones that concern us at the moment are in grains (where they are very plentiful) and legumes (where they are not quite as plentiful but are still a significant presence).

One particularly problematic type of lectin is called a "prolamin." Prolamins are found in quinoa, corn, and oats, and let me tell you, they are bad news, especially if you have celiac disease. Although, in theory, people with celiac disease can eat nongluten grains (and pseudo-grains, like quinoa), the prolamins in these supposedly safe foods damage their guts and stimulate their immune systems. Prolamins can have that effect on the rest of us too, if we have other types of autoimmune conditions or are somewhere on the spectrum.

First off, prolamins interact badly with your brush border—that all-important portion of your small intestine full of villi and microvilli. You want to protect those delicate parts of your digestive tract, not stress them with prolamins.

In addition, prolamins behave remarkably like the proteins in gluten. And if you have an autoimmune or inflammatory condition, your immune system is already pretty jumpy around gluten. An overstressed immune system—either with autoimmunity or on the spectrum—is not going to be able to tell the difference between gluten and its look-alikes, so it's best to avoid both.

THOSE AGGRESSIVE AGGLUTININS

Another type of problematic protein found in grains and legumes are "agglutinins." No, they're not actually related to gluten, but they do have the same gluey quality that gave gluten its name. They can cause red blood cells to clump together, and some are actually poisonous (though not the ones in your food).

Agglutinins have been shown to cause leaky gut and disrupt your immune system in a number of different ways. They stimulate both your innate and adaptive immune systems, and they bind with immune cells, interfering with those cells' function. Some agglutinins are deactivated by cooking—but some are not.

Agglutinins are part of the natural defense mechanism of a seed— what the seed uses to keep itself from being digested. If a seed is throwing up all sorts of obstacles to being digested, that can't be good for your digestive system, right? In the next section, I will give you a lot more facts and details, but the short version of my science lesson is this: Between prolamins and agglutinins, you're getting lots of toxic and inflammatory effects whenever you eat a grain or a legume. Completely healthy people might be able to tolerate that type of digestive stress, but if you have an autoimmune condition or are anywhere on the autoimmune spectrum, your best move is to stay away from them.

SEEDS OF INDIGESTION

Marshall was still having trouble accepting just how bad "healthy" grains and legumes could be. I think what really drove it all home for him was when I explained that seeds basically do not want to be digested. Their whole goal is to survive intact within your digestive tract, so that when you eliminate them, they still have a chance to find some fertile soil, produce another plant, and perpetuate their genes. (Obviously, they had better chances of achieving this objective throughout the millions of years when humans didn't have indoor plumbing.)

So evolution has equipped seeds with lots of protection mechanisms to keep your gut from breaking them down. And when you *do* break them down, you pay. Seeds—and therefore seed-bearing plants, such as grains and legumes—contain "amylase inhibitors," which block the enzymes your body uses to break down carbohydrates, and "protease inhibitors," which block the enzymes your body uses to break down proteins. Protease inhibitors also provoke inflammation.

These enzyme inhibitors are hardy substances that even survive cooking. Because they prevent your body from digesting large portions of the grains and legumes you consume, they end up providing a meal for unhealthy bacteria, which feast on the food your body fails to absorb. This can lead to gut dysbiosis, the overgrowth of unfriendly bacteria, promoting such conditions as small intestine bacterial overgrowth (SIBO) and yeast overgrowth.

These enzyme inhibitors can also activate your innate immune system as though they were antibodies. So besides taxing your immune system *indirectly,* by stressing your gut, they also stress your immune system *directly,* by behaving like antibodies. Again, for a perfectly healthy person, this might be tolerable, but for someone with an autoimmune condition, it's simply throwing fuel on the inflammatory fire.

The scientific term for lectins is "antinutrients," because they actively interfere with your body's ability to absorb nutrients. They also have another problematic effect: They stimulate your pancreas to produce more enzymes in order to compensate for the way they are inhibiting your digestive enzymes. It's as though your pancreas were stepping in to help your stomach and intestines do their jobs.

This creates two major problems. First, it stresses your pancreas, which is needed for other jobs, including insulin production. Insulin is the chemical that moves blood sugar, or glucose, out of your bloodstream and into your cells. When insulin production is imbalanced, you can run into all sorts of problems, including weight gain and potentially diabetes. So you don't want to give your pancreas any more work than it's already supposed to be doing.

Second, the pancreatic enzymes themselves aren't particularly gut-friendly. They tend to dissolve the tight junctions that keep partially digested food from leaking into your bloodstream, where the food provokes your immune system into considering it an invader. You've already seen how gluten induces leaky gut, but now you can see how nongluten grains and legumes can also stimulate leaky gut.

The basic rule of thumb is that it's fine to eat plants with tiny seeds, like berries or bananas, because those seeds are so small, they just survive the ride through your gut intact. You don't chew them up, they don't release their problematic chemicals, and you are able to benefit from the foods that contain them.

However, larger seeds from plants that require grinding or chewing—i.e., grains and legumes—release their digestive enzyme inhibitors when you crack them open. These are the foods that disrupt your gut integrity, stress your immune system, and keep you from absorbing all the nutrients in the other foods you consume. People without autoimmune or inflammatory conditions can manage small amounts of these other types of foods, but if you have an autoimmune condition or are anywhere on the spectrum, I'd like you to play it safe and avoid them, at least until you have healed your gut, have cooled your inflammation, are symptom-free, and are no longer taking immunosuppressants or biologic medications.

"It's a big change," Marshall told me. He wasn't happy about learning this information. "But," he went on, "I really don't think I can continue like this, with the symptoms and the side effects. If getting rid of these foods means living a normal life again, I guess it could be worth it."

THE DARKER SIDE OF NIGHTSHADES

Nightshade vegetables too have problematic effects on your body. For example, tomatoes have a particular lectin—an agglutinin—that is actually used in vaccines because it stimulates the production of antibodies. That's fine if you're asking your body to stimulate anti-polio or antiflu antibodies, but you really don't want your body making antitomato antibodies and setting off a whole inflammatory response every time you eat a salad!

FOODS TO AVOID: NIGHTSHADES

Eggplants

Peppers (avoid fresh peppers
   only; the black pepper spice
   is fine)

Potatoes (avoid white potatoes
   only; sweet potatoes are okay)

Tomatoes

Accordingly, I will be asking you to avoid foods in the inflammatory nightshade family. Remember, your goal is always to bring down inflammation, because that's what brings down symptoms and enables you to get off your medications. If you're on the autoimmune spectrum, reducing inflammation is the surest way to safeguard against developing an autoimmune condition.

The good news is that after thirty days on The Myers Way, you will find out whether you can enjoy nightshades again. (To find out more, check out the bonus chapter on my website, AmyMyersMD.com.)

SNEAKY SAPONINS

The bad news isn't over yet. Plants also contain "saponins," which potentially threaten your gut integrity and can lead to leaky gut.

All plants contain saponins, and of course I don't want you to stop eating plants. Just the ones with an especially high level of saponins: legumes, pseudo-grains (like quinoa), and nightshades. Nightshades contain a subset of saponins known as "glycoalkaloids," which, in even moderate amounts, can contribute to autoimmunity. Glycoalkaloids also feed the unfriendly bacteria, leading to gut dysbiosis. They can enter your bloodstream too and cause "hemolysis," the destruction of the red blood cell membrane.

Your most important takeaway is that grains, legumes, seeds, and nightshades contribute to leaky gut in several ways:
- by damaging intestinal cells;
- by opening the tight junctions; and
- by feeding unfriendly bacteria to create gut dysbiosis.

NOT-SO-EXCELLENT EGGS

Another inflammatory food you will be avoiding during your first thirty days on The Myers Way is the egg. Partly this is because your body often confuses eggs with gluten because of the cross-reactivity we have already discussed. Eggs are also inflammatory because they contain a substance called "lysozyme," which is intended to protect the yolk, just as lectins are intended to protect seeds. And just as lectins inflame and distress your gut, setting you up for leaky gut and other digestive problems, lysozyme produces similar ill effects.

The good news is that after thirty days on The Myers Way, you will find out whether you can enjoy eggs again. (Check out my website, AmyMyersMD.com, for a bonus chapter that will help you figure out whether eggs are safe for you.)

GMOs: A NEW KIND OF HEALTH CHALLENGE

I have never liked the idea of genetically modified plants. I figure that nature, after millions of years of evolution, has arranged for plants and animals to interact just fine. Until we know a lot more about what we're doing—and believe me, a lot of genetic modification is hit or miss—we shouldn't mess with Mother Nature.

So I wasn't surprised to find out that GMOs are particularly problematic for those of us with autoimmune issues, whether full-blown conditions or somewhere on the spectrum. The primary reason corporations modify plants is to help the plants resist pests and infections. So all the natural ways plants do that—with prolamins, agglutinins, digestive enzyme inhibitors, and saponins—are enhanced through the genetic-modifying process.

These "plant protectors" are problematic enough in their natural state. You *really* don't want to put them into your body when they have been given an extra boost in some corporate laboratory—not to mention the extra pesticides and herbicides with which many GMOs are doused. One of the major reasons that GMOs were developed in the first place is to enable farmers to use more pesticides and herbicides, guaranteeing them better yields with less work—but more poisons. The very first GMO crop was known as the Roundup Ready soybean. It was developed by the corporate giant Monsanto, which made a weed killer known as Roundup. The only problem was Roundup killed crops as well as weeds. So enter a genetically modified Roundup Ready soy plant that could enable farmers to pile on the poisons and skip the weeding.

Do you want all those poisons in *your* body? I didn't think so. Do your immune system a favor and give GMOs a pass. (For more on how to recognize and avoid GMOs, see appendix A.)

MAKING THE MOST OF THE GLUTEN SOLUTION

I remember when I first made the transition from vegetarian to meat-eater. I had come to terms with the fact that my grain- and legume-based diet was, basically, poisoning me, and I had to manage my profound regret that I hadn't discovered this before I destroyed my thyroid. Yet even though I had this new knowledge, I found it hard to apply it, at least at first.

THE MYERS WAY—MODIFIED

As a physician, I have to be honest. A vegan or vegetarian is likely not the right diet for you especially if you have an autoimmune condition. Grains, legumes, and dairy products are inflaming your body and either placing you on the autoimmune spectrum or making your disease worse. If you remove those items from your diet, there really isn't a whole lot left for you to eat, particularly when you remember how important it is for you to get protein so that your body has the amino acids you need to build muscle, replenish your brain chemicals, support all your body's functions, and therefore stay healthy.

If you feel you are able to eat some fish and other seafood, I have prepared a modified version of The Myers Way for you. It's less inflammatory than your vegetarian or vegan diet, but it's still not as nutrient-dense as the regular meal plan of The Myers Way, and you'll need to take some supplements to make up for what you're missing from your food.

On ecological grounds, I simply didn't like the idea of eating meat. I knew that raising conventional livestock takes more energy than raising grain, and, as a longtime dog lover, I hated the idea of eating an animal.

However, I had to accept that food is medicine. Our human bodies simply aren't designed to subsist on grains and legumes—they were made for meat—and my meatless, grain-based diet had made me very sick. If I wanted to get well, I would have to eat meat.

Eventually I realized that eating meat could be done in a healthy and ecologically responsible way if I ate only grass-fed and pasture-raised animals—that only the grain-fed animals were a drain on our planet's ecology. I shared this perspective with Marshall.

I also told him that my objections were not *only* about principle. As I was making the transition from vegetarian to meat-eater, I worried about what in the world I was going to eat if I couldn't rely on rice and beans or tofu stir-fries or hummus and veggies. I wondered if I could even enjoy dishes made with meat and fish or whether I could ever learn to cook that way. And since I hadn't eaten red meat in nearly thirty years, I wondered, honestly, if eating meat was going to make me sick.

Frankly, I had never liked the texture of meat. So when I finally committed to preparing a grass-fed hamburger for dinner, I had to make a last-minute switch to sautéing the "loose" meat instead of making it into a solid patty.

"You just have to take one bite," I promised myself. "You can start small."

My fork trembling, I took one bite . . . and then another . . . and then another. It was delicious. I ended up eating the whole thing. The next day, I craved meat so much, I had another serving.

I also got lots of motivation from feeling better, almost immediately. My mood swings evaporated. My brain fog lifted. My energy returned. My spirits rose. Most important, I finally felt like myself—for the first time in a long, long time.

I still don't like the texture of meat, and I often have to cover it with sauces or find other ways to disguise it. But feeling terrific is a great motivation, not to mention that cooking meat, fish, or chicken takes way less time than preparing all those grains and legumes.

I remembered that whole process, so vividly, when I watched Marshall go through it too. I saw how relieved he felt when his symptoms began to recede and we could get him off his medications. I saw how excited he was about finally losing the extra pounds that had been literally weighing him down. I saw his spirits rise and his energy soar. And I heard him say the same words I had said, or thought, so often: "I only wish I had known about this years ago, so I could have felt that good back then." I was reminded all over again of the healing power of diet and the wonderful sense of vitality that are ours for the taking—as soon as we let go of gluten, grains, and legumes.

CHAPTER 6

Tame the Toxins

CLAIRE WAS A THIRTY-YEAR-OLD graphic designer who had recently developed fibromyalgia. Like many fibromyalgia patients, she had spent months seeking the correct diagnosis, a search that in her case took her to half a dozen doctors.

Finally she found a physician who was able to tell her more than "You're just tired," "Maybe you're stressed," or "Let's give it some time and see what happens." Claire was enormously relieved to now have a name for her condition—something that explained her constant, debilitating pain. At last, she thought, her search was over.

No such luck. Claire soon discovered that conventional medical approaches to fibromyalgia are basically limited to painkillers, antidepressants, and antiseizure drugs. Nope, those aren't typos. For reasons we don't entirely understand, the last two types of medications have had some success in pain relief. They weren't satisfying options for Claire, however, because none of these treatments dealt with the underlying causes. They were simply an attempt to medicate the symptoms, which would bring, at best, temporary relief and never get to the root of the problem. In addition, Claire had avoided these types of medications all her life and she was not about to start taking them now. So she resumed her search for a physician.

Then Claire ran across an article I had written on finding the root cause of fibromyalgia. Excited, she made an appointment—and was thrilled to hear me confirm that there was indeed another approach. She told me that she was eager to start the first two pillars of The

Myers Way: *Heal your gut* and *Get rid of gluten, grains, legumes, and other foods that cause chronic inflammation.*

But when we got to the third pillar of The Myers Way, *Tame the toxins*, Claire became confused.

"I don't understand," she admitted. "I live in a nice suburb. I work in an office. I'm not near any factories. There's not much pollution out where we live, thank heavens! So, what kinds of toxins could I possibly have to worry about?"

The truth is that all of us are surrounded by toxins: in our air, food, and water; in our homes; in our workplaces; in our dry-cleaned clothes and our expensive colognes; in our pillows and mattresses. . . . The list goes on and on and on, and it is as true for those of us who live on farms, in small towns, and in idyllic suburban communities as it is for those of us who live in cities and industrial areas.

Toxins flood our water, waft through our air, and seep into our soil. We take in toxins through what we eat, drink, and breathe, and also, frighteningly, through home cleaning products, personal-care products, and cosmetics. Toxins lurk in our kitchens, our rugs, and our furniture. They are simply a fact of modern life.

And, yes, toxins affect *all* of us, even those of us who believe we live in clean and pleasant surroundings. "Toxins" literally means poisons, so let me tell you exactly what I mean by the term: I mean any substance that is significantly dangerous to the human body and is inappropriately finding its way into our bodies in large amounts (it does not need to be in large amounts—small amounts of some can be very harmful to people; it depends on the substance and the person). Toxins include heavy metals (such as arsenic, cadmium, lead, and mercury), mycotoxins (the poisons released by certain types of molds that can be found in homes, offices, and schools), and the hundreds of thousands of industrial chemicals used in just about every manufacturing process and found in just about every industrially manufactured item, from the hormone-disrupting plastic food containers in your fridge to the carcinogenic heavy metals in your water.

In 2003 the Environmental Working Group (EWG) engaged in a remarkable study in collaboration with the Icahn School of Medicine at Mount Sinai in New York City. Their mission was to discover the "body burden" carried by the average American—not Americans living next to toxic waste dumps or working in coal mines, but Americans who, like Claire, seemed to be living relatively "clean" lives.

Now, it costs a fortune to test people for industrial chemicals and heavy metals, so at first glance, the study might seem small—only nine people living in various parts of the United States. But these people were tested for 210 different substances, and frankly, the results were shocking. In each person's body was an average of 91 industrial chemicals, heavy metals, or other significant toxins, including PCBs, commonly used insecticides, dioxin, mercury, cadmium, and benzene.

Think about that for a minute: 91 toxins, not among people who worked with chemicals or lived in polluted areas, but among ordinary Americans—people like you—who assumed they were relatively safe. (Of course if you're reading this and you live in a polluted area or work in a job that involves chemicals or industrial processes, you already know that you are at risk.)

A total of 91 toxins is bad enough, but of the 91, at least 53 are known to suppress the immune system. So if you're wondering why I was talking about an autoimmune epidemic in chapter 1, now you understand one big piece of *that* puzzle.

Of course a lot of skeptics weren't too happy about such a small study. So in 2004 the Centers for Disease Control and Prevention (CDC) tested a much bigger sample: 2,500 people. They were looking for evidence of some 116 chemicals—and they found it.

Finally, in 2005 a third study was conducted—and in that study researchers found traces of 287 chemicals.

So here's what *I* wanted to know when I read about these studies: If this is how many chemicals they found, how many more chemicals are in our bodies that they *didn't* find?

These tests aren't random. You don't just take a sample of someone's blood and some machine spits out a list of all the industrial chemicals and heavy metals that show up there. To find something, you have to look for it specifically. These studies could only afford to run one or two hundred tests on each of their subjects. But as of this writing, some 80,000 chemicals are registered for use in the United States, and every year another 1,700 are added to the list. How many of *those* are *also* in our bodies?

I used to assume that if an industrial chemical has been approved for use and if there's no warning label on it, it has been carefully tested and found safe. Nope. Government agencies start with the assumption that these new chemicals *are* safe. They don't want to tell corporations—who have spent time and money developing these chemicals—that they've just wasted all that time and money.

I'll admit it. I'm angry that the Environmental Protection Agency (EPA) and the Food and Drug Administration (FDA) aren't doing a better job of protecting us. I also know that it isn't entirely their fault. The EPA alone is deluged with something like 2,000 to 2,500 applications a year for permission to use new industrial chemicals—that's 40 to 50 applications *each week*. No wonder some 80 percent of those applications are approved in three weeks or less, often without any data whatsoever.

What this means, though, is that most of the decisions regarding industrial chemicals, food additives, and the like aren't made by the government officials hired to protect us. The real decisions are made by industry lobbyists, whose main interest is in helping the corporations who hired them make money. Our protection comes second—if it counts at all.

Even when a chemical *is* studied by the FDA or EPA, the focus is usually on whether it causes cancer, not on whether it might be harmful in other ways. To make matters worse, each chemical is looked at in isolation, rather than in the context of how it functions within the product where it's used, let alone studied for how it interacts with all the other chemicals and toxins we're exposed to. As you've seen throughout this book, it's not the one-time events that are the problem. It's the *cumulative, chronic* insults that create chronic inflammation and an out-of-control immune system. This is an issue that needs further study: What effect do all these chemicals, working together, over decades, have upon our bodies—and our immune systems? Nobody really knows.

I will tell you what we *do* know. The rates of chronic illnesses are skyrocketing. So are the rates of cancer. We have an allergy epidemic. We have an asthma epidemic. And we have an autoimmune epidemic. Like I said, at least 53 of the industrial chemicals found in that first body burden study are known to suppress the immune system, and so are a lot of other toxins that those initial studies didn't have the resources to test for.

So that's the situation, folks. Nearly a hundred thousand chemicals are out there in our environment, many—if not most—are toxic, and a huge amount of them are finding their way into our bodies and making us their permanent residence. For every person, that's a huge toxic burden. For those of us with autoimmune conditions or on the autoimmune spectrum, it might be the burden that is pushing us over the edge, into a life full of symptoms, ill health, and pain.

HOW TOXINS TRIGGER AUTOIMMUNE CONDITIONS

I can attest from my clinical experience that lightening the toxic burden makes a significant difference in halting the progression of autoimmune conditions, reversing disorders, and preventing people on the autoimmune spectrum from moving deeper into autoimmunity. Exactly *how* this works, no one is quite certain, but here are a few key theories.

One hypothesis is that heavy metals, specifically, alter or damage the cells in various tissues in your body. Your immune system fails to recognize the altered tissue and attacks it as a foreign invader. It's as though heavy metals disguise the cells so that they suddenly resemble the pictures of all those bad guys posted on the walls of Command Central. (For more on where heavy metals are found, see the following sections, beginning on page 138.)

Another theory is that heavy metals stimulate the immune system so that it goes on high alert. It starts becoming unable to tell the difference between *you* and the foreign invaders; that is, it loses its "tolerance of self." (See chapter 3 for more detail.) Unable to tell self from non-self, your immune system tags your tissue for destruction, and your autoimmune condition begins. It's as though heavy metals open fire on Command Central with a whole other class of weaponry, and your poor security squad just goes nuts and starts opening fire on *everything*, the bad guys and your tissue included.

In both of these cases, as you have seen previously, inflammation is the result. In the first case, because your heavy-metal-infused tissues start resembling foreign invaders, your immune system shoots a lot of extra inflammatory chemicals into your system. In the second case, because your immune system is overstimulated, it starts shooting a lot of extra inflammatory chemicals into your system. Either way, your inflammation level goes way up . . . which is why your protocols on The Myers Way are designed to bring it down. Yeah, we want to reduce your exposure to heavy metals and help you get them out of your system (which I'll tell you more about soon), but we also want to mitigate the inflammation that inevitably results when your system and heavy metals collide.

There is a third theory about how all toxins—not just heavy metals—trigger autoimmunity, concerning the way immune cells are "educated." T cells begin life in the bone marrow, but they soon move on to the thymus, a small organ right behind your breastbone. The thymus is where T cells are "taught" to recognize foreign invaders—to identify viruses, toxins, and other dangers to your system, and to distinguish them from the friendly bacteria and healthy foods that you want to welcome into your body.

Some of the T cells get an even more specialized education. They become "regulatory T cells," with the important job of keeping the other T cells in line: making sure they do not mistake your own body for a foreign invader. It's their role to maintain tolerance of self. So when you don't have enough regulatory T cells, or when your regulatory T cells aren't properly trained, the other T cells might go rogue and start attacking your own tissue as well as genuine dangers.

What can cause this process to go off course? One huge factor is toxins, which can shrink or atrophy the thymus, keeping it from producing enough high-quality regulatory T cells. That makes it easier for your T cells to get out of line and start attacking your thyroid gland, your spinal cord, or some other crucial part of your body.

I've just thrown a lot of science at you, so let me boil it down to two key points:

- As you saw in chapter 3, the more inflammation in your body, the more likely your immune system is to become overstimulated, go rogue, and start attacking your own tissue. So let's keep the heat turned down as far as possible, which will help to counteract and maybe even prevent at least some of the toxins' ill effects.

- Low-level, chronic toxic exposure—such as what comes from pesticide-laden foods or toxic body products—is worse than a single large, acute exposure, because the cumulative burden is greater, and so is the long-term stress on your immune system.

I see it in my clinic every day: Higher levels of inflammation cause the T cells to go rogue. Turning down the flames soothes the T cells and makes it more likely that they'll stay calm and focused on their real job of attacking foreign invaders only. Heal your gut through diet and high-quality supplements, and your T cells will behave the way they are supposed to. Lighten your toxic burden, and your T cells are even more likely to "do the right thing," attacking only foreign invaders and not your own tissue.

LET'S GET PERSONAL: YOUR INDIVIDUAL BODY BURDEN

Here's what I tell my patients: Your body is like a cup, and the toxins you're exposed to are like the drops of liquid that fill that cup. You pack a healthy piece of baked chicken and some fresh veggies into a plastic container and then heat it in a microwave at work—*drip*. You buy a plastic bottle of spring water from the office vending machine—*drip*. You put on a freshly dry-cleaned outfit to go out to dinner that night—*drip*. You eat at your favorite sushi place and order a tuna roll—*drip*. You moisturize your face at night with a paraben-laden face cream—*drip, drip, drip*, all night long.

And so it goes, on and on, until, perhaps, your cup overflows with the toxins from plastics, potentially contaminated spring water, dry-cleaning chemicals, mercury-laden tuna, estrogen-mimicking parabens. . . . You've spent the entire day filling your cup, and the next day, and the day after that. Of course you hope that your cup doesn't overflow until you've lived to a ripe old age, but for many of us, it's much sooner. Those of us with autoimmune disorders may have gotten them precisely because our cups have already gotten too full—so we have even more incentive to try to empty the cup and keep it from filling again.

Now, I don't want to scare the life out of you; I don't even want to stress you out. What I *do* want is to empower you to realize that you can lighten your toxic burden and thereby support your immune system. So here's what we're going to do:

I'm going to share my four top toxin-taming strategies. If you take just these four steps, you'll have made a significant difference in relieving your toxic burden. And you can feel terrific about that.

If you are suffering from multiple autoimmune conditions, if you've been very sick for many years, or if your autoimmune condition seemed to come at you out of the blue, I'll point you to the next two areas I would explore if you were my patient: heavy metals and toxic mold.

Finally, I'll tell you how to support your body's natural ability to detoxify, so that you can continue to release the toxins from your system.

I'm excited for you to feel empowered to tame the toxins in your life—and as I've said before, knowledge is power. So let's get started.

TOXIN-TAMING STRATEGIES

When it comes to toxins, you have two main goals:

Prevention. Keep as many toxins as possible out of your system— keep the liquids from ever dripping into the cup.

Detoxification. Support your body's ability to detoxify by eating the right foods and taking the right high-quality supplements, all of which you will get during The Myers Way—pour the liquids out of the cup.

Obviously, prevention is your best friend here. The more toxins you keep out of your body, the less detox work your body has to do. However, with nearly a hundred thousand industrial chemicals in our environment, keeping toxins out of your system can be somewhat challenging, to say the least. So I'm going to share my favorite motto with you: Control what you can, and let go of what you can't.

Each of us has to figure out his or her own way of doing this. My personal strategy is to keep my home and my office toxin-free (since I'm lucky enough to control my office too). I also cook only organic food, with no plastics or toxic cookware in my kitchen. (Yeah, Teflon and other nonstick cookware are toxic. See "Toss the Teflon" starting on page 133.) Controlling my environment at home means that when I go out into the world, I have a bit more leeway.

Yeah, I'd rather choose a healthy restaurant that serves only organic veggies and pasture-raised meats, but those are hard to come by, and not all my friends want to eat there, or at least not every time. Sure, I try to pack my own lunches from the organic and pasture-raised food I have in my fridge, but if I have to stop at a health food store to pick up the lunch I didn't have time to make, I allow myself to eat the farm-raised fish they offer instead of the wild-caught salmon that I would have prepared at home. Controlling what I can—while keeping tabs on my detox pathways and supporting them at all times—makes me feel as though I have room to make a few compromises. (I'll show you how to support *your* detox pathways at the end of this chapter.)

Of course I still worry about the stressors I'm piling onto my immune system, but I have to find a way to be okay with that or else I'd never go anywhere. As you'll see in the next chapter, the stress brought on by that kind of worry and isolation can be even worse than toxins.

I understand that not everyone is in the same position as I am and that each of you has your own priorities. So here are the four strategies for taming the toxins in *your* environment and lifting a huge burden from your immune system. If you just do these four things, you're way ahead of the game:

❶ **Clean your air.** Get HEPA filters to purify your air at home—either a whole-house filter or enough individual filters to cover the entire square footage of your house or apartment.

❷ **Clean your water.** Install a whole-house water filter, or put one on every tap, so that you are drinking, bathing, and showering with toxin-free water. Also, avoid plastic water bottles.

❸ **Buy clean food.** Buy grass-fed, pasture-raised, and organic food. For extra bonus points, cook and store it in a toxin-free way.

❹ **Buy clean body products.** Over the next three months, replace all your personal-care products (shampoo, deodorant, toothpaste, moisturizer, and anything else you put on your body) with clean, toxin-free products. To look up your own cosmetics and personal-care products and find out how safe they are, go to the Skin Deep Cosmetics Database at www.ewg.org/skindeep. To learn the top toxins to watch out for in personal-care products, go to www.TeensTurningGreen.org and check out their "Dirty Thirty," which they keep updating as needed. You can even enter your own body products and find out how toxic they are.

STRATEGY ONE: CLEAN YOUR AIR

HEPA is short for "high-efficiency particulate air," and a HEPA filter is indeed highly efficient, removing 99.97 percent of all particles larger than 0.3 micrometers. You can buy a whole-house filter. If you buy the individual ones, depending on the size of your home, you might need several. If you can afford only one small HEPA filter, put it in the bedroom, because that's where you spend eight to ten hours sleeping, and you detox while you sleep. If at all possible, get a HEPA filter for your office too. Tell your supervisor you have a medical condition, if necessary, so that you get permission to have it beside your desk.

Many of my patients are surprised when they hear me recommend a HEPA filter. Certainly Claire was. "I get that there are more toxins in the environment than I realized," she told me. "But I don't see what the problem is indoors."

Actually, as I told Claire, your home air is likely *more* toxic than the outside air—anywhere from two to one hundred times more toxic. And the air in offices can be even worse. Office buildings tend to be even more airtight than homes, so they hold the toxins in, and they're full of fumes from industrial-strength cleaners, chemicals used in photocopying, and many other health hazards. Check out this warning from the EPA about indoor air in general:

> Most people are aware that outdoor air pollution can damage their health but may not know that indoor air pollution can also have significant effects. EPA studies of human exposure to air pollutants indicate that indoor air levels of many pollutants may be two to five times, and on occasion more than a hundred times, higher than outdoor levels. These levels of indoor air pollutants are of particular concern because it is estimated that most people spend as much as 90 percent of their time indoors. In recent years, comparative risk studies performed by the EPA and its Science Advisory Board (SAB) *have consistently ranked indoor air pollution among the top five environmental risks to public health.* [emphasis added]

Enough said. Get yourself some HEPA filters (I suggest some good choices in "Resources") and breathe easy.

STRATEGY TWO: CLEAN YOUR WATER

One of the most effective ways to lighten your toxic burden is to drink, shower, and bathe with filtered water only. Put filters on your home taps (see "Resources" for some suggestions), or, if you live in a house, get a whole-house filtration system. I also want you to avoid plastic water bottles at all costs.

There are three problems with those plastic bottles. First, the water itself may contain toxins or contaminants, because there is actually less regulation for bottled water than for tap water!

Second, there's the plastic. Many plastics contain a toxic substance known as BPA, or bisphenol A, a synthetic element that mimics estrogen and is considered an endocrine disrupter. Your endocrine system includes all your hormones, which means that BPAs are responsible for wreaking havoc on your thyroid, adrenals, and the glands that produce your sex hormones, putting you at risk for numerous disorders. And, yes, BPAs are used in water bottles and many other plastic containers, so they have free rein to migrate into the food or liquid inside.

The third way those plastic bottles hurt us is when they are dumped into landfills. The toxins leach into the soil and evaporate into the air, ultimately returning as rain—sometimes near the landfill, sometimes miles away. The food that's grown in toxic soil or watered with toxic rain absorbs the poisons, as do the cows that eat the grass grown in that soil or watered with that rain. Eventually, those toxins make their way back into our bodies, stressing out our immune systems and causing other health problems.

Lately there's been a certain amount of hype around BPA-free plastic, but come on, folks. Do you really think they don't have harmful chemicals in them too? Remember that BPA-free doesn't mean toxin-free. Do yourself—and the entire planet—a favor: Get yourself a stainless-steel thermos or glass bottle and keep it filled with filtered water.

The Terrible TCEs

It takes me only three letters to tell you why a water filter is so important: TCE. Trichloroethylene (TCE) is an especially deadly and common contaminant. It leaches into our groundwater from industrial runoff or from military bases, where it is used to hose down tanks, planes, trucks, and other machines. Since TCE is used by a wide range of companies—leather makers, dry-cleaning companies, and airplane and machine manufacturers—and since it can be found in household products, including glues, adhesives, paint thinners, and strippers, we're all more exposed to it than we might think.

In fact, some 10 percent of U.S. residents have TCE levels that can be detected in their blood, and TCE is frequently found in breast milk. You might breathe it in from the air around you or ingest it with your drinking water—and you might be exposed to it in your shower, since it is released when shower water converts into steam.

That's why your shower needs a filter, because it's kind of a double whammy: You breathe in TCE fumes through your lungs while absorbing liquid TCE through your skin. Multiple, chronic exposures are the worst of all—especially when you consider that TCE might work specifically to suppress your immune system.

That discovery is courtesy of Dr. Kathleen Gilbert of the Department of Microbiology and Immunology at the Arkansas Children's Hospital Research Institute in Little Rock. Dr. Gilbert has run several experiments with mice, showing that TCE can disrupt immune-system signaling, triggering the immune system to produce antibodies against its own tissue.

High doses of TCE—perhaps comparable to the type that you'd get if you worked in a plant where TCE was used—seemed to activate the mice's T cells, apparently to attack the mice's own bodies. In addition, the mice's level of inflammation rose, particularly a type of cell that has been associated with lupus and other autoimmune conditions.

Low, chronic doses of TCE—perhaps comparable to what you'd be exposed to through your shower—also triggered inflammation, as well as setting off a liver-destroying disease known as autoimmune hepatitis.

There's still a lot we don't know about TCEs, but here's what I personally conclude from Dr. Gilbert's research:

Whether you live in a big city, a pleasant suburb, or a tiny rural town, you are potentially being exposed to TCEs.

The real danger we face—especially those of us who have autoimmune conditions or are anywhere on the spectrum—is not so much a single, dramatic incident but rather the *chronic, low-level* exposure that all of us face every day. Dr. Gilbert was the first researcher to really make this clear, and we all owe her a debt of gratitude for it. Those tiny but unremitting amounts of poison keep stressing and stressing and stressing our immune systems, creating chronic inflammation and, ultimately, autoimmunity.

So check your household products and try to eliminate any that contain TCEs. And please install that water filter, so you can clean your body without poisoning it at the same time.

Frightening Fluorides

When fluoridated water was first introduced as a potential prevention against tooth decay, it was a natural product: calcium fluoride, to be exact. Now if there's fluoride in our water, it is sodium fluoride, which is literally a toxic waste product of the aluminum industry.

Yep, you read that right. The fluoride in our water today actually began life as sludge from toxic waste. Companies convert it into sodium fluoride and sell it to the government, making it profitable for them and a major health hazard for us.

To make matters worse, most public water supplies contain chlorine and bromide in addition to fluoride, and bromide frequently appears in baked goods as well. All three of those chemicals compete with iodine in our body, often displacing it. Since our thyroid gland depends on iodine, this chemical stew might well be the reason behind the rampant growth of thyroid disease.

Very few water filters get this toxic fluoride out of your water. I urge you to take action in your local community to protect your health by getting the fluoride out.

STRATEGY THREE: BUY CLEAN FOOD

Ideally, you'll eat completely organic foods. You'll buy grass-fed, pasture-raised, and organic meats and all-organic fruits and vegetables. Ideally, too, you will support local small farmers—as long as they grow organically. Not all of them do, so make sure you ask what kind of feed their animals were given—no GMO corn, soy, or alfalfa, please!—and how their vegetables were grown. (For more on GMOs, see appendix A.)

However, I know that eating organically can be expensive. So if you have to compromise, focus on the meats. Animals are at the top of the food chain, so if they're eating food laced with toxins and contaminated with heavy metals, you're getting those poisons magnified many times. Organic, grass-fed, pasture-raised meats should be your priority. (For more about heavy metals, see appendix B.)

With regard to fruits and vegetables, if you can't buy all organic, check out the website for the Environmental Working Group (www .ewg.org/foodnews) and look at their lists for the Dirty Dozen Plus and the Clean Fifteen. The Dirty Dozen Plus are the twelve foods especially likely to be contaminated with pesticides; the Clean Fifteen, even when grown conventionally, are likely to be safer. The foods on these lists can change, so I suggest checking them out regularly, just to stay on the safe side. The EWG also has good lists for picking safe fish that are less likely to be contaminated with mercury.

The Pesticide Connection

In our modern world of corporate farming, it's a pretty sure bet that if you eat conventionally farmed food, you are exposed to pesticides. To make matters worse, we now have lots of evidence that pesticides are not just toxic; they are particularly likely to trigger an autoimmune condition. Here's some evidence of what happens to farmers who work with pesticides on a daily basis:

> In one 2007 study, three hundred thousand death certificates over a fourteen-year period showed that farmers who were exposed to pesticides because of working with crops were more likely to die from an autoimmune condition.
>
> In another study, farmers who had been exposed to organochlorine pesticides throughout their lives were more likely than others to have a high "antinuclear antibody" (ANA) count—a sign of current or incipient lupus.
>
> A third study found that farmers who mixed pesticides were also more likely to have lupus.

"Okay," you might be thinking, "I'll just wash my food very carefully so that all the pesticides come off."

Sorry. Not gonna happen. Many pesticides are systemic, meaning they become an integral part of the plant and its products. An apple that has been grown in a pesticide-filled orchard, for example, has integrated the pesticides into that sweet white part that tastes so good; the poisons don't just stay on the skin. That's why I stress the importance of buying organic whenever you can, especially if your autoimmune or spectrum symptoms aren't going away as fast as you would like.

Pass on the Plastics

Oh my gosh, what *doesn't* come in plastic? Most of your food is wrapped in it—which means that you are picking up a hefty share of toxic molecules.

BPA-laden plastics are also in the coating of receipts, the lining of cans (more proximity to your food!), and sandwich bags (your food again!). So if you want to lighten your toxic load, think of some creative ways to cut down on the plastic. And please, if you can possibly help it, do not store food in plastic of any kind—including plastic bags—because the toxins migrate into your food. Use glass instead.

For a while, when people warned you about plastics, the focus was all on BPAs, but I was always certain that even BPA-free plastics were dangerous, and in March 2014 my inner certainty was confirmed. Neuroscientist George Bittner and his colleagues tested 455 products—plastic wrap, Styrofoam, the kind of plastic used in food processors and hypodermic syringes, and a frightening list of others—and found that 72 percent of them released a significant amount of estrogen-mimicking toxin into the food, medications, or personal-care products they contained. Your takeaway is simple, positive, and hopeful: Protect your immune system by avoiding plastics, especially if you already have an autoimmune condition or are anywhere on the spectrum.

Toss the Teflon

A potential immune-system disrupter called perfluorooctanoic acid (PFOA) has been found in the blood samples of 96 percent of U.S.

PLASTICS TO AVOID

We all know to stay away from BPAs, which disrupt the endocrine system and leach estrogen into the body, creating imbalances that have been linked to everything from infertility to obesity to behavioral changes in children. But there are many plastic products labeled "BPA-free" that have been shown to include chemicals that produce similar effects. Here is a guide to some of these common plastics and where they lurk in everyday products and materials. To easily identify each plastic, look for the number stamped on the packaging.

Number on Packaging / Name	Common Sources	Notes
1 Polyethylene terephthalate (PET or PETE)	Bottles of soda, water, cooking oil, mouthwash, ketchup, and salad dressing; jars of peanut butter	Used for its lightweight, versatile form, this is the main plastic used for soda and water bottles. It sometimes contains antimony, which may mimic estrogen. PET is fine for a single use, but it begins to break down when exposed to heat and harsh detergents.
2 High-density polyethylene (HDPE)	Baby bottles; bags of chips, cookies, and cereal; toys; cutting boards; ice cube trays; milk jugs; water, juice, detergent, and shampoo bottles; yogurt tubs	HDPE is marketed as a sturdy and heat-resistant material, but some environmental groups express concern over the potential hazard from the leaching of phthalates used in children's toys and bottles.
3 Polyvinyl chloride (V or PVC)	Deli containers, plastic wrap, shower curtains, and teething rings	PVC may release phthalates/carcinogens into food and drinks, especially when the containers start wearing out, are put through the dishwasher, or are heated (including in a microwave).
4 Low-density Polyethylene (LDPE)	Milk cartons, plastic produce bags, hot and cold beverage cups, frozen-food containers	
5 Polypropylene (PP)	Baby bottles, sippy cups, straws, prescription pill bottles, Tupperware, deli containers, bottle caps, yogurt cups, and some takeout containers	PP is marketed as heat-resistant, but that only means it won't melt under heat, not that it is healthy and/or won't leach chemicals.

6 Polystyrene (PS)	Takeout containers, egg cartons, meat and fish packaging, utensils, packaging peanuts	Commonly known as Styrofoam, PS contains styrene, which may mimic estrogen and, with long-term exposure to small quantities, cause fatigue, sleep difficulties, and lymphatic abnormalities, and have carcinogenic affects. It is especially dangerous when heated. PS is banned in some cities, including Portland, Oregon, and San Francisco.
7 Other, usually refers to Polycarbonate (PC) OR	Bowls, plates, cups, reusable water bottles, food packaging, blenders, syringes	PC is derived from BPA. Numerous studies have concluded that trace amounts of BPA can cause endocrine disruption, developmental conditions, and cancer.
Polylactic acid (PLA)	Takeout containers, fruit and vegetable packaging, yogurt containers, utensils	This is marketed as biodegradable and compostable but is typically made from genetically modified corn and has been shown to leach estrogen.

residents. And no wonder: PFOA is a key element in Teflon, nonstick cookware, grease-resistant boxes, and disposable coffee cups, as well as in clothing, some carpet guards, computer chips, phone cables, car parts, and flooring.

Unfortunately, we don't know all that much about how PFOA affects us. However, a paper published by Stockholm University's Unit for Biochemical Toxicology reports that investigators could not find a low enough dose at which PFOA did *not* alter our immune-cell function at every step.

So don't cook your organic vegetables and pasture-raised meats in a toxic pan. Avoid nonstick cookware and eliminate one more source of low-level daily exposure to an immune-system threat.

STRATEGY FOUR: BUY CLEAN BODY PRODUCTS

If you are maintaining even a minimum standard of hygiene, you are likely exposing yourself to a wide range of industrial chemicals. I get that most people can't go into their bathrooms, toss everything out, and just start over—though if you are really struggling with symptoms or concerned about being high on the autoimmune spectrum, that would be a great step to take.

If you feel less urgency or just can't wrap your head around such a quick change, that's okay. Do it over the next three months, buying toxin-free products to replace what runs out. Eventually, you'll have eliminated a major stressor on your immune system.

I know it's hard to see those fragrant bottles of body wash as a threat, but trust me, they are. Or, rather, don't trust me; check out the ingredients for yourself. Here are the top ingredients you need to watch out for. The list is constantly changing, but because it has approximately thirty items, it is nicknamed the "Dirty Thirty":

- aluminum zirconium and other aluminum compounds
- benzalkonium chloride and benzethonium chloride
- benzyl acetate
- bronopol
- butyl acetate
- butylated hydroxytoluene (BHT) and butylated hydroxyanisole (BHA)
- coal tar
- cocamide DEA and lauramide DEA
- diethanolamine (DEA)
- ethoxylate
- ethyl acetate
- formaldehyde
- formaldehyde-releasing preservatives (quaternium-15, DMDM hydantoin, diazolidinyl urea, and imidazolidinyl urea)
- fragrance (parfum)
- hydroquinone
- iodopropynyl butylcarbamate
- lead and lead compounds
- methylisothiazolinone (MI/MCI/MIT) and methylchloroisothiazolinone
- parabens (methyl, ethyl, propyl, and butyl)
- petrolatum

• phthalates (dibutyl phthalate, butyl benzoate phthalate, diethyl-hexyl phthalate, dimethyl phthalate)

Parabens mimic the effects of estrogen. Neither men nor women need any more estrogen in their bodies, thank you very much. Look at a list of ingredients, and if you see "paraben" anywhere—even at the end of a word (e.g., "methylparaben"), stay away! Phthalates also mimic the effects of estrogen.

You should also look out for gluten, grains, legumes, and dairy. Yep!—in your shampoo, your toothpaste, your moisturizer. If you don't believe me, spend just ten minutes checking out shampoos and moisturizers in any drugstore or even in the "personal care" aisle of your favorite "organic" grocery store. If you don't see gluten and wheat, you're almost sure to see some other foods that will inflame your system, such as oats, soy, and dairy products. It's bad enough what happens to your body when you *eat* that stuff. What do you think happens when you apply it to your skin—your largest organ—multiple times a day, in the form of shampoo, conditioner, body wash, shower gel, and moisturizer, not to mention all the other toxins you absorb through your deodorant, toner, scrubs, and cosmetics?

Don't be fooled by "organic" or "all natural" on the label, either; look at the ingredients. Luckily, there are some safer options. See the "Resources" section to find out more.

USE YOUR RESOURCES

Okay, now you know my top four toxin tamers. If you'd like to go further—if you'd like to learn more about how to get tested for heavy metals, cope with the problem of toxic mold, explore biological dentistry, or rid your home environment of toxins—check out appendixes B, C, D, and E.

I want to make The Myers Way as easy for you as possible, so I've also put together a resources section full of helpful websites and products. If you're looking for water filters, organic cleaning products, safer cosmetics, or any of the other products referred to in this chapter, check out "Resources" for some recommendations.

LIGHTENING THE HEAVY-METAL BURDEN

Many of my patients face an additional toxic burden: heavy metals. This is something I consider with patients who've had a lot of exposure to heavy metals: silver dental fillings; a diet rich in tuna, swordfish, and other large, mercury-laden fish; or some other type of environmental exposure. Heavy metals are also something I look into if diet alone isn't moving a patient as far as we would like. I routinely test many of my autoimmune and spectrum patients for aluminum, arsenic, cadmium, mercury, and lead.

If you want to get tested for heavy metals, find a functional medicine practitioner (see "Resources"). For more information on the kinds of tests you might consider, see appendix B.

At this point you might be thinking, "Heavy metals? How would I ever get exposed to them?" Well, let's look at some of the most common heavy metals and find out.

Lead

I also test for lead, because it too is common. Back in the 1970s lead was banned from being used in gasoline, but it took twenty years for it to be completely removed. Lead was formerly used in paint and can still be found in old pipes. Although water treatment plants check to make sure their water is lead-free, you can pick up a considerable dose if the pipes leading to your home are the old-fashioned kind. (New pipes are lined with plastic that contains PCBs, which poses other types of health problems, so check out "Resources" and then go install that water filter!)

Here's a nifty place for a toxic heavy metal: right on your lips. Some four hundred shades of lipstick contain trace amounts of lead. Battles over lead in lipsticks have been raging since the 1990s. If the prospect of poison on your lips bothers you, check out the "Resources" section for some safer choices.

Pottery and toys from China are another source of lead, since their standards for toxic products are even lower than ours. I can attest personally to the widespread presence of lead in the U.S. population; when I test, I'm always finding elevated lead levels. By the way, researchers have found lots of links between lead and lupus, which leads me to suspect that lead is implicated in other autoimmune conditions as well.

Mercury

So many people are exposed to mercury that I routinely test for it too. Just consider how many places mercury shows up:

- cosmetics
- dental fillings
- fish
- pesticides
- skin lighteners
- vaccinations

Mercury is also found in the air near coal-burning plants (check www.epa.gov to find out if there are any in your area). Then it settles on the ground and waterways, where it makes its way into plants and water systems . . . and from there into fish and small animals that eat those plants and drink or swim in that water . . . and from there into larger fish and animals that eat the small ones . . . and from there into those of us who eat fish and meat. (You might want to know that wild king salmon don't eat other fish, so they are likely to be less full of mercury than other species.)

Arsenic

If you're a mystery fan, you might think that arsenic only shows up in old British murder mysteries, the kind set in cozy English villages with tea shops and duchesses. Sadly, arsenic is so prevalent in our modern world that I test for it routinely. (Technically, arsenic is not a heavy metal, but a heavy metal *alloy*: the mix of a metal and other elements. However, it's still a major factor in the toxicity that can trigger or worsen an autoimmune condition, which is why I am including it here.)

In some areas you might be exposed to arsenic in your drinking water. It's also found in the soil, where it makes its way into rice, vegetables, and fruits. Recently there were even reports of arsenic in apple juice. Arsenic is also found in the treated woods used for decks, and in India and China, it works its way into herbs. Oh yes, and industrial farms actually put arsenic in their chicken feed, *deliberately.* So now, besides mercury-laden fish, we're exposed to arsenic-laced chicken.

It still blows my mind to think that arsenic is used in animal feed, but it's been in use since the 1940s; apparently, it saves on the feed. As a powerful poison, arsenic fights some common poultry diseases, and it supports tissue and vascular development—counterintuitive, I know, but true. Historically, according to a 2013 report by Bloomberg .com, about 70 percent of U.S. poultry has been given arsenic-based drugs. The FDA did ban three arsenic drugs used in poultry and pig feeds, but who knows how many more are out there.

By the way, the arsenic residue in rice comes from the water in which rice crops stand, but it also comes from the poultry feces used as fertilizer. And if that doesn't upset you enough, consider that many infant rice cereals—a major food for many children—contain something like five times the levels of arsenic found in oatmeal.

ELECTRONIC HAZARDS

A growing area of concern is electromagnetic fields (EMFs), the charged area produced by electric and electronic devices, including computers, televisions, cell phones, microwaves, and the like. Although electric devices have been around for quite a while, we've only had electronic devices for a couple of decades, so there aren't many long-term studies about their effects. The few that are beginning to emerge are pretty scary, however, especially for those of us with autoimmune conditions or who are high on the spectrum.

Now, I'm going to be very honest with you: I never give advice that I can't follow myself. The part of me that reads the latest science wants to shut off all the electronic devices in my home forever. The part of me that lives in the real world says, "Live without a computer and a cell phone? Not gonna happen!"

So here are the best compromises I can suggest to you, the ones that feel doable and that I practice myself:

- Turn your router off every night. You're not using it then, and why expose yourself to more electronic radiation while you sleep?

- Never carry an "on" cell phone on your body. Carry it in a bag, or keep it in airplane mode while it is in a pocket or bra.

- Never hold a cell phone by your head. Use speaker mode or headsets.

- If you want your cell phone by your bed at night, put it in airplane mode. That way you can still use it as your alarm clock, as I do.

WHAT'S IN YOUR MOUTH?

Heavy metals and other potential sources of inflammation are not just "out there" in the environment. They also lurk in your mouth, exposing you to exactly the type of chronic, low-grade assault we need to be most concerned about:

Root canals. These can become infected, an ongoing source of inflammation that stresses your immune system.

Wisdom teeth. If you've had them removed, cavitation (a hole in the bone below) might remain, and it too can become inflamed or filled with infections.

Bridges, posts, and porcelain crowns. In a variety of ways, each of these dental additions to your mouth can expose you to toxins, heavy metals, and inflammation.

Silver fillings. These are made with an amalgam of copper, silver, and mercury, which leach toxins into the bloodstream, so I recommend you have your metal fillings replaced with composite fillings by a biological dentist—a type of dentist who knows about the dangers of heavy metals and has learned to remove them safely. A regular dentist could theoretically make this switch, but he or she probably won't know how to do it safely, so as to keep mercury vapors from penetrating the blood–brain barrier and making their way into your brain. See appendix D for more information and "Resources" for suggestions on how to find a biological dentist.

MOLDS AND MYCOTOXINS

One of the most serious problems I run across in my practice is mycotoxins, volatile organic compounds (VOCs) that are given off by certain types of molds. Yet most people don't even realize that myco-toxins are affecting them.

How can mycotoxins stay so far under the radar?

First of all, three-fourths of the population have genes that can withstand the effects of mycotoxins without symptoms. You might be suffering from mycotoxins while the rest of your family is just fine—even other family members with autoimmune conditions.

Then, too, it's hard to believe that something is a problem if you can't see it, and most molds don't show themselves out in the open. They lurk under the floorboards, behind the walls, or in the cracks between windows and window frames. It's hard enough detecting them if they're in your home; if they're somewhere in a school or office building, you might never have access to them. Yet the toxins they release into the air are affecting you, every single day.

Finally, molds are underrated as a problem because most doctors don't know about them. Even most functional medicine physicians are ignorant about molds and mycotoxins. I myself only became familiar with the topic after the office I used to rent became infested due to a heavy rainstorm, and I realized that it was affecting me and another staff person enough that we had to move.

So if you show up at your doctor's office with a mycotoxin prob-lem, you'll very likely not get properly diagnosed. Even I don't usually bring up the topic the first time a patient comes to see me, because the vast majority of the people I treat get better simply by following The Myers Way—cleaning up their diets, healing their guts, and sup-porting their immune systems. However, I do start wondering about mycotoxins when

- diet alone doesn't seem to be doing a good enough job;
- a patient has really strange symptoms that don't add up;
- the patient suddenly develops an autoimmune condition out of the blue; or

- the patient has recurrent yeast overgrowth, despite remaining on The Myers Way and being promptly treated.

People are often skeptical about mold in the home if only one family member is getting sick, but remember, only one-quarter of the population have the genes that make them vulnerable.

Nevertheless, I have seen many cases where molds made more than one family member sick. I once treated twin two-year-old boys who came to me with the worst eczema I had ever seen, their arms and legs raw from scratching. They were so reactive that the only foods they could digest were meat and rice. After several bouts of yeast overgrowth, which further exacerbated their eczema, we finally figured out that mold in the home was the problem, and the family managed to get it cleaned up. The boys improved quickly, to the point where they were eating a full complement of The Myers Way–approved meats, fruits, and vegetables for the first time ever. (I was happy to get them off the rice, which wasn't ideal for them in the long term but had been what they could tolerate in the short term.)

Lo and behold, when the mold disappeared, the boys' mother was able to get off antidepressants (with the supervision of her doctor, of course). She had never related her "psychological" problem to the physical effect of mycotoxins, but clearly the toxic mold was a major factor in her disorder as well as her sons'.

If you suspect toxic mold is causing your symptoms, see appendix C for more information on what to do next. This could make a huge difference in reversing your condition or in keeping you from moving further up the spectrum.

YOUR BODY'S NATURAL DETOX PROCESS

Ideally, you want to keep the toxins from going in. But once they're *in*, you need to pee, poop, and sweat them out.

This detoxification is a two-phase process that requires converting your toxins from *lipid*-soluble (dissolving in fat, so they get stored in your body) to *water*-soluble (dissolving in water, so you can excrete them). If your body goes through just phase one and does not proceed

> ### SWEATING IN YOUR SAUNA
>
> Infrared saunas are a great way to get your daily sweat in, especially if you can't easily exercise. Many companies now make infrared saunas you can have installed in your own home; they even make collapsible "solo saunas" designed to fit in a small apartment. Check out "Resources" for more.

on to phase two, you're in worse trouble than if your body had never started detoxing at all, because phase one actually exposes you to the toxins that otherwise would have been safely stored in your fat.

Most of this process takes place through your liver, which needs "cofactors," specific chemicals that enable your body to move on to phase two. I've made sure that The Myers Way supplies you with the cofactors you need via nutrient-dense foods and high-quality supplements.

Your body also needs a lot of energy to complete phase two. Accordingly, The Myers Way provides you with plenty of protein.

I never recommend prolonged fasting or juice fasts. As you just saw, your body needs energy and other vital nutrients to detox. If you're fasting, your detox process could get stalled in phase one, leaving you worse off than before.

Your small intestine is another crucial part of detox: Many toxins are processed in the gut, so they never have to enter the rest of your body. You need a healthy gut for the process to work well, but luckily, The Myers Way takes care of that too. We also make sure you get the right kind of exercise, drink lots of filtered water, and take high-quality supplements to support your detox pathways.

GLORIOUS GLUTATHIONE

Glutathione is your body's biggest detoxifier. Every cell in your body has some of this vital nutrient, but it's most highly concentrated in your major detox organ: your liver. Glutathione helps to carry the toxins out of your body by binding itself to the free radicals—molecules that damage your tissue. Glutathione binds to mercury also.

If you don't have enough glutathione, toxins hang around in your body longer, or they get stored in your fat cells, where they might wreak havoc on your immune system. The Myers Way helps your body make its own glutathione by having you eat plenty of garlic, onions, and cruciferous veggies (broccoli, kale, cauliflower, cabbage). You also take a special glutathione supplement.

Now, here's where you have to be careful. Most glutathione is not absorbed well in the gut because it gets broken down before it can penetrate into your cells. The "liposomal" form of glutathione is advertised as being able to penetrate into your cells, but I have not found it to be effective, either personally or in my clinic. However, the "acetylated" form of this supplement does not break down. So when you take the glutathione supplements I recommend, please use one of the forms recommended in "Resources"; we have one that is acetylated and produced with nanotechnology to make it even easier for your body to absorb. Yeah, you can buy cheaper versions of glutathione, but they'll be virtually ineffective. When it comes to supplements, you definitely get what you pay for.

THE IMPORTANCE OF GENETICS

Functional medicine is personalized medicine—the treatment of every single patient as an individual. Never do I see this more vividly than when I am looking at my patients' genetics, particularly their "SNPs."

SNP—pronounced "snip"—is short for single-nucleotide polymorphism, which is a fancy way of saying "genetic mutation" (a variation in the way DNA is sequenced along a gene). SNPs can affect us in all sorts of ways, including when it comes to detox.

For example, the *MTHFR* (methylenetetrahydrofolate reductase) gene helps us "methylate" heavy metals, a process that enables us to get them out of our bodies. You need B6, B12, and folate for this process to work, but mutations in the *MTHFR* gene can get in the way.

I know this problem very well, because I have two of these mutations, and many of my patients have one or two of them as well. As a result, we detox a far smaller percentage of heavy metals than we should. To compensate, we need to take extra-large doses of special *pre*-methylated B6, B12, and folate. Since detoxing heavy metals is so much harder for us than for the general population, we also need to be even more careful to avoid exposure.

About 50 percent of the population have one *MTHFR* mutation, and about 20 percent have two. If you have an autoimmune condition or are high on the spectrum, I highly recommend you have your physician test you for this mutation so you can protect yourself with the right supplements.

Another key SNP occurs on the *GSTM1* gene. This gene enables us to process glutathione, which, as I mentioned, is a key support for detoxification. If you have a *GSTM1* SNP, you need to increase your intake of cruciferous vegetables and take extra detox supplements: glutathione, alpha-lipoic acid (ALA), milk thistle, NAC (n-acetylcysteine), and magnesium.

Finally, the *COMT* gene codes the protein known as COMT (catechol-O-methyltransferase). COMT is the enzyme that enables us to process several key brain chemicals, including dopamine, epinephrine, and norepinephrine, all of which energize and excite us. People with the *COMT* SNP seem to find life more rewarding—but they also seem to have more difficulties metabolizing estrogen (putting them at greater risk for breast cancer), alcohol, and some other toxins. The COMT enzyme also helps detoxification in the liver and the gut, and, like the *MTHFR*, it relies on B vitamins. So if you have the *COMT* SNP, you should also be taking pre-methylated doses of vitamin B.

THE SKINNY ON SUPPLEMENTS

As you have seen by now, we live in a toxic world. We can't afford to detox just once or twice a year; we need to support our detox pathways every single day.

If you're fairly low on the autoimmune spectrum, you might be able to detox through the nutrients you get just from food. But if you have an autoimmune condition, are high on the spectrum, or have any of the SNPs just discussed, you need to take supplements.

I should caution you that supplements are an unregulated industry, so you want to be sure to always buy high-quality products. I have included in the "Resources" section recommendations for companies I have looked into, so you can rely on them. If you go with a different brand, make sure it is third-party tested, follows good manufacturing practices, and produces only high-quality, gluten- and dairy-free products.

HOW CLAIRE TAMED HER TOXINS

When Claire first realized how many toxins she was being exposed to and how great a toxic burden she likely carried, she felt overwhelmed and discouraged. "I feel surrounded," she told me. "Like everything is just waiting to leap out at me and make me sick."

I encouraged her to turn her feelings of fear into a commitment to take action, and I reminded her that it was okay to start small and take things one step at a time. After all, as you'll see in the next chapter, stress is also bad for your autoimmune condition. Let's not let anxiety about the toxic burden create a whole new kind of problem!

Claire was already committed to following The Myers Way for diet, including the 4Rs protocol for gut healing. When she began the diet, she decided to undertake the four key steps I had suggested: HEPA filters for her home and work; water filters for all her taps plus a stainless-steel thermos; organic food, cooked without Teflon and stored without plastic; and a gradual replacement of her personal-care products. "These are all things I do every day, sometimes several times a day," she told me. "I eat, drink, shower, and use body products all the time, so I'd like those choices to support my immune system rather than weaken it."

Claire thought that after thirty days on The Myers Way, she might find another burst of energy to make some additional changes. At that point, she told me, she might consider replacing her home cleaning products, switching to an eco-friendly dry cleaner, and maybe even buying an organic mattress (see appendix E). Starting small and going step-by-step helped Claire to feel empowered rather than overwhelmed.

Claire saw an immediate reward for combining the eating plan and the 4Rs with these important detox steps. Within a few weeks, she experienced a dramatic drop in symptoms and an equally dramatic boost of energy. For the first time in a long while, Claire told me, she felt "normal again—like the self I used to be. It's so good to get that self back again!"

"I wish I didn't have to deal with all of this," she said at the end of our last visit. "But since I do, at least I have the information and the resources I need. And it's amazing how even small changes can make such a big difference."

CHAPTER 7

Heal Your Infections and Relieve Your Stress

My patient Jasmine was concerned.

A woman in her early forties with one son, a commuter marriage, and a demanding job as a professor at a local university, she had come to me six months ago full of hope. Although she had been struggling for several months with her Graves' disease—the same autoimmune condition that I have—she had finally found some relief through our work together. No longer did she have to cope with disabling panic attacks that might strike at any moment, even while she was teaching a class or having dinner with her son. Her hands no longer trembled when she picked up a fork or a pen. And after months of persistent insomnia, which had kept her continually frustrated and exhausted, she was finally able to sleep through the night.

Yet Jasmine was still on medication to stop her thyroid gland's overactive production of thyroid hormone—and that medication had side effects. Ironically, as the medication reduced the effects of too much thyroid, Jasmine was now having the opposite experience: the dry and cracking skin, fatigue, and constipation associated with low levels of thyroid hormone. Despite her healthy diet, she had also started to gain weight.

"These side effects are so hard to take," Jasmine told me. "I want to lose that extra weight. I want my old energy back. And I want to get off medications entirely!"

So far, despite Jasmine's diligent commitment to The Myers Way eating plan and healing her gut, we hadn't been able to achieve those goals. "Dr. Myers," she asked me, respectfully but urgently, "is this the best I can hope for?"

"Absolutely not," I told her. "I know we can make more progress." To do so, I explained, we would need to turn to the fourth pillar of The Myers Way: *Heal your infections and relieve your stress.*

I explained to Jasmine that while diet and intestinal healing can lead to radical improvements for many patients, sometimes they are not enough. Sometimes we need to look at the infections that are frequently associated with multiple sclerosis, lupus, and other autoimmune diseases.

Jasmine looked at me with confusion. "But I thought we took care of my infections," she said. "The yeast overgrowth and the SIBO—they cleared up months ago!"

"Yes," I explained, "but there are other infections caused by viruses or different types of bacteria that can also cause problems. For example, the herpes virus or the virus that causes mononucleosis, Epstein–Barr, can also trigger problems with autoimmunity, as can the bacteria *E. coli*."

I went on to explain to Jasmine that these kinds of infections can bring on an autoimmune disorder or trigger a flare in someone who has been symptom-free. In addition, stress can retrigger infections and worsen autoimmune conditions—as well as cause you to develop one—whether or not an infection is involved. Stress can also provoke weight gain, which itself is inflammatory . . . and the extra inflammation was putting a further strain on Jasmine's immune system.

Jasmine nodded as I spoke about stress. A strong woman from an immigrant family, she was used to facing challenges, and she had faced a great many in the past few months. At work, her department's funding had just been reduced. Her long-distance marriage was not easy. And her son had just been diagnosed with learning disabilities.

"All right, then," I told Jasmine. "It's great that you have healed your gut and are still following a healthy diet—and you have seen the good results. Now we're going to take it to the next level. Our next steps are to heal your infections and lighten your burden of stress."

THE FOURTH PILLAR

So far you have heard about the first three pillars of The Myers Way:

1. *Heal your gut.*
2. *Get rid of gluten, grains, legumes, and other foods that cause chronic inflammation.*
3. *Tame the toxins.*

Now it's time to explore the fourth pillar:

4. *Heal your infections and relieve your stress.*

Some of you, like Jasmine, may need to address lingering bacterial or viral infections. (Most common gut infections are addressed in chapter 4, "Heal Your Gut," with the 4Rs protocol, pages 86–89.) Stress is also part of this pillar because it can become a vicious cycle with infection: Stress frequently triggers or retriggers an infection, while infections create added stress for the body. Even those of us without infections need to find sane and healthy ways of coping with our stress, since stress is so challenging for our immune systems. So let's take a closer look at both how infections and stress make autoimmunity worse and how healing infections and relieving stress can make us all healthier.

AUTOIMMUNITY AND INFECTIONS

Like many teenagers, Jasmine had developed a bad case of mononucleosis when she was fourteen. She still remembered vividly the runny nose, sore throat, aching head, and high fever she struggled with for three weeks, and the debilitating fatigue that lingered throughout the spring and summer.

"Mono" is caused by the Epstein–Barr virus, which, once it burrows its way inside you, never actually leaves. Even though Jasmine would never again come down with mononucleosis, she would always be infected with Epstein–Barr.

Epstein–Barr is just one of many viruses—along with other bacterial and viral infections—that have been associated with autoimmune conditions. Infections can often bring on an autoimmune condition, or they can make a condition worse or trigger a flare.

As with so much about autoimmune conditions, there is simply a lot that we do not know about how this happens. Scientists have come up with a few theories, though, so let me share the most important ones with you. Infections affect our immune system in multiple ways; therefore, all these hypotheses hold some truth.

Molecular mimicry. You have already heard of molecular mimicry with regard to your immune system's responses to reactive foods, such as dairy and gluten. But molecular mimicry can be triggered by infections as well. Suppose you have been infected with a virus or bacterium. Rogue T cells and B cells in your immune system can't distinguish between the virus and your own tissue, so they attack both. They also recruit other parts of your immune system and "instruct" them to attack you too.

Bystander activation. According to this theory, an infection destroys some of your tissue, and your immune system rushes to the scene to put out the fire. It attacks the infection, just as it's supposed to. But it also attacks your own tissue, the innocent bystander in this scenario. Bystander activation can occur with both bacterial and viral infections. However, since a virus burrows right into your cells, it is even more likely to provoke this type of attack: Your immune system rushes in to attack the virus, which is surrounded by your own cellular tissue, an innocent bystander in the line of fire.

Cryptic antigens. Okay, that is a *very* science-heavy term, so if you prefer, just think of this theory as "hijacking." This one typically applies to viruses, such as the herpes virus or Epstein–Barr, which might hijack your cells' DNA, trying to hide from your immune system by imitating your cells. Your immune system isn't fooled, though. It recognizes that an infection is present in your body and mobilizes an attack—which extends both to the virus and to the cells that the "invader" has hijacked.

Now let's look at some of the infections that are most commonly associated with autoimmune disorders. These are by no means the only infections that might trigger autoimmunity, but they are the ones I see most often and the ones most frequently studied.

VIRAL INFECTIONS: HERPES

There are a lot of viruses in the herpes family, and they all seem to be implicated in autoimmune conditions. However, herpes simplex (types 1 and 2) and Epstein–Barr are the most studied, so we're going to focus on them.

Herpes simplex is the virus that gives you cold sores and/or genital herpes. If you have herpes, you likely know it, but you can always ask your doctor to test you for it. However, close to 90 percent of all people living in the United States have antibodies to one or both of the herpes simplex viruses, so even if you don't think you have it, you might simply never have realized you do. There is no cure for herpes—once it gets into your system, it stays there. Sometimes, though, it's active, while other times it's dormant.

When herpes is active, your immune system makes antibodies for it—and those antibodies can trigger an autoimmune response. When herpes is dormant, it's less likely to be involved in an autoimmune response; however, you might not necessarily know whether it's active or not, since the signs can be subtle and easy to miss.

Active herpes can be treated with antiviral medications, which can be prescribed by your doctor. You can also take two supplements: lysine, an amino acid, and monolaurin, most commonly derived from coconut oil (see "The Myers Way Autoimmune Program Supplements," pages 197–200).

VIRAL INFECTIONS: EPSTEIN–BARR

The infection that has been most extensively studied in connection with autoimmunity is caused by the Epstein–Barr virus, the virus that infected Jasmine. (I had mono as a teenager, so Epstein–Barr infected me too.) Epstein–Barr is in the herpes family, the same group of viruses that can give you genital herpes, cold sores, chicken pox, and shingles. Since 95 percent of all U.S. adults have picked up this virus by age forty, you very likely have it. Half of all children have the condition by age five, so if you live in the United States, Epstein–Barr is pretty much a fact of life.

At this point you might be saying, "Wait a minute! I'm *sure* that

95 percent of the people I know have not had mono." However, you can be exposed to Epstein–Barr, develop mononucleosis, and simply never show any symptoms. Or you can be misdiagnosed as having had the flu. But 95 percent of the U.S. population does have the antibodies for Epstein–Barr, which means they were once somehow infected with it. And once you've caught the virus, it remains within your body for the rest of your life, whether you feel sick or not.

Epstein–Barr has been strongly correlated with a number of auto-immune conditions, including multiple sclerosis, lupus, chronic fatigue syndrome, fibromyalgia, Hashimoto's, and Sjögren's, as well as Graves' disease. The correlations with multiple sclerosis and lupus are especially strong. For example, some 99 percent of children with lupus have Epstein–Barr antibodies, as compared to only 70 percent of children in a healthy nonlupus control group.

Likewise, while 95 percent of all U.S. residents have Epstein–Barr antibodies, 100 percent of people with MS have them. Basically, people with MS test positive for Epstein–Barr, while people *without* the virus don't seem to get MS. We also know that high levels of Epstein–Barr antibodies seem to predict MS symptoms and flares, and a history of infectious mononucleosis doubles the risk for MS.

It's not simply that people with autoimmune conditions are some-what more likely to be infected with Epstein–Barr. Their viral load is also much higher than that of healthy individuals. "Viral load" is the level of the virus in your blood. Once you get a viral infection, some level of the virus might remain in your blood even when you are not showing any symptoms. The degree of the virus's presence is measured in terms of how many viral "copies" exist in every milliliter of your blood. You don't need to remember all the technical detail; just know that having a higher viral load means that the virus is more active and present within your body than in someone with a lower viral load, even if you don't have any symptoms.

Two studies, whose results have recently been reconfirmed, found that lupus patients had a viral load from fifteen to forty times higher than that of people without autoimmune conditions. Indeed, when I tested Jasmine, her Epstein–Barr viral load was unusually high.

There are two ways to treat Epstein–Barr. Conventional medical doctors tend to rely on prescription antivirals. Unfortunately, most of these medications are not very effective, and the one that is has caused some dangerous side effects. Honestly, prescription medication is just not an effective treatment.

I prefer to take another approach. First, support your immune system by following the protocols of The Myers Way, which I lay out for you in chapter 8: Eat immune-friendly foods; take high-quality supplements; heal your gut; drink lots of filtered water; get the right kind of exercise (see page 189 to find out when you might need to take it easy); sleep seven and a half to nine hours each night, or more if needed; support your detox pathways; detoxify your personal environment as much as possible; and reduce and/or manage your stress. Second, those of you who are concerned about infections can also consume lots of coconut oil and coconut derivatives (see page 181 and "Resources"). You'll be happy to learn that lots of our Myers Way recipes include healthy amounts of coconut oil, so that will give you a good start.

BACTERIAL INFECTIONS AND AUTOIMMUNITY

Here's a list of the most common associations between bacterial infections and autoimmune conditions:

Type of Microbe	Associated Disorder
Campylobacter	Guillain–Barré syndrome
*Chlamydia pneumoniae**	Multiple sclerosis
Citrobacter, Klebsiella, Proteus, Porphyromonas	Rheumatoid arthritis
E. coli, Proteus	Autoimmunity in general
Klebsiella	Ankylosing spondylitis
Streptococcus pyogenes	Rheumatic fever
Yersinia	Graves' disease, Hashimoto's thyroiditis
* This is *not* the same bacterium that causes the sexually transmitted disease, though obviously it is from the same family.	

This list is by no means comprehensive, but it should be a good starting point for you and your physician. If you're not getting better rapidly enough—say, after three months of following The Myers

Way—consider asking your doctor to test you for the type of microbe associated with your condition. If your doctor does not see the necessity, explain that you have read that microbes are implicated in auto-immune conditions, and your mind would rest easier if you knew microbes were not making your problem worse.

If you test positive, you may need to take antibiotics to heal the infection. I hope by now I don't need to remind you: Always take probiotics while you are taking antibiotics, to replenish your friendly bacteria. You should also take caprylic acid and an enzyme called Candisol that breaks down the yeast cell wall, which will prevent yeast overgrowth while you are taking antibiotics (just follow the Yeast Overgrowth / SIBO Dietary Protocol on pages 195–96). To prevent and/or repair the leaky gut that antibiotics can bring on, make sure you are also taking the supplements listed on pages 197–200.

THE INFECTIOUS EFFECT OF LYME DISEASE

Another type of infection commonly implicated in autoimmunity is Lyme disease, which is caused by bacteria known as *Spirochaetes*. These creatures are spread through the bites of ticks and seem to be found mainly in the northeastern United States. Some 60 percent of untreated Lyme disease patients develop arthritis that persists for years, leading scientists to speculate that the arthritis might be caused by either a bystander activation or molecular mimicry.

This close connection between Lyme disease and arthritis frequently leads to confusion. Many people are diagnosed with autoimmune conditions when they actually have Lyme disease, and vice versa. And of course some people might have both—in which case, each condition needs to be treated; it's not enough to treat just one.

If you think you might have either Lyme disease or arthritis, make sure your physician has done a thorough and accurate job of diagnosing you so you get the correct treatment. The most efficient thing to start with is to find out whether or not you have Lyme disease.

There is a conventional test for Lyme disease, which you can request, but I have found that it isn't very accurate because you get a lot of false negatives; that is, the test can say that you don't have Lyme disease when you really do. I prefer a more sophisticated test known as iSpot Lyme. You can either get a functional medicine physician to order this test or ask your conventional doctor to order it for you through one of the sources I list in "Resources." Even if your conventional doctor is skeptical, he or she should be willing to rule out Lyme disease by using this test.

THE VITAMIN D CONNECTION

Vitamin D is absolutely vital to your immune system. You get it from oily fish and from exposure to the sun, or you can take it as a supplement, which I recommend.

However, the vitamin D that you get from these sources has to be metabolized by the body. Your liver makes 25-hydroxyvitamin D, while your kidneys make 1,25-dihydroxyvitamin D, which is the active version.

Many people are by now aware that they want normal or high-normal levels of 25-hydroxyvitamin D, which seems to have a protective function against breast and colon cancer. However, most physicians—even in functional medicine—are not checking levels of 1,25-dihydroxyvitamin D. Researcher Trevor Marshall has found that having high levels of 1,25-dihydroxyvitamin D and low levels of 25-hydroxyvitamin D can actually suppress your immune system, which might lead to autoimmunity. Have your physician check your levels of both types of D and then work with you to restore a healthy balance.

THE STRESS PARADOX

"All right," Jasmine said after we had discussed her Epstein–Barr viral load. "I will continue to support my immune system through The Myers Way, and I will take the monolaurin coconut derivatives you have recommended. Is there anything else I can do to make progress?"

Yes, I told her, there was. Her next step was to look at her burden of stress. Stress often triggers infections, and it generally has ill effects on the immune system. The challenges Jasmine faced at home and work were part of the rich, satisfying life she had chosen. But they were also part of the stress burden that was making it more difficult to resolve her autoimmune disease.

Jasmine was surprised to learn that stress was such a significant factor in her condition. Jasmine's family had raised her to believe that stress is something you simply "shake off"—an inevitable by-product of hard work. Jasmine was more used to ignoring her stress burden than thinking of what she might do to lighten it.

Many of us view stress in this way. Yet stress has an enormous impact on both our immune systems and our health—something that most people, and even most physicians, don't realize. Considering the significant role stress plays in our health and daily lives, there remain an awful lot of misconceptions about it. So let's clear up the misunderstandings and find out just how big a role stress plays in autoimmunity.

Here's the first and maybe even the most important point I'd like to share with you: The way you think, feel, and respond to situations doesn't only affect your stress level. *It also affects your immune system.*

Yep, you read that right. When you're upset, stressed out, anxious, or on edge, your immune system is affected. When you're feeling calm, peaceful, or quietly content, your immune system is affected by that too.

Now, here's where it gets complicated. Stress does affect your immune system, but it doesn't do so in a linear, one-directional, or easy-to-understand way. The effects of stress on your immune system are real but complex. Sometimes they are downright paradoxical, which means they can seem to be doing two opposite things at the same time. You have to look closely to figure out exactly what's going on. Luckily, I'm right here to walk you through it.

When scientists first discovered the relationship between stress and immune function, they thought it was a lot simpler than it actually is. Some sixty years ago, the pioneering researcher into stress, Hans Selye, found that upsetting or difficult experiences appeared to suppress the immune system. In experiments he conducted on rats, he discovered that the tissues of their thymus gland actually atrophied when the rats were subjected to "nonspecific unpleasantness"—i.e., stress.

As I mentioned, the thymus gland's ability to produce, regulate, and balance your T cells is crucial to your immune system. So if stress affects the thymus, you know that's going to be an important relationship for anyone with an autoimmune condition.

Of course stress doesn't just affect the thymus. It disrupts many different types of immune function through many different pathways.

When I say "stress," by the way, I'm not just talking about emotional stress. Physical stress has the same effect. Undergoing surgery, training for a marathon, or pulling an all-nighter are all significant stressors. So are eating gluten, consuming reactive foods, and coping with a toxic burden. Of course stress also includes such emotional challenges as worrying about your finances, facing deadline pressure, or having a painful argument with a loved one.

Your body responds to stress of any kind by releasing a cascade of stress hormones—biochemicals intended to help your body gear up for a challenge. Chief among these is cortisol, a powerful chemical with a wide variety of effects. Cortisol is what you need to mobilize your energy—physical, mental, and emotional—to respond to an important demand. Cortisol helps you stay focused and motivated. It can also cause you to feel wired, edgy, and "stressed."

Another thing about cortisol is that it's highly inflammatory. This makes sense when you remember why we need inflammation in the first place. Inflammation is your immune system's response to a wound, injury, or infection—a threat to your body's safety and integrity. If you're facing a stressor, cortisol helps you rev up to meet the challenge, but it also alerts your immune system. If your challenge involves an attack or injury, cortisol ensures that your inflammatory chemicals are standing by, ready to rush to the wound.

So, early on in the stress response, contrary to what scientists initially thought, stress doesn't *suppress* the immune system; it actually *activates* it.

This response may not make much sense if your challenge is more emotional than physical. However, your immune system evolved back in the day when "challenge" meant arduous physical exertion and/or danger. For good or ill, your body has just *one* stress response, which it brings forth whether the stress is physical (fleeing a saber-toothed tiger, trekking across the tundra to a new village), mental (doing a complicated equation, trying to evaluate which of three household appliances gives you the best value), or emotional (helping your learning-disabled son do his homework, worrying about your career).

Those early scientists were also right: Stress *does* activate your immune response—but it also suppresses it. That very same inflammatory stress hormone—cortisol, which pushed your immune system into high gear—then goes on to suppress your immune response. In other words, stress stimulates your immune system, which in turn mobilizes a chain reaction, which triggers cortisol release, which then suppresses your immune system.

In a healthy immune system, the process takes about an hour. So you get sixty minutes of activation followed by a gradual suppression of the immune system.

Why would your immune system start a chain reaction whose end point is to suppress itself? The answers have special relevance to anyone who has or might develop an autoimmune condition, so read on.

STRESSFUL SUPPRESSION

Okay, it makes sense why stress would activate your immune system, right? Most of the time a healthy immune system just hangs out at baseline. Then, under stress (which your body interprets as potential danger), your immune system kicks into high gear. Clearly it can't be on high alert *all* the time; that would use up too many of your body's resources.

However, as you saw in chapter 3, if your immune system stays on hyperalert for too long, it becomes like an overworked security squad that cracks under pressure. It goes rogue and begins firing not just at the bad guys but at your own tissue.

In other words, acute stress (a short-term deadline, a quick disagreement with your spouse, a thirty-minute workout) revs up your immune system so you get that extra protection during a time of crisis. Then your immune system falls back down to baseline when the stress is over. That's one good thing about acute stress: It contains its own built-in "stop" mechanism.

In chronic stress, by contrast, the immune system is activated—and because the stress never really turns off, your immune system *keeps* being activated. Your immune system never really has a chance to return to baseline. The result is a body full of inflammation and, eventually, perhaps an autoimmune condition.

Of course your body is designed to keep this from happening. This is why your body tries to *suppress* your immune response—precisely to keep it from going over the top into overactivation and autoimmunity. Major stressors—either extremely intense stress or a stress that goes on for a long time—normally return your immune system not just to baseline but to 40 to 70 percent *below* baseline, to a state where you are really immunosuppressed.

This is why conventional medical doctors frequently treat autoimmune conditions with corticosteroids, which are a form of cortisol. They know that stress suppresses your immune system, and they're trying to get your overactive immune system to calm down. The problem is once your immune system has been suppressed, it can no longer protect you against actual threats.

Okay, but here's the *really* paradoxical part: Even though stress seems to suppress the immune system, *stress can also make autoimmune diseases and inflammatory conditions worse*. Studies have shown that for many autoimmune disorders, including multiple sclerosis, rheumatoid arthritis, ulcerative colitis, inflammatory bowel disease, and Hashimoto's thyroiditis, stress is what triggered the disease in the first place, and stress is also what makes it flare up. And guess what. This stress connection also holds true for Jasmine's condition (and mine), Graves' disease, as I discovered when the combined stress of my mother's death and my first year in medical school pushed me over the edge into Graves' disease.

THE STRESS TRIGGER

To understand the paradoxical nature of stress—the way it can both modify your autoimmune symptoms *and* make your condition worse—we have to distinguish between acute and chronic stress, and between different types of chronic stress.

As you just saw, a healthy stress response is acute: It goes up, stimulates your immune system, goes down, and returns your immune system to baseline.

By contrast, chronic stress—stress that never seems to end—will eventually suppress your immune system somewhere between 40 and 70 percent below baseline (think of how students always get sick during exam week or how you often catch a cold after a couple of tough months at work).

However, if your stress levels keep going up and down—chronic stress with some breaks—or if your stress levels keep going up and up and up (just when you think things can't get worse, they do), *then* you are at risk for an overactivation of your immune system and, eventually, autoimmunity.

So the type of steady, prolonged stress you get from taking those steroids the doctor prescribed for you will indeed suppress your immune system, putting you at risk for other problems but frequently lessening the symptoms of your autoimmune disease. However, stress that includes more ups and downs, or that keeps going up, overactivates your immune system. That can trigger an autoimmune condition if you don't actually have one, or set off a flare or a relapse if you do.

This seems to be a design flaw in our immune systems. In the words of Robert M. Sapolsky, professor of neurology and biology at Stanford University, MacArthur genius, and author of *Why Zebras Don't Get Ulcers*, "The system apparently did not evolve for dealing with numerous repetitions of coordinating the various on-and-off switches."

This makes sense. In more primitive times, humans faced either relatively brief challenges (like an attack from a predator or hauling a heavy boat out of the water) or steady, prolonged challenges (like a long migration or a famine). We didn't evolve to deal with a lot of ups and downs, so our complicated network of stress hormones and immune-system chemicals doesn't know how to cope with them. If we're faced with too varied an experience of chronic stress, Sapolsky writes, "ultimately something uncoordinated occurs, increasing the risk that the system becomes autoimmune."

STRESS AND INFECTION

Here's another layer to the way stress either triggers or worsens an autoimmune condition: through infection, specifically viral infection. As you saw earlier, both the Epstein–Barr and the herpes viruses are dormant, or "latent," a lot of the time. The herpes virus is latent whenever you don't have cold sores or an outbreak. The Epstein–Barr virus is latent as soon as you have recovered from your mono. Back in its active days, the virus burrowed inside some of your cells. Then it went into hibernation and became latent: It just lies there, not replicating itself, not colonizing your cells, just sort of hiding out.

Eventually, though, something comes along to trigger the virus, reactivating it. The virus's first response is to replicate itself, so it grows more numerous and more powerful, colonizing more and more of your cells. Then it goes latent again. The cycle can keep repeating.

Often, when viruses replicate, they burst open the cells they are taking over. Naturally that triggers an immune response. As Sapolsky describes it, "just as those activated immune cells are about to pounce, [the viruses] burrow into another round of cells. While the immune cells are cleaning up, the virus goes latent again."

So, as you can see, if you have a virus lurking in your system, every time that virus is reactivated, it provokes your immune system. That internal stressor can lead to overstimulation of the immune system . . . and that in turn can lead to autoimmunity.

Okay, but what reactivates the virus? A depressed immune system. Those clever viruses seem to know just when it's safe for them to reactivate, because the immune system will be at its most depleted and unable to effectively shoot them down.

At this point you might be asking, "How in the world does the virus know when my immune system is depleted?" Well, since stress depresses the immune system, those sneaky viruses are actually cued to respond to your stress hormones, specifically to a form of cortisol known as a glucocorticoid. So, many viruses flare up during times of physical or psychological stress, including herpes, Epstein–Barr, and varicella zoster, which causes chicken pox and shingles.

But the process doesn't stop there. When either herpes or Epstein–Barr infects your nervous system, it *triggers* a stress response. The virus itself triggers the response, which then *activates* the virus, which at the same time suppresses your immune system. And of course your suppressed immune system gives the virus even more leeway to provoke symptoms without being destroyed by all those killer chemicals.

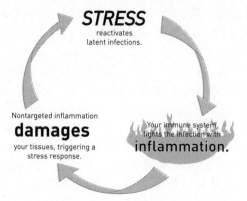

Here is the mechanism through which stress plus a viral infection can either bring on or reactivate an autoimmune condition:

- The stress reactivates your infection.
- Your immune system comes in to destroy the source of the infection.
- While the infection is being attacked, your body's tissue also takes a hit, because of either molecular mimicry, bystander activation, or hijacking.

CORTISOL, INFLAMMATION, AND WEIGHT GAIN: A VICIOUS CYCLE

The cortisol generated by your stress response has another unwanted side effect: It provokes weight gain. Many animal studies have shown that when animals are stressed, they gain weight, even when they're consuming the same number of calories they did before they were stressed. They also gain more weight than control groups of unstressed animals eating the same amount of calories. Studies have shown that if given the opportunity, animals also tend to eat more when they're stressed, but they gain weight even when their calories are restricted.

These studies are significant because they show that stress is not "all in your head"; it's in your metabolism, your adrenal glands, and your immune system. Likewise, your stress-induced weight gain is not a matter of willpower; it's a matter of biology. Animals don't eat because their favorite comfort foods remind them of childhood or because they're substituting food for love. They eat because their biology drives them to do so. The facts that they eat more under stress, and they gain weight even when they *don't* overeat, prove that these issues have a profound biological basis.

This makes sense if you think about animals—or early humans— whose stress responses enable them to hold on to precious body fat while facing challenging conditions in the wild. If you're an early human facing cold and hunger during a long, northern winter or joining your village in a mass trek across the desert to find a new home, your stress response helps you to retain body fat, get the most calories possible from your food, and remain on high alert for danger. That inflammatory, fat-retaining stress response could actually save your life.

However, if you're a present-day human whose stress, like Jasmine's, consists of painful phone calls to your child's school, anxious meetings with an underfunded department, and troubling conversations with your long-distance spouse, holding on to body fat is not so functional. In fact, it could make a dangerous disorder even worse, setting you up for diabetes, heart disease, and other conditions, including a worsening of your autoimmune condition.

Stress-induced body fat adds another twist to the vicious cycle because that extra fat is also inflammatory. Contrary to our previous belief that body fat was metabolically inert—that it just lay there and didn't do anything—body fat is actually a chemical factory that plays an intricate role in your body's endocrine, hormonal, and nervous systems. Among other things, it releases cytokines and other inflammatory chemicals, raising your overall level of inflammation and provoking all the related symptoms we have been talking about. (For a full list of symptoms, see page 7.)

Again, for early humans, that makes sense. Body fat's role in the levels of inflammation is part of the same stress-immune response. Stressful times were by definition times for gaining weight while a person mobilized a high level of inflammatory chemicals to combat any wounds, injuries, or infections.

Now, however, gaining weight just turns up the inflammatory heat in an already stressed body, potentially triggering the development of a new autoimmune condition or provoking the flare-up of an existing one. This was Jasmine's experience, as her many life stresses led to weight gain and created inflammatory responses that prevented her from taking her healing to the next level.

ADRENAL FATIGUE: ANOTHER STRESS-RELATED PROBLEM

Stress doesn't only affect your immune system. It also affects your endocrine system, the system that produces and regulates your hormones, including your stress hormones. As you have seen, when you are stressed—either physically, mentally, or emotionally—your body responds with a cascade of stress hormones, including cortisol. If you are subjected to chronic stress, you are at risk of "adrenal fatigue," a dysregulation of your endocrine system in which your stress hormone levels are too high, too low, or both. You respond by feeling wired or exhausted, or a combination of both.

Stressors include many of the factors I want you to avoid on The Myers Way: gluten and other reactive foods, which stress your gut; irregular meals, which stress your blood sugar; too little sleep; and infections. All these things can stress your body, along with psychological challenges at work and in your personal life. Accordingly, all types of stress put you at risk of adrenal fatigue, which in turn stresses your gut, your other hormones (including your thyroid and sex hormones), and many other aspects of your physiology.

Adrenal fatigue is also associated with lowered levels of the hormone known as DHEA—and when DHEA falls too low, that becomes a risk factor for autoimmunity. So addressing adrenal fatigue is crucial for your immune health as well as your overall health.

Conventional physicians don't really recognize adrenal fatigue. They do recognize an autoimmune disease known as Addison's, in which your adrenals are putting out extremely low levels of stress hormone. If you're not at that level of distress, conventional physicians will tell you that nothing's wrong.

I see it differently. In my view, adrenal fatigue lies on a spectrum. At one end, you're completely fine—full of energy and with optimal adrenal function. I'm assuming that if you're in my office, or if you're reading this book with any health concerns at all, you're not at that end. At the other end is Addison's. In between is a wide range of adrenal distress, all of which puts at least some stress on your body's other systems and some of which significantly raises your risk of developing autoimmune disorders.

One reason conventional doctors see adrenal fatigue in such black-and-white terms is because they look for it with a blood test, which gives a less nuanced set of results. I do a saliva test, in which patients take samples of their own saliva four times during the course of a day, enabling me to track the flow of their hormone levels.

THE MYERS WAY ADRENAL FATIGUE TEST

Check all the boxes that apply to you.

- ☐ I am frequently tired.
- ☐ I feel tired even after eight to ten hours of sleep.
- ☐ I am chronically stressed.
- ☐ It is difficult for me to handle stress.
- ☐ I am a night-shift worker.
- ☐ I work long hours.
- ☐ I have little relaxation time during my days.
- ☐ I get headaches frequently.
- ☐ I don't exercise consistently.
- ☐ I am or have been an endurance athlete (or participate in CrossFit).
- ☐ I have erratic sleep patterns.
- ☐ I wake up in the middle of the night.
- ☐ I crave salt.
- ☐ I crave sugar.
- ☐ I have high sugar intake.
- ☐ I have difficulty concentrating.
- ☐ I carry weight in my midsection (an apple-shape body).
- ☐ I have low blood sugar issues (hypoglycemia).
- ☐ I have irregular periods.
- ☐ I have a low libido.
- ☐ I have PMS or perimenopausal/menopausal symptoms.
- ☐ I get sick frequently.
- ☐ I have low blood pressure.
- ☐ I have muscle fatigue or weakness.
- ☐ I rely on caffeine for energy (coffee, energy shots, etc.).

THE MYERS WAY ADRENAL FATIGUE TEST, *continued*

Scoring

Fewer than 2 boxes checked: Great! Continue to manage your stress to support your adrenals and minimize the strain on your immune system.

From 2 to 5 boxes checked: Good. Follow The Myers Way to support your adrenals. You don't need any additional supplementation, but do follow the de-stressing strategies offered in this chapter.

From 6 to 10 boxes checked: Follow The Myers Way to support your adrenals and take the adaptogenic herbs recommended for adrenal fatigue in the supplements chart on page 200. Also follow the de-stressing strategies offered in this chapter.

More than 10 boxes checked: Follow The Myers Way to support your adrenals, and take the adaptogenic herbs recommended for adrenal fatigue in the supplements chart on page 200. Also follow the de-stressing strategies offered in this chapter, and consult a functional medicine practitioner if your symptoms don't resolve within two or three months. Adrenal fatigue can be a complex and challenging problem to treat, so make sure to get the support you need.

Readings can vary wildly from high to low to normal throughout the day, so you really need a complete picture before making a diagnosis.

To get a sense of your own degree of adrenal fatigue, take the test on page 167 and above. I treat adrenal fatigue by figuring out what's stressing the body and then helping my patient remove or modify the stressors, including dietary factors, toxins, and life challenges. Usually these include the same stressors that are creating the autoimmune condition, so if you are following The Myers Way, you have already made a good start in discovering and treating them. I also recommend adaptogenic herbs, which help boost levels of stress hormones when they are low and lower them when they are high.

DE-STRESSING STRATEGIES

Jasmine listened carefully as I explained all the ways that stress provoked her immune system, her inflammation, and her weight gain. She thought for a moment, then shook her head. "I don't know what to do about this, Dr. Myers. The problems I have cannot be fixed right away. So then it seems that my stress will continue."

On the contrary, I told her. She might not be able to make changes in the problems themselves, but there were two other things she could do: She could change the way she handled the problems, and she could find ways to let go of stress when a stressful circumstance was over. For example, Jasmine might feel stressed when she was talking with her son's teachers about his learning disabilities or when she was sitting in a meeting at work, trying to figure out how to handle departmental business on a limited budget. But her immune system, her weight, and her overall health would benefit if she could let that stress go as soon as she ended the conversation or left the meeting.

I went on to tell Jasmine about the situation that had given its name to the book *Why Zebras Don't Get Ulcers*—a situation that I personally had witnessed as well. Zebras don't get ulcers, Sapolsky writes, because they let go of stress as soon as the challenge that provoked it is over. They don't spend time or energy worrying about a lion catching them—they ran from the lion when the lion was there, and they focused on other things when the lion was gone.

I had seen exactly the same incident when I was on a safari in Africa. From the safety of our jeep, I could see a lion pouncing on a zebra that had wandered a few steps away from the herd. The zebra managed to evade the lion's grasp . . . and as soon as it had reached safety, it trotted along calmly with the other zebras. Most humans in the same situation would almost certainly have felt shaken and upset for at least a few hours after the life-threatening incident, and they would have been anxious and edgy for days afterward. "Wow, I almost got killed," a human would be thinking. "The lion could have ripped my arm off—that would have really hurt. What if the lion comes back? What if next time I'm slower and it actually does kill me? I hate thinking that a lion has that kind of power over me. But I'm just a

STRESS-RELIEVING STRATEGIES

Acupuncture

Art: either making it or looking at it

Breathe: It's physiologically impossible to be anxious when you are breathing deeply!

Conversations: Talk to the people you love. Even a brief conversation can bring those cortisol levels down!

Counseling: psychodynamic therapy, cognitive behavioral therapy, art or music therapy

Dance: Put on a favorite song and dance your stress away.

Exercise: but don't overdo it!

Eye movement desensitization and reprocessing (EMDR): a form a therapy that can help you let go of traumatic events or upsetting feelings

Hot tub, whirlpool, or Jacuzzi

Martial arts

Massage

Meditation or prayer

Music: Studies show that just half an hour's worth of listening can cause your cortisol levels to drop.

Nature: a long walk, a hike, or just time spent sitting in a natural setting

Passion: Make some time for whatever you're passionate about.

Pets

Play

Saunas

Sex

Shake it off: Literally shake your arm, leg, or head, and envision shaking off the worry or stress, especially after having an upsetting conversation or hearing a difficult piece of news.

Spiritual practice: time in a church, synagogue, mosque, zendo, or other spiritual center

Tai chi

Tapping: a practice that is an integral part of emotional freedom technique (EFT), a way of letting go of stressful thoughts or emotions

Tea: Take even five minutes to sit quietly with a fragrant cup of caffeine-free herbal tea, focusing on the smell, the warmth, and the taste.

Yoga

puny human. What can I do about it?" That's how you get chronic stress—and chronic inflammation—and autoimmune conditions.

A zebra doesn't have any of those thoughts. Its stress response is always acute, never chronic. When danger threatens, the zebra reacts. When danger does not threaten, the zebra is calm. So, I told Jasmine, we have to learn to be a little bit more like zebras.

Jasmine laughed at that image, but she saw my point. I went on to suggest some strategies that might be helpful both for letting go of stressful thoughts and for physically letting go of stress. If Jasmine could alleviate even a portion of her daily stress, releasing that stress throughout the day or at least at the end of the day, her immune system as well as her weight would benefit.

Just as animal studies have proven that stress biologically induces weight gain, studies have also proven that de-stressing strategies affect your biological stress response and, therefore, your immune system. For example, several scientific studies have shown that listening to music for half an hour lowers your cortisol levels. And a very intriguing recent study showed that meditation affected the expression of inflammatory genes.

Since we humans are *not* zebras, I told Jasmine, we have to work a bit at adopting a zebra-like approach to stress: living in the moment, not worrying about what might happen next or what we can't control. Yes, it takes a bit of practice. But it can be *so* worth it in the end.

DE-STRESSING YOUR DAY

De-stressing is a personal thing, and it requires you to make space to uncover how you best quiet your mind and relax your body. I always tell my patients that the single most important thing they can do is create time in the day—starting with fifteen minutes minimum. This window will expand over time, but it is essential that you actually start by stopping. That's right—stop doing and start being. It doesn't matter what it is you do, but when it is over, you will know it is de-stressing if you feel relaxed, energized, calmer, and happier. Some patients exercise, some meditate, some walk, some nap . . . find what works for you, and make sure you do it daily.

JASMINE'S TRIUMPH

Jasmine really took to heart the conversations we had about stress and its relationship to her immune system. She decided that she, her husband, and her son needed to see a family therapist to help them work through the challenges in her son's newly identified learning disabilities and the commuter relationship with her husband. "It is not easy talking about our problems with a stranger," she told me, "but I think, in the end, it helps."

Jasmine decided that she also needed more "me time." She found a tango dancing class offered at a local community center and began going once a week. Jasmine enjoyed the combination of exercise and self-expression so much that soon once a week turned into twice a week, with an occasional weekend afternoon.

Slowly but surely, Jasmine's efforts paid off. The fourth pillar was working. She lost the extra weight she had put on, looked better, and felt better. We were able to get her completely off her suppressive medication, and her thyroid worked just fine. Her antibodies even returned to normal. Finally, Jasmine felt energized, vital, and excited about her life, even though challenges remained both at home and at work.

I was especially pleased to see Jasmine completely recovered from Graves' disease, because I had suffered from the same condition and I knew how debilitating it could be. Conventional medical treatments are so harsh—often you have to either ablate your thyroid or have it surgically removed. I was so glad that I could spare Jasmine that fate. To me, her story is a testament to the power of stress relief—and the power of thinking like a zebra.

Part Three

Learn the Tools

CHAPTER 8

Putting The Myers Way into Practice

So HERE IS WHERE the rubber finally meets the road. Roughly 80 percent of the healing that happens in my clinic comes from following The Myers Way, the very same journey you are about to embark on yourself. I am excited for you, because I know that you are going to begin feeling much better very soon.

By the end of the first week you should be feeling energized, focused, and clear. Your mood will likely improve as your ability to concentrate expands. Your skin will begin to glow. (No kidding—that's what happens when you ease the inflammation that has been plaguing your system.) Based on what many patients have told me, your sex life might even improve.

This thirty-day protocol is "science in a box"—a simple, step-by-step program that can be easily followed by anyone and yet embodies all the brilliance and complexity of a functional medicine view of the human body. By the way, you don't have to do this program alone. You can do it with a partner, with a support group of friends who also want to get healthier, or with your entire family. Your friends and family might like to know that I have seen this program dramatically help people with migraines, fatigue, irritable bowel syndrome, constipation, and skin issues, as well as anxiety, depression, brain fog, and simple fatigue. When you consider how many people are on the auto-immune spectrum without even realizing it—suffering from symptoms and disorders triggered by inflammation—you can imagine how help-ful this anti-inflammatory protocol will be to virtually everyone.

So let's get started. In this chapter, I take you through the basic principles, helping you along every step of the way. In chapter 9, I provide you with a thirty-day meal plan and recipes that will give you a terrific boost for your first month.

THE BASIC PRINCIPLES

The Myers Way is based on one simple idea: Food is medicine. If you eat the foods that your body craves and avoid the foods that are not suited to your body, you can achieve the vibrant, energetic state of health that is your birthright.

Basically, the foods you will avoid are either toxic or inflammatory. Everyone should avoid toxic foods and minimize their exposure to inflammatory foods. People with autoimmune conditions or who are on the autoimmune spectrum need to go to extra lengths to avoid inflammatory foods that might intensify their symptoms, provoke an autoimmune condition, or perhaps even stimulate a second autoim-mune condition. Remember, if you are on the autoimmune spectrum (pages 22–25), you are at risk of developing an autoimmune condition. And if you have an autoimmune condition, you are three times more likely to develop another.

The foods you will eat are healing and nutrient-dense. The proteins will supply you with the amino acids you need to support your immune system, among other functions. The fats will help heal the cells of your gut wall, providing further immune support. And the complex carbohydrates, fruits, and vegetables will provide the fiber you need to support the friendly bacteria that inhabit your gut and the rest of your body—bacteria that are absolutely crucial to a healthy immune system.

The Myers Way also incorporates nutritional supplements to pro-mote gut healing, immune support, and a good balance of friendly bacteria. Many are also anti-inflammatory. Since lifting your toxic burden is one of the pillars of The Myers Way, the supplements will also help your cells detoxify; in fact, they are a crucial part of that process.

You may be wondering why, if your diet will be so healthy and nutritious, you also need supplements. In an ideal world, of course, you would be able to rely on food alone for all the healing support you need. But our food system is compromised by over-farming and genetically modified crops, so the foods we eat are lacking the nutrition they used to provide. As we have discussed, our environment is filled with untested chemicals, unfiltered water, contaminated foods, and polluted air, so we are exposed to more toxins than ever before. We need supplements to compensate for that environmental damage.

In addition, most of us lead high-stress lives with far too little space for restoration, relaxation, familial nurturing, and community support. We need more nutrients than if we lived healthier, more balanced lives.

Remember, as you saw in chapter 6, some of us have mutations of three key genes: *MTHFR, GSTM1,* and *COMT* (pages 145–46). If you do, you need special detox support. Because of the way your body works, you will never get everything you need from your diet, and you'll have to take supplements to compensate. We are not cookie-cutter people. Each of us is genetically unique, and each of us is coping with his or her own particular degree of stress at the moment. We need different types of supplements to respond to both our genes and our environment.

IF YOU'RE PREGNANT OR POSTPARTUM

A lot of autoimmune diseases actually can be set off by pregnancy or giving birth. And if you have a sensitivity to gluten or dairy, you can pass those antibodies on to your baby, either through the placenta while you are pregnant or through your breast milk while you are breast-feeding. I've seen children who have never themselves ingested gluten but who picked up antibodies to gluten from their mom.

So if you're pregnant or postpartum, please don't give in to your cravings for wheat or dairy. And if you want to *start* The Myers Way while you are pregnant or breast-feeding, it's not only safe, it's probably the healthiest choice you could make for yourself and your child. (If you are pregnant or breast-feeding, please consult your physician.)

And don't be misled by USDA minimum daily requirements. They really are just what they sound like: *minimum*. The USDA daily minimum recommendation for vitamin C, for example, is based on what you need to prevent the disease of scurvy, not what is ideal for optimal health.

Finally, if you have an autoimmune condition or are on the autoimmune spectrum, your system is already in distress, fighting the pressures of inflammation and struggling to overcome the damage wrought by leaky gut. Supplements can quickly help bring that inflammation down, heal your leaky gut, and provide your immune system with the extra support it needs to reverse course and head back down the autoimmune spectrum toward a more balanced, healthier state. Once your symptoms resolve, we will begin to reduce some of the supplements.

HOW TO FOLLOW THIS PROGRAM

Look, we all want to keep things simple. So I've made following The Myers Way as simple for you as possible. Basically, all you have to do is follow the instructions in chapter 9. There, I tell you exactly what to eat and which supplements to take for every day of the monthlong program. Here's what you'll find:

- a thirty-day meal plan and all the recipes you need

- a seven-day seafood plan that shows you how to do a modified version of The Myers Way without red meat or poultry

- tests to see whether you are likely to have yeast overgrowth, SIBO, or parasites, and instructions that you may need to make modifications you'll be making to your diet and supplements if you have any of these conditions

With brilliant registered dietitian Brianne Williams, R.D., L.D., who works side by side with me at my functional medicine clinic in Austin, we have even organized the thirty days to be as nutritious, delicious, and user friendly as possible.

But if you're anything like me, you'll do better following the plan if you understand how it works and why it benefits you. So in this

AN IMPORTANT WORD ABOUT MEDICATIONS

To the extent you can, avoid all nonessential medications during your thirty days on The Myers Way, because they can make it harder for your liver to detoxify your body and can in some cases create new problems, as you saw with acid blockers and antibiotics in chapter 4.

However, *do not stop your essential medications* (any medications for the heart, diabetes, blood pressure, thyroid, hormones; antianxiety medications; antidepressants; etc.) without consulting your primary-care practitioner first. Even if our goal is to get you completely off your medications, you *must not stop taking any prescription medication* without the supervision of your health-care provider.

You do want to more frequently monitor your blood pressure and blood sugar levels, especially if you are treating yourself for yeast overgrowth. I find that most patients are able to reduce the medications they are taking for high blood pressure and high blood sugar while they are following The Myers Way.

Ideally, you will take only the supplements suggested for you on The Myers Way, but if a primary-care physician or practitioner has prescribed or recommended supplements, again, check with that person before discontinuing anything.

chapter I'm going to explain exactly which foods to eat, which to avoid, which supplements to take, and what they'll do for you. This information is embodied in the thirty-day program, so you don't really need to remember it. But when you continue on the next month, devising your own meal plans and perhaps enjoying a few restaurant meals, you'll be glad to know which foods to enjoy and which to avoid.

I'll also help you figure out how to set up your kitchen: which foods to toss and which to stock up on. I'm a working woman myself, so I get it. Life is rushed, there's never enough time, and why cook when you can pick up something on the way home? But there are ways to make The Myers Way work for you, and I'm here to help you, every step of the way.

After I help you learn what to eat and drink, I'll tell you the kinds of exercise that will best support your immune system and offer you some suggestions for lightening your stress burden. Finally, I'll help you figure out how to evaluate your results on The Myers Way so you can decide whether it will be possible for you to add in some of the foods you're avoiding now, and if so, which ones.

GETTING READY

Before you begin The Myers Way, prepare your family, kitchen, mind, body, and schedule. This is an opportunity for an incredibly healing and energizing experience that will be enhanced with the proper planning and preparation. The changes you will be making to your diet may not always seem easy—eating habits are deeply ingrained, after all—but they can be simple.

So begin by stocking your kitchen with those foods to enjoy.

FOODS TO ENJOY

Quality Proteins

- Organic, grass-fed beef
- Organic, grass-fed lamb
- Organic, grass-fed pork
- Organic, pasture-raised poultry (chicken, duck, turkey)
- Water-packed fish (sardines)
- Wild-caught fresh fish (cod, halibut, Pacific salmon, pollack, sole, trout)
- Wild game

Organic Vegetables

- Artichokes
- Asparagus
- Bamboo shoots
- Beets
- Bok choy
- Broccoflower
- Broccoli
- Broccolini
- Brussels sprouts
- Cabbage
- Carrots
- Cauliflower
- Celery
- Chives
- Cucumbers
- Kale
- Leeks
- Lettuce
- Mushrooms
- Okra
- Olives (canned in water)
- Onions
- Parsnips
- Sea veggies (seaweed, kelp)

- Spinach (all leafy greens)
- Squash (acorn, butternut, spaghetti, kabocha)
- Sweet potatoes
- Turnips
- Yellow squash
- Zucchini

Healthy Fats

- Avocado
- Avocado oil
- Coconut oil
- Grapeseed oil
- Olive oil
- Safflower oil

Organic Fruits

- Apples
- Applesauce (unsweetened)
- Apricots
- Avocados
- Bananas
- Blackberries
- Blueberries
- Cherries
- Coconut
- Cranberries
- Figs
- Grapefruits
- Grapes
- Kiwis
- Kumquats
- Lemons
- Limes
- Mangos
- Melons
- Nectarines
- Oranges
- Peaches
- Pears
- Raspberries
- Strawberries
- Tangerines

Flavorful Seasonings

Special note: Please avoid seasonings labeled just "spices." They could contain anything, including gluten.

- Apple cider vinegar
- Basil
- Bay leaf
- Black pepper
- Cacao (100%)
- Cardamom
- Carob
- Cilantro
- Cinnamon
- Clove
- Cumin
- Dandelion
- Dill
- Fennel seed
- Garlic
- Ginger
- Mustard
- Nutmeg
- Oregano
- Parsley
- Rosemary
- Sea salt
- Tarragon
- Thyme
- Turmeric

Refreshing Beverages

- Homemade fruit and vegetable juices
- Teas (caffeine-free herbal tea; organic green tea in moderate amounts, if needed)
- Water (filtered water, mineral water, seltzer)

So get the following foods out of your kitchen and prepare to let them go. If you can't stand the idea of letting them go for life, make a deal with yourself that you'll reevaluate after thirty days on The Myers Way. Once you see your symptoms disappear, your energy increase, and your health return, I'm betting you'll be motivated to continue.

TOXIC FOODS TO TOSS

- Alcohol

- Fast foods, junk foods, processed foods

- Food additives: any foods that contain artificial colors, flavors, or preservatives

- Genetically modified foods (GMOs), including canola oil and beet sugar

- Processed meats: canned meats (such as SPAM; canned fish is okay), cold cuts, hot dogs; sausage is okay, but make sure it's gluten-free

- Processed and refined oils: mayonnaise, salad dressings, shortening, spreads

- Refined oils, hydrogenated fats, trans fats, including margarine

- Stimulants and caffeine: chocolate, coffee, decongestants, yerba maté

- Sweeteners: sugar, sugar alcohols, natural sweeteners (such as honey, agave, maple syrup, molasses, and coconut palm sugar), sweetened juices, high-fructose corn syrup; stevia in moderation is okay

- Trans fats and hydrogenated oils, which are frequently found in packaged and processed foods

CONDIMENTS AND SPICES TO TOSS

- Barbecue sauce
- Cayenne pepper (black pepper is okay)
- Chocolate (100 percent cacao is approved)
- Ketchup
- Paprika
- Red pepper flakes
- Relish
- Soy sauce
- Tamari
- Teriyaki sauce

INFLAMMATORY FOODS TO TOSS

- Corn and anything made from corn (corn flour, cornmeal, grits) or containing high-fructose corn syrup
- Dairy: butter, casein, cheese, cottage cheese, cream, frozen yogurt, ghee, goat cheese, ice cream, milk, nondairy creamer, whey protein, yogurt
- Eggs
- Gluten: anything that contains barley, rye, or wheat
- Gluten-free grains and pseudo-grains: amaranth, millet, oats, quinoa, rice
- Legumes: beans, garbanzos, lentils, peas (dried and fresh), snow peas
- Nightshades: eggplant, peppers, potatoes, tomatoes; sweet potatoes are okay
- Nuts, including nut butters
- Peanuts
- Seeds, including seed butters
- Soy
- Sweetened fruit juices

CRAVING CARBS?

To satisfy those starchy cravings, enjoy sweet potatoes, acorn squash, summer squash, spaghetti squash, pumpkin, and (mashed or riced) cauliflower.

LETTING GO OF CAFFEINE

If you typically consume two or more cups of caffeinated beverages (such as coffee, tea, energy drinks, soda) and/or caffeinated treats (such as chocolate), your body is likely used to relying on caffeine as a stimulant for artificial energy. This is a very powerful habit that is difficult to break. You are not alone! I will show you how to get real and sustained energy from wholesome and nutrient-dense foods.

Meanwhile, if you're concerned about withdrawal symptoms, you might want to start the program on a weekend. That will give you some time to relax and allow your body to adjust. It is normal to feel tired since your body has been relying on caffeine.

Because coffee is so acidic, I'd like you to avoid it for your thirty-day program—yes, even decaf. Choose alkaline herbal teas such as ginger or decaffeinated green tea.

So take a deep breath and put down the coffee cup. You have two choices:

Cold Turkey

Begin the first day of The Myers Way, and be prepared for some uncomfortable withdrawal symptoms, including headaches and fatigue, especially if you are used to drinking two or more caffeinated drinks a day.

Gradual Withdrawal

Or start gradually reducing your intake the week before your program begins, which can help you minimize withdrawal symptoms.

Five-day reduction
- Day 1: 2 cups caffeinated beverage
- Day 2: 1 cup caffeinated beverage
- Day 3: ½ cup caffeinated beverage
- Day 4: ¼ cup caffeinated beverage
- Day 5: 100 percent caffeine-free

Three-day reduction
- Day 1: 1 cup 50 percent decaf and 50 percent caffeinated
- Day 2: 100 percent decaf
- Day 3: No coffee at all, either caffeinated or decaf

Tea replacement
- Replace 1 cup coffee or tea with green tea for a week

CRAVING DAIRY?

Full-fat coconut milk makes a fabulous substitute if you're looking for a creamy texture or flavor in your herbal tea.

LETTING GO OF SUGAR

Can I make a confession? This was a tough one for me. I've always liked sweets, and I found letting go of sugar to be one of the harder parts of this program. Though when you have achieved the results you want, you might occasionally be able to indulge in small amounts of sugar.

At least for the first thirty days of The Myers Way, it's crucial that you completely rid your body of sugar to give the program a chance to work. Almost certainly the more upsetting you find it to let go of sugar, the more important it is for you to do so. You might be relying on sweets for your energy, but the problem with that is you get a false, temporary burst of energy—and then you crash. And then you need to load up on sugar again to overcome the effects of the crash, and there you are, on a glucose roller coaster, with every crash sending you rushing for a soda, cookie, or piece of candy. Sugar feeds yeast overgrowth and SIBO as you saw in chapter 4. Sugar and sweeteners also suppress your immune system, as you saw in chapter 3, and stress your adrenals, contributing to the adrenal fatigue you read about in chapter 7.

What I want you to do—before you ever go back to sugar—is feel the kind of energy you get from real, whole-food sources. I can say this, a few days after you stop eating sweets, your sugar cravings should disappear. So toss out sweets cold turkey on Day 1 of The Myers Way, and if you can, get all the following foods completely out of your house:

- Agave nectar
- Artificial sweeteners (includes aspartame, saccharin, sucralose)
- Beet sugar
- Brown rice syrup
- Brown sugar
- Cane sugar

- Coconut palm sugar
- Corn syrup
- Dehydrated cane juice
- Dextrose
- Glucose
- High-fructose corn syrup
- Honey
- Lactose
- Maltose
- Maple syrup
- Molasses
- Refined (white) sugar
- Sucrose
- Sugar alcohols (includes maltitol, mannitol, sorbitol, xylitol)

If you're looking for some added sweetness, fruits and berries are good options. A little coconut butter can be used to sweeten your caffeine-free herbal tea. Your taste buds will adapt as you cut out added and artificial sweeteners, and you'll be amazed at how much sweeter an apple or a strawberry will taste.

We do have a few recipes with a small amount of stevia, a plant native to Paraguay whose leaves are three hundred times sweeter than sugar. I actually grew this with farmers in Paraguay during my time in the Peace Corps and helped them export it to Japan and the United States.

By the way, all beet sugar has been made from genetically modified plants, so please avoid it.

SKIP THE SALT . . . UNLESS IT'S SEA SALT

Research indicates a link between a diet high in salt and autoimmune disorders. In one study, mice fed a high-salt diet developed an increased number of inflammatory T cells, which led to autoimmunity.

This research was conducted with table salt and packaged food—and of course we already know that packaged and processed foods contribute to inflammation and possibly autoimmunity. However, sea salt is full of essential trace elements, and based on my clinical observation of patients and my understanding of the importance of these trace elements, I believe its benefits—when consumed in small amounts—outweigh the risks. During The Myers Way, therefore, you will be consuming some sea salt.

EMBRACING THE PROMISE OF THE MYERS WAY

These simple, clean foods aren't just "good for you" and full of nutrients; they offer you rich, interesting flavors, a wide variety of textures, and a rainbow of colors, which will satisfy all your senses when you sit down to eat. Your body will spring to life as it finally gets the nourishment it craves in a form that actually suits it, and your immune system will breathe a sigh of relief as the burden of toxic and inflammatory food is lifted. You'll find this approach to food a source of abundance and pleasure, as well as health and vitality—as long as you give yourself time to get used to this new way of eating and to let go of the cravings, addictions, spikes, and crashes that might have been part of your earlier diet.

KNOWING WHAT TO EXPECT

Depending on how many toxic and inflammatory foods your diet included before beginning The Myers Way, you might experience some of the symptoms listed on the next page during the first two or three days of your thirty-day program.

Some of the symptoms are the result of withdrawal. If you're used to consuming lots of sweet or starchy foods, drinking lots of caffeinated beverages, and otherwise loading up on "quick-fix" foods, you might feel a drop in energy and focus when you pull those unhealthy but stimulating foods out of your diet. Your symptoms could also result from the hunger pangs of yeast overgrowth and the bacteria you are starving out.

Likewise, if you have developed a lot of food sensitivities, you might feel some withdrawal as you stop eating those unhealthy but attractive foods. In addition, if you suffer from yeast overgrowth, the yeast cause you to crave sugar, and you might have to struggle a bit to resist. Luckily, the Yeast Overgrowth / SIBO Dietary Protocol on pages 195–96 is there to support you while on The Myers Way, so take the tests and find out if you need that extra boost.

The other reason you might notice some symptoms is because you are detoxing—cleansing the poisons from your system. While purging

**Some possible symptoms you may experience
during your first few days:**

- bad breath
- body aches
- body odor
- brain fog
- changes in bowel movements
- changes in mood
- changes in sleep
- cravings
- fatigue
- headaches
- hunger
- joint pain
- rash

Within a week, you might notice:

- improved concentration, mental focus, clarity
- improved digestion
- improved mood
- improved sleep
- increased energy
- less fluid retention
- less joint and muscle pain
- regular bowel movements
- resolutions of skin issues (acne, eczema, rashes)
- weight loss

yourself of toxins will ultimately make you feel much better, these toxins can cause symptoms on their way out. If you can, view the symptoms as signs that your body is letting go of toxic and inflammatory foods, and look forward to a burst of healthy energy coming soon.

Happily, within a week on The Myers Way, you are likely to start feeling better—maybe even better than you have felt in a long time. And by the end of the thirty days, you should notice significant improvement in gut health, energy, mood, brain function, and even appearance, with clearer skin, healthier hair, and perhaps even some weight loss. You'll sleep better, you'll find pain relief if you need it, and you'll feel the relief as well of your inflammation being soothed and your system returning to balance.

Meanwhile, you might find it helpful to start on a weekend or during time off so you can get in a little extra rest if you have trouble adjusting. Also, stay hydrated. Drinking six to eight glasses of filtered water each day can help relieve your withdrawal headaches and flush the toxins being released into your system.

EXERCISE

Moving your body is always important, so I want you out in the world, talking walks, snowshoeing, skiing, hiking, running. Or, if you prefer, go to a gym, a dance studio, or a yoga studio and get moving there.

Now, I don't want you to overdo it. I'd like you to exercise, but if you were relatively sedentary before you began The Myers Way, start slowly and build up your strength gradually. Remember, too, that cleansing and detoxifying can cause you to feel sluggish and tired at first, so give your body a break if that is what it's asking for.

You should also keep in mind your score on the Adrenal Fatigue Test on pages 167–68. Your adrenal glands are the organs that produce stress hormones, support your energy levels, and keep you going even when you're tired. Some exercise is good for adrenal and autoimmune conditions, but if you overdo it, you can really set back your healing. You should exercise to the point that you feel good and energized afterward and also the next day. If you feel exhausted or worse after exercise, you are doing too much. And if your symptoms get worse, decrease your exercise or stop it altogether.

For example, if you feel some joint pain after walking two miles, and the next day you are exhausted, cut back. Try just one mile and see what happens. If that feels good, that's what you should aim for. If you're still in pain and feeling fatigued, drop down to half a mile. Feeling good should be your guide.

The following are some recommended activities to keep your body moving during The Myers Way.

Low Energy

Dancing	Playing with	Stretching
Household cleaning	your kids	Swimming
Pilates	Restorative yoga	Walking

High Energy

Biking	Running	Weight lifting
Hot yoga	Swimming	
Interval training	Tennis	

SLEEP

Sleep is when your body heals, and if you have an autoimmune condition, sleep is even more important for your rest and recovery. While on The Myers Way, give yourself the best possible shot at rejuvenating your energy and healing your symptoms: Get seven and a half to nine hours of deep, refreshing sleep each night—or even more if you need it. Cutting out the caffeine, sugar, and high-fat foods should help, and so should some gentle exercise.

If you have trouble sleeping, I've also included appendix F to give you a start in solving any sleep problems that might be getting in your way. Food and sleep are your medicines; don't skimp on either one.

DE-STRESSING

Hey, I get it. You're busy, your life is full of pressing obligations, you have loved ones who need you, and now you're trying this whole new way of cooking, eating, and thinking about food. Of *course* you're stressed. Who wouldn't be?

Somewhere in your busy day, though, if you can find just fifteen minutes to sit and breathe or meditate . . . if you can find time in your week for just one yoga class, one acupuncture session, or one massage . . . if you can get creative about trading child care with a neighbor or a relative and give yourself some time off every couple of weeks . . . if you and your significant other can plan a relaxing date night even once a month, you'll be amazed at the health benefits that can result. We talked about stress relief in chapter 7, and I have some suggestions in "Resources" also, so do yourself and your body a favor and find some time for stress relief. I promise you'll be way more efficient when you do go back to work or to your family obligations— and your immune system will reward you a hundredfold.

MOVING FORWARD

If you want to take it one step further, you can join our website community, along with hundreds of others who have already completed

The Myers Way. We have a very active, supportive community where you can ask questions, share suggestions, and maybe even come up with some new recipes! If you're looking for more personalized counseling, you can also set up a phone call through my website with one of my registered dietitians.

CHAPTER 9

Your Thirty-Day Protocol

Meal Plans and Recipes

I RECOMMEND STARTING on a day when you have some extra time to get a few basic recipes made so you can enjoy the first week. I've assumed that you're doing your meal prep on weekends and will be more crunched for time during the week, but obviously, adjust the plan to fit your own schedule.

The recipes and meal plans are two servings per meal to accommodate two people—and the servings are rather large. Please adjust as needed for your own situation. Throughout the meal plans you'll see instructions for how to save and use leftovers, so all you have to do is follow the instructions, day by day.

Be flexible, though. Every person and family is different; you might run out of food more or less quickly than outlined. If you love any of the recipes and want to eat them more frequently on the meal plan or want to personalize any of the recipes to better suit your tastes, feel free to do so as long as you don't include any of the toxic or inflammatory foods on pages 182–83. The main focus to remember here is to avoid the foods I have asked you to cut out. Finally, for those of you who want to create your own meals, you can use the "Create Your Own Meal" alternative on page 263.

Before you plunge into the meal plans, take a moment to go through the tests for yeast overgrowth, small intestine bacterial overgrowth (SIBO), and parasites. If you test positive for yeast overgrowth or SIBO, you will need to follow the protocol and adjust your meal plan accordingly. Following the tests is a supplements chart that tells you which supplements to take each day and how to customize them based on those three conditions, as well as on the results of your Adrenal Fatigue Test (pages 167–68). We're all individuals with different needs, so I'm happy to share this personalized approach with you.

And now your thirty days of healing begins. Enjoy.

DO I HAVE YEAST OVERGROWTH, SIBO, OR PARASITES?

Take each test and adjust your dietary protocol as needed. Then see pages 197–200 for a chart that will help you customize your supplements.

YEAST OVERGROWTH

_____ I have an autoimmune disease, such as Hashimoto's thyroiditis, rheumatoid arthritis, ulcerative colitis, lupus, psoriasis, scleroderma, or multiple sclerosis.

_____ I have skin or nail fungal infections, such as athlete's foot, ringworm, or toenail fungus.

_____ I suffer from chronic fatigue or fibromyalgia, or I am tired all the time.

_____ I have digestive issues, such as bloating, constipation, or diarrhea.

_____ I have difficulty concentrating, poor memory, lack of focus, ADD, ADHD, or brain fog.

_____ I have skin issues, such as eczema, psoriasis, hives, rosacea, or an unexplained rash.

_____ I am easily irritated and/or have frequent mood swings, anxiety, or depression.

_____ I get vaginal yeast infections, have rectal itching, or have vaginal itching.

_____ I suffer from seasonal allergies or itchy ears.

_____ I have sugar and refined carbohydrate cravings.

If you checked three or more items above, you have tested positive for yeast overgrowth. I recommend you follow the Yeast Overgrowth / SIBO Dietary Protocol that follows.

SMALL INTESTINE BACTERIAL OVERGROWTH (SIBO)

_____ I have been diagnosed with irritable bowel syndrome or inflammatory bowel disease.

_____ I get bloated after meals or feel bloated a lot of the time.

_____ I have gas, abdominal pain, or cramping.

_____ I have odorous, loose stools.

_____ I have food intolerances, such as gluten, dairy, soy, or corn.

_____ I have histamine intolerance.

_____ My joints ache.

_____ I feel tired all the time.

_____ I have skin issues, such as eczema, psoriasis, hives, rosacea, or an unexplained rash.

_____ I have asthma or other respiratory problems.

_____ I feel depressed and hopeless.

_____ I have been diagnosed with a B12 deficiency.

If you checked three or more items above, you have tested positive for SIBO. I recommend you follow the Yeast Overgrowth / SIBO Dietary Protocol below.

YEAST OVERGROWTH / SIBO DIETARY PROTOCOL

You will be treating your yeast overgrowth and/or SIBO by taking specific supplements, which are indicated in the chart on pages 197–

200, as well as by starving the yeast and bacteria of the sweet and starchy foods they crave. Accordingly, you will need to be conscious of reducing your carbohydrate intake as you follow The Myers Way over the next thirty days. I recommend no more than two cups of starchy vegetables (such as sweet potatoes, butternut squash, acorn squash, spaghetti squash) and no more than one cup of fruit a day. You will also want to eliminate all vinegars other than apple cider vinegar. But don't worry. We took that into account when creating the meal plans. As long as you follow the meal plans and recipes, you should be fine; just keep these guidelines in mind when you eat out or dine at someone else's home.

PARASITES

_____ I have constipation, diarrhea, or gas.

_____ I have traveled internationally.

_____ I remember getting "traveler's diarrhea" while outside the country.

_____ I have had what I believe was food poisoning and my digestion has not been the same since.

_____ I have trouble falling asleep and I wake up multiple times during the night.

_____ I have skin issues, such as eczema, psoriasis, hives, rosacea, or an unexplained rash.

_____ I grind my teeth in my sleep.

_____ I have pain or aching in my muscles or joints.

_____ I feel exhausted, depressed, or apathetic almost all the time.

_____ I never feel satisfied after I eat.

_____ I have iron-deficiency anemia.

_____ I have been diagnosed with irritable bowel syndrome, ulcerative colitis, or Crohn's disease.

If you checked three or more items, you would benefit from taking the supplements recommended for parasites in the following chart.

THE MYERS WAY AUTOIMMUNE PROGRAM SUPPLEMENTS

For Everyone

Supplement	Supplement Used in My Clinic	Recommended Company	How to Take	Alternatives
Probiotic*	Complete Probiotic Capsules or Powder OR Prescript-Assist Broad Spectrum Probiotic	**Klaire/ProThera** (Ther-Biotic Complete) OR **Prescript-Assist**	1 capsule twice daily or ¼ teaspoon daily OR 1 capsule twice daily	50+ billion IU, 10+ strains of probiotic (avoid probiotics that are grown on any avoided foods such as soy, dairy, wheat) daily OR 1240 mg soil-based probiotic blend daily
Omega 3 Fish Oil	Complete Omega 3 Capsules	**Metagenics** (OmegaGenics EPA-DHA 500)	1–4 capsules twice daily	1000–4000 mg omega 3 (EPA and DHA) daily
L-Glutamine OR Gut Repair Powder	L-Glutamine OR GI Repair Powder	**Designs for Health** OR **Xymogen** (GlutAloeMine)	4 capsules daily OR 1 scoop daily	3000 mg L-glutamine daily OR Blend of L-glutamine, deglycyrrihizinated licorice, and aloe vera
Acetyl-Glutathione OR N-Acetyl-Cysteine + Vitamin C + Liver Support Supplement	Glutathione OR N-Acetyl-Cysteine + Complete Vitamin C + Liver Support	**CitriSafe** OR **Designs for Health** **Xymogen** **Klaire/ProThera** (HepatoThera Forte)	1–2 capsules in the morning and the afternoon OR 1 capsule twice daily on empty stomach 2 capsules twice daily 1 capsule twice daily on empty stomach	600–1200 mg acetyl-glutathione daily OR 1800 mg N-acetyl-cysteine daily 2000 mg vitamin C daily Liver support blend including: alpha-lipoic acid and milk thistle
Vitamin D3	Vitamin D 1000 IU Drops	**Pure Encapsulations**	2 drops under the tongue per day	2000 IU vitamin D daily

Depending on your checklist results or where you perceive your issues lie after reading through the book, you may choose to take some of the supplements that follow.

Supplement	Supplement Used in My Clinic	Recommended Company	How to Take	Alternatives
Inflammation/Immune Support				
Curcumin Phytosome	Meriva-SR Curcumin	**Thorne Research**	2 capsules twice daily	1000 mg curcumin daily
Resveratrol	CitriSafe Resveratrol	**CitriSafe**	Dissolve 1 under tongue twice daily	50 mg resveratrol daily
Acetyl-Glutathione OR N-Acetyl-Cysteine + Vitamin C + Liver Support Supplement	Glutathione OR N-Acetyl-Cysteine + Complete Vitamin C + Liver Support	**CitriSafe** OR **Designs for Health** **Xymogen** **Klaire/ProThera** (HepatoThera Forte)	1–2 capsules in the morning and the afternoon OR 1 capsule twice daily on empty stomach 2 capsules twice daily 1 capsule twice daily on empty stomach	600–1200 mg acetyl-glutathione daily OR 1800 mg N-acetyl-cysteine daily 2000 mg vitamin C daily Liver support blend including: alpha-lipoic acid and milk thistle
Gut Health				
Probiotic*	Complete Probiotic Capsules or Powder OR Prescript-Assist Broad Spectrum Probiotict	**Klaire/ProThera** (Ther-Biotic Complete) OR **Prescript Assist**	1 capsule twice daily or ¼ teaspoon daily OR 1 capsule twice daily	50+ billion IU, 10+ strains of probiotic (avoid probiotics that are grown on any avoided foods such as soy, dairy, wheat) daily OR 1240 mg soil-based probiotic blend daily
L-Glutamine OR Gut Repair Powder	L-Glutamine OR GI Repair Powder	**Designs for Health** OR **Xymogen** (GlutAloeMine)	4 capsules daily OR 1 scoop daily	3000 mg L-glutamine daily OR Blend of L-glutamine, deglycyrrihizinated licorice, and aloe vera
Collagen	Great Lakes Collagen Hydrolysate	**Great Lakes Gelatin**	1–2 tablespoons twice daily	Grass-fed beef collagen
Digestive Enzymes	Complete Enzyme capsules**/ chewables	**Klaire/ProThera** (Vital-Zymes Complete/ Chewable)	2 capsules/chewables with each meal	800 mg of a broad spectrum enzyme blend including: amylase, protease, and lipase with every meal
Betaine Hydrochloride with pepsin	Betaine HCL & Pepsin	**Thorne**	1–2 capsules with meals—discontinue if you feel minimal heartburn, indigestion, or warmth in your stomach or chest	500–1300 mg betaine hydrochloride with pepsin with each meal

Supplement	Supplement Used in My Clinic	Recommended Company	How to Take	Alternatives
Detoxification Support				
Acetyl-Glutathione OR N-Acetyl-Cysteine + Vitamin C + Liver Support Supplement	Glutathione OR N-Acetyl-Cysteine + Complete Vitamin C + Liver Support	**CitriSafe** OR **Designs for Health** **Xymogen** **Klaire/ProThera** (HepatoThera Forte)	1–2 capsules in the morning and the afternoon OR 1 capsule twice daily on empty stomach 2 capsules twice daily 1 capsule twice daily on empty stomach	600–1200 mg acetyl-glutathione daily OR 1800 mg N-acetyl-cysteine daily 2000 mg vitamin C daily Liver support blend including: alpha-lipoic acid and milk thistle
Infections (EBV, Herpes, etc.)				
L-Lysine	Lysine	**Designs for Health** (L-Lysine)	1 capsule a day to prevent outbreak—if you are having an outbreak, you can take 1 capsule three times a day	750–2250 mg L-lysine daily
Lauricidin	Lauricidin	**Lauricidin** (Monolaurin Supplement)	Start with ¼ teaspoon two to three times a day with food, and slowly work up to 1 teaspoon two to three times a day with food	
Humic Acid	Humic Acid	**Allergy Research Group**	Start with 1 capsule twice daily and work up to 2 capsules twice daily	750–1500 mg humic acid daily
Yeast Overgrowth				
Caprylic Acid	Caprylic Acid	**Pure Encapsulations**	2 capsules twice daily on an empty stomach	1600 mg caprylic acid daily
Candisol	Candisol	**Bairn Biologics**	2 capsules twice daily on an empty stomach	
SIBO				
Herbal supplement*	MicrobClear	**Designs for Health** (GI Microb-X)	1 capsule twice daily	Herbal formula including at least four of the following: Tribulus Extract, Wormwood Extract, Berberine Sulfate, Grapefruit Extract, Barberry Extract, Bearberry Extract, Black Walnut Extract

Supplement	Supplement Used in My Clinic	Recommended Company	How to Take	Alternatives
Parasite				
Herbal Supplement*	Microb-Clear	**Designs for Health** (GI Microb-X)	1 capsule twice daily	Herbal formula including at least four of the following: Tribulus Extract, Wormwood Extract, Berberine Sulfate, Grapefruit Extract, Barberry Extract, Bearberry Extract, Black Walnut Extract
Adrenal Support				
Adaptogenic herbal blend	AdrenoMend	**Douglas Laboratories**	2 capsules daily with food for 1 to 2 weeks, then increase to 4 capsules each day with food for 2 to 4 months	Herbal formula including at least five of the following: Schisandra chinensis, Bacopa monnieri, Rhodiola rosea, Eleutherococcus senticosus, Magnolia officinalis, Rehmannia glutinosa, Panax ginseng, Coleus forskohlii

*Take probiotics at least 2 hours away from herbal supplement for parasite/SIBO.

**The Complete Enzyme capsules contain an ingredient derived from egg white. Individuals with known egg-white allergy should consult their physician before using this product.

THE THIRTY-DAY MEAL PLAN

Remember that this meal plan is based on the idea that you will be cooking for two people, so each meal accounts for two servings to be enjoyed. Feel free to adjust to fit your family's needs. If you are cooking for one, simply cut in half the number of servings you are instructed to make. That still leaves you plenty of leftovers. I've listed the recipe titles in boldface on the days you need to cook them and without boldface when you are enjoying leftovers. If you would like a detailed plan walking you through exactly how many servings to make, when to prep recipes, and when to enjoy leftovers, you can find a chart on pages 267–77. This will allow for your thirty days to run as smoothly and deliciously as possible.

Prep Day

The day before you begin the meal plan, make the following recipes to enjoy throughout the first week. This day is crucial: Prepping before you begin will really help you start off the program smoothly. If you have a typical workweek, I recommend prepping on a Saturday and beginning the program on a Sunday when you still have some extra time for cooking. After you prep, enjoy some Lemon Garlic Oven-Roasted Chicken (page 247) to get a sneak peak before you begin!

> **Lemon Garlic Oven-Roasted Chicken** (page 247)
> **Gut Healing Broth** (page 226)
> **Sweet Apple Breakfast Sausage** (pages 256–57)

Day 1

Breakfast
> **Sweet Apple Breakfast Sausage** (pages 256–57)
> **Hearty Sweet Potato Hash** (page 217)
> **Spring Green Veggie Juice** (page 259)
> **Chai Tea Latte** (page 259) or decaf green tea, if desired

Lunch
> **Organic Citrus Kale Salad with Cranberries** (page 231)
> **Organic Farm Five-Veggie Soup** (page 229)

Dinner
Creamy Basil Pesto Sauce over Spaghetti Squash (page 254)
Enjoy ½ cup organic mixed berries, such as raspberries,
 strawberries, blueberries, or blackberries

Day 2

Breakfast
Sweet Apple Breakfast Sausage
Hearty Sweet Potato Hash
Reheat and sip on Gut Healing Broth
Chai Tea Latte (page 259) or decaf green tea, if desired

Lunch
Creamy Basil Pesto Sauce over Spaghetti Squash

Dinner
Roasted Wild-Caught Salmon with Tangy Mango Salsa
 (page 238)
Sautéed Organic Mixed Greens with Garlic (page 218)
Simple Organic Roasted Asparagus (page 224)

Day 3

Breakfast
Roasted Wild-Caught Salmon with Tangy Mango Salsa
Spring Green Veggie Juice (page 259)
Reheat and sip on Gut Healing Broth

Lunch
Tropical Nicaraguan Salad (page 232)
Organic Farm Five-Veggie Soup

Dinner
**Organic Baby Kale and Spinach Salad with Rosemary and Basil
 Grass-Fed Burgers** (page 231)
Creamy Acorn Squash (page 218)
Enjoy ½ cup organic mixed berries, such as raspberries,
 strawberries, blueberries, or blackberries

Day 4

Breakfast
Savory Breakfast Sausage (page 256)
Coconut Cream Berry Parfait (page 265)
Reheat and sip on Gut Healing Broth

Lunch
Organic Baby Kale and Spinach Salad with Rosemary and
    Basil Grass-Fed Burgers
Creamy Acorn Squash

Dinner
Spicy Fish Tacos (page 246)
Brussels Sprouts with Dark Organic Cherries (page 224)

Day 5

Breakfast
Wild-Caught Seafood, Kale, and Zucchini Scramble (page 243)
Reheat and sip on Gut Healing Broth

Lunch
Arugula, Blood Orange, and Fennel Salad (page 233)

Dinner
Chicken Coconut Curry (page 248)
Cauliflower "Pilaf" (page 220)
Enjoy ½ cup organic mixed berries, such as raspberries,
    strawberries, blueberries, or blackberries

Day 6

Breakfast
Savory Breakfast Sausage
Hearty Sweet Potato Hash (page 217)

Lunch
Chicken Coconut Curry
Cauliflower "Pilaf"

Dinner

    Wild-Caught Halibut with Caramelized Sweet Onions (page 239)

    Organic Broccolini with Garlic and Lemon (page 225)

    Sautéed Organic Mixed Greens with Garlic (page 218)

Day 7

Breakfast

    Sweet Apple Breakfast Sausage (pages 256–57)

    Hearty Sweet Potato Hash

    Spring Green Veggie Juice (page 259)

    Chai Tea Latte (page 259) or decaf green tea, if desired

Lunch

    Clean Cobb Salad (page 230)

    Simple Organic Roasted Asparagus (page 224)

Dinner

    Creamy Basil Pesto Sauce over Spaghetti Squash (page 254)

    Gut Healing Broth (page 226)

    Enjoy ½ cup organic mixed berries, such as raspberries,
        strawberries, blueberries, or blackberries

Day 8

Breakfast

    Sweet Apple Breakfast Sausage

    Coconut Cream Berry Parfait (page 265)

    Reheat and sip on Gut Healing Broth

    Chai Tea Latte (page 259) or decaf green tea, if desired

Lunch

    Creamy Basil Pesto Sauce over Spaghetti Squash

Dinner

    Thai Green Curry with Shrimp (pages 240-41)

    Organic Broccolini with Garlic and Lemon (page 225)

Day 9

Breakfast

Savory Breakfast Sausage (page 256)
Hearty Sweet Potato Hash (page 217)
Reheat and sip on Gut Healing Broth
Chai Tea Latte (page 259) or decaf green tea, if desired

Lunch

Thai Green Curry with Shrimp

Dinner

Chinese Spice Slow-Cooked Pork (page 258)
Cauliflower "Pilaf" (page 220)
Enjoy ½ cup organic mixed berries, such as raspberries,
strawberries, blueberries, or blackberries

Day 10

Breakfast

Savory Breakfast Sausage
Coconut Cream Berry Parfait (page 265)
Reheat and sip on Gut Healing Broth

Lunch

Chinese Spice Slow-Cooked Pork
Cauliflower "Pilaf"

Dinner

Spicy Turkey Cabbage Wraps (page 251)
Zucchini "Noodle" Salad (page 232)

Day 11

Breakfast

Sweet Apple Breakfast Sausage (pages 256–57)
Hearty Sweet Potato Hash
Reheat and sip on Gut Healing Broth

Lunch

Spicy Turkey Cabbage Wraps
Zucchini "Noodle" Salad (page 232) or **Create Your Own
Organic Mixed Salad** (pages 261–62)

Dinner
>   Sweet Citrus Salmon Salad (page 239)
>   Brussels Sprouts with Dark Organic Cherries (page 224)

Day 12

Breakfast
>   Wild-Caught Seafood, Kale, and Zucchini Scramble (page 243)

Lunch
>   Organic Citrus Kale Salad with Cranberries (page 231)

Dinner
>   Garlic Oven-Roasted Cabbage (page 222)

Day 13

Breakfast
>   Sweet Apple Breakfast Sausage
>   Coconut Cream Berry Parfait (page 265)

Lunch
>   Tropical Nicaraguan Salad (page 232)

Dinner
>   Organic Baby Kale and Spinach Salad with Rosemary and
>   Basil Grass-Fed Burgers (page 231)
>   Crispy Sweet Potato Fries (page 222)

Day 14

Breakfast
>   Free-Range Organic Chicken and Veggie Scramble (page 250)
>   Chai Tea Latte (page 259) or decaf green tea, if desired

Lunch
>   Creamy Pesto "Pasta" with Shrimp (page 242)
>   Simple Organic Roasted Asparagus (page 224)

Dinner
>   Slow-Cooked Moroccan Lamb Curry (page 253)
>   Roasted Kabocha Squash with Cinnamon (page 219)
>   Enjoy ½ cup organic mixed berries, such as raspberries,
>   strawberries, blueberries, or blackberries

Day 15

Breakfast
Free-Range Organic Chicken and Veggie Scramble
Roasted Kabocha Squash with Cinnamon

Lunch
Spicy Fish Tacos (page 246)
Cucumber Seaweed Salad (page 234)

Dinner
Creamy Pesto "Pasta" with Shrimp
Simple Organic Roasted Asparagus (page 224)

Day 16

Breakfast
Slow-Cooked Moroccan Lamb Curry

Lunch
Spicy Fish Tacos
Cucumber Seaweed Salad (page 234) or
   Create Your Own Organic Mixed Salad (pages 261–62)

Dinner
Lemon Garlic Oven-Roasted Chicken (page 247)
Grandma's Hearty Chicken "Noodle" Soup (page 228)
Gut Healing Broth (page 226)

Day 17

Breakfast
Grandma's Hearty Chicken "Noodle" Soup
Chai Tea Latte (page 259) or decaf green tea, if desired

Lunch
Cilantro Salmon Stuffed Avocado (page 241)
Arugula, Blood Orange, and Fennel Salad (page 233)

Dinner
Creamy Basil Pesto Sauce over Spaghetti Squash (page 254)
Crispy Kale Chips (page 225)
Enjoy ½ cup organic mixed berries, such as raspberries,
   strawberries, blueberries, or blackberries

Day 18

Breakfast
Savory Breakfast Sausage (page 256)
Coconut Cream Berry Parfait (page 265)
Reheat and sip on Gut Healing Broth

Lunch
Clean Cobb Salad (page 230)

Dinner
Spicy Chicken and Sausage Gumbo (page 252)
Organic Broccolini with Garlic and Lemon (page 225)

Day 19

Breakfast
Savory Breakfast Sausage
Coconut Cream Berry Parfait (page 265)
Reheat and sip on Gut Healing Broth

Lunch
Spicy Chicken and Sausage Gumbo
Organic Broccolini with Garlic and Lemon (page 225)

Dinner
Wild-Caught Halibut with Caramelized Sweet Onions (page 239)
Creamy Butternut Squash Soup with Cinnamon (page 227)

Day 20

Breakfast
Sweet Apple Breakfast Sausage (pages 256–57)
Creamy Butternut Squash Soup with Cinnamon
Reheat and sip on Gut Healing Broth
Chai Tea Latte (page 259) or decaf green tea, if desired

Lunch
Wild-Caught Halibut with Caramelized Sweet Onions
Organic Citrus Kale Salad with Cranberries (page 231)

Dinner
- **Tropical Nicaraguan Salad** (page 232)
- **Brussels Sprouts with Dark Organic Cherries** (page 224)
- **Cinnamon Apple Crisp** (page 265)

Day 21

Breakfast
- Sweet Apple Breakfast Sausage
- **Hearty Sweet Potato Hash** (page 217)
- **Spring Green Veggie Juice** (page 259)
- Reheat and sip on Gut Healing Broth

Lunch
- **Lemon Garlic Oven-Roasted Chicken** (page 247)
- **Clean Cobb Salad** (page 230)
- **Organic Farm Five-Veggie Soup** (page 229)
- **Gut Healing Broth** (page 226)

Dinner
- **Saturday Night Sushi** (page 244)
- **Crispy Coconut Shrimp** (pages 244–45)
- **Roasted Veggies** (page 224)

Day 22

Breakfast
- Cinnamon Apple Crisp
- **Spring Green Veggie Juice** (page 259)
- Reheat and sip on Gut Healing Broth

Lunch
- **Artichokes with Ume Plum Vinaigrette** (page 223)
- **Arugula, Blood Orange, and Fennel Salad** (page 233)

Dinner
- **Chicken Coconut Curry** (page 248)
- Artichokes with Ume Plum Vinaigrette

Day 23

Breakfast
   Savory Breakfast Sausage (page 256)
   Coconut Summer Squash (page 223)
   Reheat and sip on Gut Healing Broth
   Chai Tea Latte (page 259) or decaf green tea, if desired

Lunch
   Chicken Coconut Curry
   Organic Citrus Kale Salad with Cranberries (page 231) or
      Create Your Own Organic Mixed Salad (pages 261–62)

Dinner
   Loaded Sweet Potatoes (pages 250–51)
   Organic Farm Five-Veggie Soup

Day 24

Breakfast
   Savory Breakfast Sausage
   Coconut Cream Berry Parfait (page 265)
   Reheat and sip on Gut Healing Broth

Lunch
   Loaded Sweet Potatoes
   Zucchini "Noodle" Salad (page 232) or
      Create Your Own Organic Mixed Salad (pages 261–62)

Dinner
   Cilantro Salmon Stuffed Avocado (page 241)
   Simple Organic Roasted Asparagus (page 224)

Day 25

Breakfast
   Sweet Apple Breakfast Sausage (pages 256–57)
   Hearty Sweet Potato Hash (page 217)
   Reheat and sip on Gut Healing Broth

Lunch
   Tropical Nicaraguan Salad (page 232)

Dinner
> **Chinese Spice Slow-Cooked Pork** (page 258)
> **Cauliflower "Pilaf"** (page 220)

Day 26

Breakfast
> Sweet Apple Breakfast Sausage
> Hearty Sweet Potato Hash
> **Spring Green Veggie Juice** (page 259)

Lunch
> Chinese Spice Slow-Cooked Pork
> Cauliflower "Pilaf"

Dinner
> **Spicy Fish Tacos** (page 246)
> **Cucumber Seaweed Salad** (page 234)
> Enjoy ½ cup organic mixed berries, such as raspberries,
> strawberries, blueberries, or blackberries

Day 27

Breakfast
> **Savory Breakfast Sausage** (page 256)
> **Coconut Cream Berry Parfait** (page 265)
> **Chai Tea Latte** (page 261) or decaf green tea, if desired

Lunch
> Spicy Fish Tacos
> **Cucumber Seaweed Salad** (page 234) or
>> **Create Your Own Organic Mixed Salad** (pages 261–62)

Dinner
> **Seared Grass-Fed Steak and Sweet Potatoes** (pages 254–55)
> **Sautéed Organic Mixed Greens with Garlic** (page 218)
> **Banana Cream Mini Cake Bites** (page 266)

Day 28

Breakfast
> Seared Grass-Fed Steak and Sweet Potatoes
> **Spring Green Veggie Juice** (page 259)

Lunch
    Lemon Garlic Oven-Roasted Chicken (page 247)
    Easy Chicken Lettuce Wraps (page 255)
    Organic Broccolini with Garlic and Lemon (page 225)
    Gut Healing Broth (page 226)

Dinner
    Saturday Night Sushi (page 244)
    Oven-Roasted Cod in Coconut Oil with Spinach (pages 242–43)
    Cucumber Seaweed Salad (page 234)

Day 29

Breakfast
    Wild-Caught Seafood, Kale, and Zucchini Scramble (page 243)
    Spring Green Veggie Juice (page 259)
    Reheat and sip on Gut Healing Broth

Lunch
    Easy Chicken Lettuce Wraps

Dinner
    **Organic Baby Kale and Spinach Salad with Rosemary and Basil
       Grass-Fed Burgers** (page 231)

Day 30

Breakfast
    Savory Breakfast Sausage
    Hearty Sweet Potato Hash (page 217)
    Reheat and sip on Gut Healing Broth
    Chai Tea Latte (page 259) or decaf green tea, if desired

Lunch
    Arugula, Blood Orange, and Fennel Salad (page 233)

Dinner
    Creamy Basil Pesto Sauce over Spaghetti Squash (page 254)
    Brussels Sprouts with Dark Organic Cherries (page 224)

THE SEVEN-DAY SEAFOOD MEAL PLAN

This Seven-Day Seafood Meal Plan is a modified version of The Myers Way for those of you who are not currently eating poultry, beef, lamb, or pork. Remember, as discussed on page 115, this protocol is less inflammatory than your vegetarian or vegan diet, but it's still not as nutrient-dense as the regular meal plan of The Myers Way. If you would like to use this seafood plan as a transition, or if it is as far as you want to go, that is your decision. Just like the regular meal plan this seafood meal plan is based on the idea that you will be cooking for two people, so each meal accounts for two servings to be enjoyed. Feel free to adjust to fit your family's needs. If you are cooking for one, simply cut in half the number of servings you are instructed to make. That still leaves you plenty of leftovers. If you would like a detailed plan walking you through exactly how many servings to make, when to prep recipes, and when to enjoy leftovers, you can find a chart on pages 278–80. This will allow for your thirty days to run as smoothly and deliciously as possible.

Prep Day

The day before you begin the meal plan, make the following recipes to enjoy throughout the first week. This day is crucial: Prepping before you begin will really help you start off the program smoothly. If you have a typical workweek, I recommend prepping on a Saturday and beginning the program on a Sunday when you still have some extra time for cooking. After you prep, enjoy some Creamy Butternut Squash Soup with Cinnamon (page 227) to get a sneak peak before you begin!

> **Creamy Butternut Squash Soup with Cinnamon** (page 227)
> **Chicken Coconut Curry** (page 248) without chicken

Day 1

Breakfast
> **Coconut Cream Berry Parfait** (page 265)
> **Spring Green Veggie Juice** (page 259)
> **Chai Tea Latte** (page 259) or decaf green tea, if desired

Lunch

Organic Citrus Kale Salad with Cranberries (page 231)

Chicken Coconut Curry without chicken

Dinner

Lemon and Mushroom Baked Trout (page 245)

Organic Broccolini with Garlic and Lemon (page 225)

Day 2

Breakfast

Wild-Caught Seafood, Kale, and Zucchini Scramble (page 243)

Creamy Butternut Squash Soup with Cinnamon

Lunch

Lemon and Mushroom Baked Trout

Organic Citrus Kale Salad with Cranberries (page 231)

Dinner

Wild-Caught Halibut with Caramelized Sweet Onions (page 239)

Sautéed Organic Mixed Greens with Garlic (page 218)

Spiced Butternut Squash with Turmeric (page 219)

Enjoy ½ cup organic mixed berries, such as raspberries, strawberries, blueberries, or blackberries

Day 3

Breakfast

Chicken Coconut Curry without chicken

Lunch

Wild-Caught Halibut with Caramelized Sweet Onions

Creamy Butternut Squash Soup with Cinnamon

Sautéed Organic Mixed Greens with Garlic

Dinner

Creamy Pesto "Pasta" with Shrimp (page 242)

Enjoy ½ cup organic mixed berries, such as raspberries, strawberries, blueberries, or blackberries

Day 4

Breakfast
  Coconut Cream Berry Parfait (page 265)
  Spring Green Veggie Juice (page 259)

Lunch
  Creamy Pesto "Pasta" with Shrimp

Dinner
  Roasted Wild-Caught Salmon with Tangy Mango Salsa
    (page 238)
  **Twice-Baked Perfect Sweet Potatoes with Cinnamon and
    Nutmeg** (page 221)
  Simple Organic Roasted Asparagus (page 224)

Day 5

Breakfast
  Coconut Cream Berry Parfait (page 265)
  Spring Green Veggie Juice (page 259)

Lunch
  Roasted Wild-Caught Salmon with Tangy Mango Salsa
  Tropical Nicaraguan Salad (page 232)

Dinner
  Oven-Roasted Cod in Coconut Oil with Spinach (pages 242–43)
  Cauliflower "Pilaf" (page 220)

Day 6

Breakfast
  Wild-Caught Seafood, Kale, and Zucchini Scramble (page 243)

Lunch
  Oven-Roasted Cod in Coconut Oil with Spinach
  Cauliflower "Pilaf"

Dinner
  Crispy Coconut Shrimp (pages 244–45)
  Arugula, Blood Orange, and Fennel Salad (page 233)
  Cinnamon Apple Crisp (page 265)

Day 7

Breakfast
    Coconut Cream Berry Parfait (page 265)
    Spring Green Veggie Juice (page 259)
    Chai Tea Latte (page 259) or decaf green tea, if desired

Lunch
    Spicy Fish Tacos (page 246)
    Artichokes with Ume Plum Vinaigrette (page 223)

Dinner
    Saturday Night Sushi (page 244)
    Cucumber Seaweed Salad (page 234)

The Myers Way Recipes

VEGETABLES

Hearty Sweet Potato Hash

SERVES 4

What a wonderful way to start your day! This warm and hearty dish is everything you're looking for in a comfort food. Since you will be enjoying this hash for breakfast, I recommend prepping your ingredients beforehand if you want to save time in the morning.

2 to 4 teaspoons coconut oil
2 medium sweet potatoes, finely diced
1 yellow onion, diced
¼ teaspoon ground cinnamon
⅛ teaspoon ground nutmeg
Pinch of sea salt
Pinch of ground black pepper

Set a large pan over medium heat. Add the coconut oil, sweet potatoes, and onions. Cover and simmer the mixture for 7 to 10 minutes, stirring frequently. Add the cinnamon, nutmeg, salt, and pepper. Cook the mixture uncovered for an additional 2 to 3 minutes, stirring frequently, or until the sweet potatoes are soft and slightly browned.

Creamy Acorn Squash

SERVES 4

This squash melts in your mouth, thanks to the creamy coconut and sweet spices.

    1 acorn squash
    2 teaspoons coconut oil or coconut manna, plus more coconut oil for
        greasing the baking dish
    Pinch of ground cinnamon
    Pinch of ground nutmeg

Preheat the oven to 375°F.

Cut the squash in half from top to bottom. Remove the seeds with a spoon and discard them.

Grease a medium-size baking dish with coconut oil. Place the squash halves facedown in the baking dish, then bake them for 30 minutes. Then turn each squash half faceup with tongs. Spoon 1 teaspoon of the coconut oil or manna over each half, and sprinkle them with the cinnamon and nutmeg. Cook for another 10 minutes before serving.

Sautéed Organic Mixed Greens with Garlic

SERVES 2 TO 4

You'll never complain about eating your greens after trying these fantastic greens, drizzled with sweet coconut oil.

    1 bunch greens, or about 4 to 5 cups according to your taste, of kale,
        rainbow chard, collards, or mustard greens
    2 teaspoons coconut oil, or more if needed
    1 garlic clove, minced
    Pinch of sea salt

Rinse the greens and pat them dry. Separate the stems from the leaves, and chop the stems into 2-inch segments. Chop the leaves into 1-inch strips.

Heat the coconut oil and garlic in a medium pan and add the chopped stems. Sauté the mixture for about 5 minutes, then add the leaves and a pinch of salt. Add 1 more teaspoon of oil if greens are sticking, and sauté for another 2 to 3 minutes. Enjoy warm.

Roasted Kabocha Squash with Cinnamon

SERVES 4 TO 6

When I finally tried this squash, I wished I had been making it for years. It has such a rich flavor that goes well with anything. It looks like a little green pumpkin and likely can be found close to the spaghetti squash at your grocer.

2 tablespoons coconut oil, melted, plus more for greasing the baking sheet
1 kabocha squash
Pinch of sea salt
Pinch of ground black pepper
⅛ teaspoon ground cinnamon
Pinch of ground nutmeg

Preheat the oven to 350°F.

Grease a baking sheet with coconut oil. Carefully slice the squash in half from top to bottom. Remove the seeds with a spoon and discard them. Slice each half into 1-inch-thick wedges and place them in a large bowl. Drizzle the slices with the melted coconut oil and sprinkle them with the salt, pepper, cinnamon, and nutmeg. Spread the slices on the baking sheet and roast them for about 20 minutes, then turn them over and roast them for another 20 minutes. The peel is edible, but you can remove it before serving if you prefer.

Spiced Butternut Squash with Turmeric

SERVES 2

1 butternut squash, peeled, seeded, and chopped into ½- to ¾-inch cubes
1 to 2 tablespoons coconut oil, melted, plus more for greasing the baking sheet
¼ teaspoon ground turmeric

Preheat the oven to 375°F.

In a large bowl, toss the squash cubes with the oil and turmeric. Then arrange them on a greased baking sheet and bake for 30 minutes—the longer longer you bake it, the crispier it gets!

Slow-Roasted Carrots and Beets with Turmeric

SERVES 2 TO 4

You can just see the amazing nutrition in the bright colors of these carrots and beets.

4 carrots, peeled
2 golden beets, peeled
2 to 3 teaspoons coconut oil, melted
Pinch of sea salt
Turmeric to taste

Preheat the oven to 350°F.

Chop the carrots into thin disks or into 2-inch segments and then quarter them lengthwise. Chop the beets into bite-size pieces, about 1 inch long and ½ inch wide.

In a medium bowl, toss the veggies in the melted coconut oil, salt, and seasonings of your choice. Spread the veggies on a baking sheet, then roast them for about 20 minutes, depending on the desired texture.

Cauliflower "Pilaf"

SERVES 4

This recipe is one of my favorites. It's incredibly easy and feels like I'm eating rice again. I love to make a lot of this to enjoy for the whole week in different dishes, especially curries!

1 head cauliflower, chopped coarsely
1 yellow onion, diced
2 tablespoons coconut oil
¼ teaspoon sea salt

Rinse the cauliflower heads and break them apart into florets. Working in batches, place the florets into a food processor with an S-shaped blade and process the cauliflower until it begins to resemble rice. Another option is to use a ricer instead of a food processer.

In a skillet set over medium heat, sauté the onion in the coconut oil. When the onions become translucent, add the processed cauliflower to the skillet. Stir to combine and sauté the mixture until it is soft. Season the "pilaf" with salt and any other preferred seasonings to taste.

Simply Delicious Baked Sweet Potatoes

SERVES 2 (1 POTATO PER PERSON)

Every time I eat a sweet potato I'm amazed at how delicious it is all by itself. This is also a great recipe to make in bulk and enjoy throughout the week to save time. They are even great cold, on the go!

Coconut oil for greasing the baking sheet
2 medium sweet potatoes

Preheat the oven to 400°F.
Grease a baking sheet with coconut oil. Wash and cut the sweet potatoes in half lengthwise and place them facedown on the sheet. Bake them for 45 to 60 minutes, or until they are soft.

Twice-Baked Perfect Sweet Potatoes with Cinnamon and Nutmeg

SERVES 2 (1 POTATO PER PERSON)

Okay, I know I said sweet potatoes are wonderful all by themselves, but this recipe is to die for! You will feel like you are eating dessert. Enjoy this special treat!

Simply Delicious Baked Sweet Potatoes (recipe above)
2 tablespoons coconut oil
⅛ teaspoon ground cinnamon
Pinch of ground nutmeg
Pinch of sea salt
Pinch of ground black pepper
¼ cup full-fat coconut milk (optional)
2 teaspoons sliced scallions (optional)

Preheat the oven to 375°F.
Scoop out the flesh of each baked potato half from its skin with a spoon, and place the flesh in a medium bowl. Reserve the skins on a baking sheet.
Add the coconut oil, cinnamon, nutmeg, salt, pepper, and the optional coconut milk to the bowl with the potato flesh. Mash to combine the mixture with a potato masher or a fork. Spoon the filling back into the reserved skins, and bake them for 10 to 15 minutes. Top each with the optional scallions before serving.

Garlic Oven-Roasted Cabbage

SERVES 4

    Coconut oil for greasing the baking sheet

    1 head green cabbage

    2 garlic cloves

    2 tablespoons extra-virgin olive oil

    Pinch of sea salt

    Pinch of ground black pepper

    1 large avocado, sliced

    1 Rosemary and Basil Grass-Fed Burger (page 257)

Preheat the oven to 400°F.

Grease the baking sheet with coconut oil.

Place the cabbage on a cutting board with the root on the bottom. Cut the cabbage into about 1-inch-thick slices. Smash the garlic cloves with the side of a chef's blade to soften them, and rub all the sides of the cabbage slices with the garlic. Drizzle olive oil on the top and bottom of each cabbage slice, and sprinkle them with salt and pepper.

Place the cabbage slices on the baking sheet and roast them for about 25 minutes, then flip them and roast for another 25 minutes.

Serve topped with avocado slices and a Rosemary and Basil Grass-Fed Burger.

Crispy Sweet Potato Fries

SERVES 2

You'll feel anything but deprived enjoying these crispy fries.

    2 medium sweet potatoes

    Coconut oil

Wash and peel the sweet potatoes. Chop them into thin "fries" about 2 inches long and ¼ to ½ inch thick.

Heat enough coconut oil in a large pan to cover the fries. When the oil is hot, add half the potatoes to the pan with a slotted wok spoon. Fry them for about 7 minutes, removing them from the oil before they turn brown (the fries will crisp up after they are taken out of the oil). Fry the remaining potatoes in the same manner.

Artichokes with Ume Plum Vinaigrette

SERVES 2 TO 4

2 artichokes
½ lemon
1 garlic clove, peeled and smashed
Ume Plum Vinaigrette (pages 236)

Fill a large pot with enough water to cover the artichokes, and bring the water to a boil.

In the meantime, on a cutting board chop the stems off the artichokes so they can sit flat (flower side up) on the bottom surface of the pot. Trim the pointed tips off each leaf with a kitchen scissors and discard them. Cut the top inch off each artichoke too and discard those. Rub all cut areas of both artichokes with the juicy lemon half.

Add the lemon half, garlic, and each artichoke carefully to the boiling water with a slotted wok spoon. Place a lid, small enough to fit inside the pot, on top of the artichokes to keep them submerged in the boiling water. Simmer them for about 30 to 35 minutes, or until they are tender. Remove the artichokes with the slotted spoon and let them drain and cool in a strainer upside down so all the water can drip out.

To eat, pull each petal off the artichoke one at a time, dip the leaf in the prepared Ume Plum Vinaigrette, and place it in your mouth, skimming the base of the petal through your teeth to strip off the tender flesh. When you get to the heart of the artichoke, scrape off the fuzzy top layer and discard it before enjoying the artichoke heart.

Leftover artichokes can be steamed to reheat them.

Coconut Summer Squash

SERVES 2

1 zucchini
1 yellow squash
2 teaspoons coconut oil

Wash the squash and cut off the ends. Grate the zucchini and the yellow squash with a grater.

Heat the coconut oil in a medium pan, then add the grated squash and sauté the mixture for 1 to 2 minutes.

Roasted Veggies

SERVES 2

   4 cups chopped veggies of your choice (asparagus, beets, broccoli,
       cauliflower, carrots, celery, zucchini, sweet potatoes, etc.)
   1 to 2 tablespoons coconut oil, melted
   ¼ teaspoon sea salt
   Optional seasonings: turmeric, cinnamon, nutmeg, cumin, black pepper

   Preheat the oven to 350°F.
   In a bowl, combine the chopped veggies, coconut oil, salt, and optional
seasonings, stirring until the veggies are evenly coated. Spread the veggies on
a baking sheet and roast them for 15 to 25 minutes. The cooking time will de-
pend on the choice of vegetable and the desired texture. Keep an eye on them
to determine the best cooking time.

Simple Organic Roasted Asparagus

SERVES 2

   24 organic asparagus stalks, end discarded
   1 tablespoon coconut oil or olive oil
   Pinch sea salt
   1 lemon wedge

   Preheat oven to 375°F. Wash asparagus and place in oven safe baking dish.
Drizzle with oil and sprinkle with salt. Roast for 20 to 25 minutes.
   Squeeze juice from lemon wedge over asparagus before serving.

Brussels Sprouts with Dark Organic Cherries

SERVES 2

   3 cups organic Brussels sprouts, stems chopped off
   ½ cup fresh organic cherries, pitted
   2 to 3 tablespoons olive oil or coconut oil, melted plus extra for greasing
   ¼ teaspoon salt

   Preheat oven to 375°F. Grease baking sheet with coconut oil. Cut Brussels
sprouts in half. Mix with cherries, oil, and salt. Roast 15 to 20 minutes depending on desired crispiness.

Organic Broccolini with Garlic and Lemon

SERVES 2

Any of these great organic green side recipes can be doubled to enjoy the next day.

8 stalks organic broccolini, ends trimmed
1 tablespoon coconut oil or olive oil, more as needed
½ sweet onion, diced
3 cloves garlic, minced
½ lemon

Heat medium sized pan with oil. Add onion and cook for 2 minutes. Add garlic and broccolini. Let cook for 5 to 7 minutes, stirring frequently. When broccolini is tender, squeeze with lemon and serve.

Variation: Use 1 head of broccoli instead of broccolini.

Crispy Kale Chips

SERVES 2

1 head curly kale
2 tablespoons coconut oil
¼ teaspoon sea salt
¼ teaspoon turmeric

Preheat oven to 400°F. Wash kale and pat dry. Place kale in large bowl. Tear the leaves into 2 to 3 inch pieces and separate leaves from stems. Discard stems. Drizzle with oil and massage oil into leaves to coat thoroughly. Add salt and turmeric, and mix well. Bake for about 10 minutes, until kale is crispy, in batches or on multiple baking sheets. During baking, keep an eye out to prevent burning the thin chips.

SOUPS AND BROTHS

Gut Healing Broth

Makes approximately 16 4-ounce servings (8 cups)

The gelatin in Gut Healing Broth protects and heals the mucosal lining of the digestive tract and helps aid in the digestion of nutrients. This broth is great in soups or to just sip from your favorite mug.

1 organic, pasture-raised chicken carcass (left over from Lemon Garlic
    Oven-Roasted Chicken on page 247) or 1 pound bones (marrow bones,
    chicken bones, knuckle bones)
2 tablespoons apple cider vinegar
1 teaspoon sea salt
2 garlic cloves, peeled and smashed with the flat side of a knife
8 cups water
Chopped carrots, celery, onions (optional)

Put the chicken carcass or bones in a slow cooker with the vinegar, salt, garlic, water and vegetables. Depending on the bones you use and the size of your slow cooker, you can add more water to cover the bones. Cook the mixture on low for at least 24 hours before cooling. (You can use the broth at any time after 8 hours of cooking, but I recommend cooking it for at least 24 hours.)

When the broth is ready, use a slotted spoon to remove the bones. Then pour it through a fine-mesh strainer to separate the fat. It may still be greasy, but after it's stored in the fridge, the fat will rise to the top and you can skim it off.

Heat individual portions for drinking or using in recipes. Use for 4 to 5 days then freeze.

Creamy Butternut Squash Soup with Cinnamon

SERVES 4 TO 6

You'll love this sweet and creamy soup the first time you taste it and maybe even more the second time! Note, you can peel and chop up butternut squash and sweet potatoes at any time and freeze the flesh to keep on hand for this recipe or to use later.

- 2 garlic cloves (keep whole)
- 2 to 3 tablespoons extra-virgin olive oil
- 1 butternut squash, peeled, seeded, and cut into chunks (or you can use frozen chunks)
- 2 medium sweet potatoes, peeled and cut into chunks (or you can use frozen chunks)
- 1 large sweet onion, diced
- ½ teaspoon ground cinnamon
- ¼ teaspoon ground nutmeg
- 4 cups Gut Healing Broth (previous recipe, page 226) or gluten-free, low sodium packaged broth (Pacific Natural Foods has some good organic broths)
- 1 13.5-ounce can full-fat coconut milk
- Sea salt to taste
- Ground black pepper to taste

In a large soup pot, sauté the garlic in the olive oil until it is aromatic. Add the squash, sweet potatoes, onion, cinnamon, and nutmeg, and sauté for 3 to 5 minutes, stirring the mixture frequently. Add the broth and bring the soup to a boil, then turn the heat down and simmer, partially covered, for about 20 minutes until the potatoes and squash are tender.

Remove the pot from the heat. Blend the mixture with an immersion blender or in a standard high-speed blender, working in batches, until it's completely smooth.

Return the soup to a burner set on low heat and stir in the coconut milk. Continue to heat the soup on a low flame, stirring well. Season with salt and pepper.

Variation: Top individual servings of the soup with pomegranate seeds for some crunch.

Grandma's Hearty Chicken "Noodle" Soup

SERVES 4

The zucchini "noodles" transform this soup into a classic chicken noodle soup. This is the perfect dish to bring back some warm childhood memories.

    1 tablespoon coconut oil (more if needed)
    1 garlic clove, minced
    1 yellow onion, chopped
    ¼ teaspoon ground turmeric
    ½ sweet potato, chopped
    4 carrots, chopped
    4 stalks celery, chopped
    1 bay leaf
    20 ounces (2.5 cups) Gut Healing Broth (page 226) or gluten-free,
        low-sodium packaged broth
    2 cups chopped or shredded cooked organic, pasture-raised chicken
    2 teaspoons chopped fresh basil
    2 teaspoons chopped fresh cilantro or parsley (or both)
    ¼ teaspoon sea salt
    ⅛ teaspoon ground black pepper
    2 zucchini, spiral-cut into "noodles" using a spiral slicer or julienne peeler

In a large soup pot set over medium heat, warm the coconut oil. Add the garlic and sauté until it is slightly browned. Add the onions and turmeric, and continue to sauté for about 3 minutes. Add the potato, carrots, celery, and bay leaf. If the vegetables seem dry, add another 2 to 3 teaspoons of coconut oil. Cook the mixture for about another 10 minutes. Add the broth, chicken, basil, parsley and/or cilantro, salt, and pepper. Bring the soup to a boil, then simmer it covered for an additional 40 minutes.

Turn the heat off and remove the bay leaf. Stir in the zucchini "noodles," cover the pot, and let the soup sit for 5 to 10 minutes before serving hot.

Organic Farm Five-Veggie Soup

SERVES 4

1 cup chopped yellow squash

1 cup chopped zucchini

1 cup chopped broccoli

1 cup chopped cauliflower

1 cup chopped yellow onions

1 garlic clove, minced

2 teaspoons extra-virgin olive oil

1 cup Gut Healing Broth (page 226) or gluten-free, low-sodium packaged
broth

¼ teaspoon fresh dill

Sea salt to taste

Ground black pepper to taste

Steam the squash, zucchini, broccoli, and cauliflower. Set them aside.

In a pan, caramelize the onions and garlic in the olive oil. Set them aside.

In a high-speed blender, working in batches, puree some of the broth
with the steamed veggies, onions and garlic, dill, salt, and pepper. When the
mixture is smooth, pour it into a large soup pot. Add any remaining broth and
simmer the soup until it's hot.

SALADS

Clean Cobb Salad

SERVES 2

2 cups chopped romaine lettuce

1 cup chopped baby kale

½ cucumber, chopped

1 organic, pasture-raised chicken breast, cooked and chopped

½ apple, chopped

½ large avocado, sliced

1 tablespoon olive oil

Juice from ½ lemon

2 teaspoons full-fat coconut milk (optional)

1 clove garlic, minced

Pinch of sea salt

Pinch of ground black pepper

In a medium bowl, toss together the lettuce, kale, cucumber, chicken, apple, and avocado. Set the mixture aside.

Put the oil, lemon juice, coconut milk, garlic, salt, and pepper in a food processor or a high-speed blender and mix until the dressing is smooth. Drizzle the salad with the dressing and serve. If you are preparing the salad for leftovers, wait to chop the apple and avocado to maintain freshness, and keep the dressing on the side.

Variation: Use Organic Herb Roasted Chicken Tenders (page 249) for salad in place of chicken breast.

Organic Citrus Kale Salad with Cranberries

SERVES 2

The citrus in this recipe helps to soften the crispy kale leaves, and the fruit brings a pop of sweetness. You'll be asking for seconds!

1 bunch kale (about 4 to 5 cups)

Juice of ½ orange

Extra-virgin olive oil

1½ cups shredded, cooked chicken (can use leftover Lemon Garlic Oven-Roasted Chicken, page 247)

½ cup unsweetened dried cranberries or fresh pitted cherries (optional)

1 small cucumber, chopped (optional)

Wash and pat dry the kale leaves, then chop them. In a medium bowl, toss the chopped kale with the orange juice and olive oil to coat the leaves. Add the chicken, as well as the optional cranberries or cherries and cucumber. Let the salad sit for at least 30 minutes before serving, to meld the flavors.

Variation: Leave out chicken if already enjoying animal protein in a meal.

Organic Baby Kale and Spinach Salad with Rosemary and Basil Grass-Fed Burgers

SERVES 2

4 to 5 cups organic baby kale and spinach mix

1 to 2 tablespoons coconut oil

1 small sweet onion, sliced thinly in strips

2 to 4 Rosemary and Basil Grass-Fed Burgers/Meatballs (page 257)

½ cup Super Guacamole (page 236)

Wash the greens and pat the leaves dry. Slice the leaves into 1-inch strips and divide them between two serving bowls.

Heat the coconut oil in a medium pan. Sauté the onion until it caramelizes (let the onions stick to the pan to allow for caramelization, then stir them before they burn).

Top each serving of greens with 1 to 2 burgers, a spoonful of guacamole, and the caramelized onions.

Tropical Nicaraguan Salad

SERVES 2

4 to 6 cups organic mixed field greens
¼ to ½ small mango, peeled and grated
½ cup strawberries, thinly sliced
½ cucumber, thinly sliced
1 avocado, diced
¼ teaspoon sea salt
2 tablespoons olive oil
2 teaspoons balsamic vinegar (use apple cider vinegar on the Yeast Overgrowth / SIBO Dietary Protocol)

In a large salad bowl combine greens, mango, berries, cucumber, and avocado. In a small bowl mix together salt, oil, and vinegar. Drizzle desired amount of dressing over salad and serve.

Variation: Serve with Organic Herb Roasted Chicken Tenders (page 249), left over chicken, or salmon if you are enjoying as a meal.

Zucchini "Noodle" Salad

SERVES 2

1 zucchini, spiral-cut into "noodles" using a spiral slicer or grated
2 medium avocados, chopped
½ cup pitted and chopped olives
¼ cup sliced scallions
2 tablespoons fresh lemon juice
2 tablespoons extra-virgin olive oil
⅛ teaspoon sea salt
Pinch of ground black pepper

Combine the zucchini "noodles," avocados, olives, and scallions in a medium bowl. In a small bowl, whisk the lemon juice, olive oil, salt, and pepper, then drizzle the dressing over the veggies. Toss the salad to coat everything evenly.

Variation: Serve with leftover salmon.

Arugula, Blood Orange, and Fennel Salad

SERVES 2

This salad is delicious the next day, and the dressing can be doubled to enjoy later on Create Your Own Organic Mixed Salad (pages 261–62).

4 cups arugula

1 blood orange, peeled and sectioned, white pith removed

½ small fennel bulb, thinly sliced

1 red beet, peeled, sliced, and baked according to the Roasted Veggies recipe (page 224)

¼ red onion, thinly sliced

2 tablespoons chopped fresh cilantro

For the Dressing

Juice of ½ blood orange

2 teaspoons fresh lemon juice

2 teaspoons fresh lime juice

1 tablespoon extra-virgin olive oil

Pinch of sea salt, or to taste

Pinch of ground black pepper

Put the arugula in a large bowl. Slice each blood orange wedge in half. Scatter the oranges on top of the arugula. Add the fennel bulb slices, along with the beet and onion slices. Top the salad with the cilantro.

Whisk together in a bowl all the dressing ingredients and drizzle the dressing over the salad, tossing to coat everything evenly.

Variation: Serve with Organic Herb Roasted Chicken Tenders (page 249), leftover chicken, or grilled shrimp if you are enjoying it as a meal.

Cucumber Seaweed Salad

SERVES 2

> 1 cup wakame or arame
>
> 1 small cucumber, seeded and cut into quarters lengthwise, then into ½-inch slices

For the Dressing

> 1 tablespoon coconut aminos (avoid on Yeast Overgrowth / SIBO Dietary Protocol)
>
> 1 tablespoon apple cider vinegar
>
> 1½ teaspoons extra-virgin olive oil
>
> 1 teaspoon fresh lemon juice
>
> ½ teaspoon freshly minced ginger root
>
> Sea salt to taste

If you are using wakame, cut it with scissors into 1-inch pieces. Soak the pieces 5 to 10 minutes, then remove any hard pieces.

If you are using arame, soak it in cold water for 5 to 10 minutes, then drain it. Using a scissors, cut it into 1-inch pieces.

In a large bowl, toss together the seaweed and the cucumber. Set the mixture aside.

To make the dressing, place all the dressing ingredients into a high-speed blender and pulse them a few times until the dressing is smooth. Or just gently beat the mixture with a whisk or fork in a bowl. Drizzle a desired amount over the seaweed and cucumbers, and serve.

CONDIMENTS

Creamy Basil Pesto Sauce

MAKES ¾ TO 1 CUP

This sauce is easy to make in bulk and adds some zest to any dish.

2 cups tightly packed fresh basil
¼ cup plus 1 tablespoon extra-virgin olive oil
2 garlic cloves
Pinch of sea salt
Pinch of ground black pepper
¼ cup water

Blend all the ingredients together in a high-speed blender until the mixture is smooth. Store the sauce in the refrigerator for up to a week.

Olive Tapenade

MAKES ABOUT 1 CUP

1 cup pitted olives
2 garlic cloves, minced
2 tablespoons capers
2 tablespoons chopped fresh parsley
Leaves from 3 sprigs fresh thyme, finely chopped
1 tablespoon fresh lemon juice
1 tablespoon apple cider vinegar
2 tablespoons extra-virgin olive oil
Pinch of sea salt
Pinch of ground black pepper

Place all the ingredients into a food processer or high-speed blender. Pulse or blend the mixture until it is well combined, adding extra oil or water to reach a desired consistency.

Ume Plum Vinaigrette

MAKES ABOUT ¼ CUP

1 tablespoon ume plum vinegar
3 tablespoons extra-virgin olive oil
2 teaspoons minced fresh parsley or basil
Pinch of garlic powder

Place all the ingredients into a high-speed blender or a bowl and blend or whisk them until the vinaigrette is well combined. Double or triple the recipe and store the extra in the fridge for up to a week.

Super Guacamole

MAKES APPROXIMATELY 3 CUPS

This guacamole is packed with five different veggies to ramp up the nutrition and fiber. It's one of The Myers Way favorites.

Flesh of 2 avocados
½ yellow onion, diced
½ cucumber, julienned
½ yellow squash, grated
½ zucchini, grated
2 carrots, peeled and julienned
1 garlic clove, grated or minced
2 tablespoons chopped fresh cilantro
Juice of ½ lemon or lime
Sea salt to taste
Lemon or lime wedge, as a garnish

In a medium bowl, mash the flesh of the avocados. Stir in the onions, cucumber, squash, zucchini, carrots, garlic, cilantro, lemon or lime juice, and salt. Garnish the guacamole with a lemon or lime wedge.

Tangy Mango Salsa

MAKES APPROXIMATELY 3 CUPS

Delicious! In Texas, we can't go without our salsa, and this dish is a wonderful combination of flavors.

1 mango, chopped
1 avocado, chopped
½ red onion, chopped
3 tablespoons chopped fresh cilantro
Juice of 1 small lemon
2 to 3 teaspoons lemon zest
1 tablespoon extra-virgin olive oil
Pinch of sea salt, or to taste
Pinch of ground black pepper, or to taste

In a large bowl, stir together all the ingredients until they are well combined. Season with salt and pepper to taste.

Whipped Avocado and Lemon Dressing

MAKES APPROXIMATELY ½ CUP

Flesh of 1 medium avocado
Juice of 1 medium lemon
1 tablespoon extra-virgin olive oil
Water (adjust amount for desired consistency)

Place all the ingredients into a high-speed blender or a bowl and blend or whisk them until the dressing is smooth.

SEAFOOD

Roasted Wild-Caught Salmon with Tangy Mango Salsa

SERVES 4

For the salmon sauce, look for a prepared brown mustard made with apple cider vinegar. Eden Food makes a great organic mustard of this type.

> 2 8-ounce wild-caught Alaskan salmon fillets
> 1 tablespoon extra-virgin olive oil
> Sea salt to taste
> Ground black pepper to taste
> 6 tablespoons Tangy Mango Salsa (page 237)

> *For the Salmon Sauce*
> 2 tablespoons extra-virgin olive oil
> 1½ tablespoons chopped fresh parsley
> 1½ tablespoons chopped fresh dill
> 3 tablespoons prepared brown mustard
> 1 garlic clove, minced
> 1 to 2 tablespoons fresh lemon juice

Preheat the oven to 400°F.

Coat both sides of each salmon fillet with olive oil and a sprinkling of salt and pepper. Place the fillets on a large rimmed baking sheet in a cold oven on the bottom rack. Roast the salmon for about 25 minutes, or until it is heated through and flaky.

In a small bowl, combine all the ingredients for the salmon sauce, then drizzle it over the fillets before serving. Top each with the Tangy Mango Salsa.

Wild-Caught Halibut with Caramelized Sweet Onions

SERVES 4

4 8-ounce wild-caught halibut fillets (or substitute another fish of your preference)

Sea salt to taste

Ground black pepper to taste

2 tablespoons extra-virgin olive oil, plus additional oil for greasing the baking dish

4 yellow or sweet onions, thinly sliced into rings

2 tablespoons fresh lemon juice

Preheat the oven to 400°F.

Season each halibut fillet with salt and pepper. Place the fillets into an oiled baking dish and bake them for 10 to 15 minutes, or until the fish is flaky. Halfway through the cooking, add more olive oil to the dish if necessary.

Heat 2 tablespoons of olive oil in a medium pan. Sauté the onions in the oil until they caramelize, then spoon the mixture on top of the cooked fish and drizzle with lemon juice before serving.

Sweet Citrus Salmon Salad

SERVES 2

Buy and prep enough ingredients to make this recipe for the next couple days. You can wait to chop certain ingredients, such as the cucumber, avocados, and basil, to maintain their freshness.

8 to 10 ounces fresh wild-caught or canned salmon, cooked

1 cucumber, chopped into small pieces

2 avocados, chopped into small pieces

Juice of 1 medium orange

2 tablespoons chopped fresh basil

Sea salt to taste

Flake the salmon into a medium bowl. (If you are using canned salmon, drain any excess water before flaking it.) Stir in the cucumber, avocados, orange juice, basil, and salt. Enjoy!

Thai Green Curry with Shrimp

SERVES 4 TO 6

I'm especially excited for you to try this dish. This curry tastes like you ordered it from your favorite Thai restaurant. It will be well worth the extra effort the recipe requires. You can easily make the green curry paste in bulk and store it in the freezer to cut your prep time in half the next time you make this dish.

2 large heads cauliflower

1 tablespoon coconut oil

2 teaspoons anchovy paste

1 13.5-ounce can coconut milk, minus 2 tablespoons reserved for the curry paste

1½ pound large wild-caught shrimp, peeled and deveined

2 cups sliced mushrooms (eliminate on Yeast Overgrowth / SIBO Dietary Protocol)

5 scallions, sliced

2 tablespoons fresh lime juice

1 cup chopped fresh basil

4 stalks fresh lemongrass, cut into 1-inch segments, ends discarded

1 teaspoon sea salt

Fresh basil leaves and lime zest, as a garnish (optional)

For the Green Curry Paste

1 shallot, sliced

4 garlic cloves

¾-inch piece ginger root, peeled

½ cup packed fresh cilantro leaves

½ cup packed fresh basil leaves

½ teaspoon ground cumin

½ teaspoon ground black pepper

3 tablespoons gluten-free fish sauce (eliminate on Yeast Overgrowth / SIBO Dietary Protocol)

2 tablespoons fresh lime juice

2 tablespoons coconut milk

First, make the green curry paste. Blend all the curry paste ingredients in a food processor or a high-speed blender until the mixture is smooth. Set it aside.

Rinse the cauliflower heads and break them apart into florets. Working in batches, place the florets into a food processor with an S-shaped blade and process the cauliflower until it begins to resemble rice. Another option is to use a ricer instead of a food processor.

Heat the coconut oil in a large pan. Add the curry paste and the anchovy paste. Stir the pastes for about 30 seconds, then add the coconut milk and simmer the mixture to thicken it for a few minutes. Stir in the cauliflower and cook it for 3 minutes. Add the shrimp and mushrooms, and cook for 2 to 3 additional minutes, or until the shrimp are almost cooked through. Add the scallions, lime juice, basil, lemongrass, and salt. Continue to cook the mixture until the shrimp are ready and the mushrooms are soft.

Serve garnished with the fresh basil and lime zest.

Note, the lemongrass segments are not intended for consumption, so eat around them or discard them before serving.

Variation: Serve over julienned cucumbers and diced avocado.

Cilantro Salmon Stuffed Avocado

SERVES 2

This is a Myers family favorite. My dad texted me right after he tried this recipe to share how much he loved it!

    5 ounces wild-caught salmon, cooked and cut into small chunks (you can
        also use packaged boneless salmon)
    ½ cup chopped lettuce, any variety
    2 tablespoons chopped fresh cilantro
    3 tablespoons fresh lemon juice
    2 tablespoons extra-virgin olive oil
    ½ teaspoon ground cumin
    Sea salt and ground black pepper to taste
    2 avocados, sliced in half and pitted, making sure to keep the flesh
        in the peel

In a medium bowl, gently combine by hand the salmon, lettuce, cilantro, lemon juice, olive oil, cumin, salt, and pepper. Spoon the mixture into each avocado half and serve.

Creamy Pesto "Pasta" with Shrimp

SERVES APPROXIMATELY 4

Another one of my favorites. These zucchini "noodles" are quicker to make than boiling regular pasta, and you'll love the noodle texture!

4 large zucchini, ends chopped off, spiral-cut into "noodles" using a spiral slicer or julienne peeler

2 teaspoons coconut oil

2 garlic cloves, minced

⅛ teaspoon sea salt, plus more to sweat the zucchini

Pinch of ground black pepper

1 pound jumbo wild-caught shrimp, peeled and deveined

4 tablespoons Creamy Basil Pesto Sauce (page 235)

5 to 6 tablespoons full-fat coconut milk

½ cup chopped fresh basil

Place the zucchini in a large bowl and generously salt them to let the "noodles" sweat for about 20 minutes.

Meanwhile, heat the coconut oil in a large pan. Add the garlic, ⅛ teaspoon salt, and pepper, and sauté the garlic until it begins to brown. Then add the shrimp and cook them for about 3 minutes, stirring frequently.

Squeeze the zucchini "noodles" between clean towels to absorb the excess moisture. When the shrimp begins to turn pink, add the zucchini to the pan, along with the Creamy Basil Pesto Sauce and the coconut milk. Stir to evenly coat everything with the sauce, and heat the mixture for about another 30 seconds to 1 minute. Sprinkle each serving with the chopped basil.

Oven-Roasted Cod in Coconut Oil with Spinach

SERVES 4

9 ounces fresh spinach leaves

1½ cups matchstick carrots, freshly chopped or purchased precut

2 red onions, sliced into rings

4 8-ounce wild-caught cod fillets, fresh or frozen

12 thin avocado slices

2 teaspoons coconut oil

Juice of 2 lemons

Pinch of fresh or dried dill

Pinch of sea salt

8 to 12 thin lemon slices

Preheat the oven to 350°F.

Layer the spinach in two 8 × 8 oven-safe oiled baking dishes. Spread each layer of spinach with a layer of carrots and red onions. Place the fillets on top of the bed of veggies, pressing them down. Dribble 2 tablespoons of water into each dish if you are using fresh fish. Place 3 avocado slices over each fillet, dab each with ½ teaspoon coconut oil, and sprinkle each with lemon juice, dill, and salt. Top each fillet with 2 to 3 lemon slices. Cover the dishes with foil, and cook them for 15 to 20 minutes, or until the cod is flaky (longer if you are using frozen fish).

Wild-Caught Seafood, Kale, and Zucchini Scramble

SERVES 2

This is the perfect breakfast recipe to use leftover animal protein and to get your veggies in right when the sun comes up. To prepare this recipe easily in the morning, substitute salmon for any fish you have on hand.

8 ounces wild-caught Alaskan cooked salmon or leftovers of any fish of
    your choice

1 large zucchini, cut into thin half moons

4 cups kale, washed and chopped

1 tablespoon coconut oil

Pinch of sea salt

Pinch of ground black pepper

1 large avocado, halved

Heat large pan over medium heat with coconut oil. Add cooked salmon, zucchini, and kale and sauté for about 5 minutes until salmon is crispy and veggies are tender. Add salt and pepper. Mix well and serve hot with a side of avocado.

Saturday Night Sushi

SERVES 2

It can take some practice to make the perfect sushi roll, but no matter what it looks like, it will still taste great! You will need a lot fewer ingredients than you think in order to make your sushi roll tight and compact. There are great videos online to help you learn how to make your Saturday Night Sushi!

6 sheets nori
Flesh of 1 large avocado, mashed
6 ounces smoked salmon
1 mango, thinly sliced
1 cucumber, thinly sliced
3 steamed asparagus spears, sliced in half lengthwise (optional)
3 scallions, sliced in half lengthwise (optional)

Place 1 nori sheet on a sushi mat or cutting board. With a flat spoon, spread the avocado very thinly over the entire surface of the nori sheet. Place a 1-ounce strip of smoked salmon along the bottom edge of the avocado-covered nori sheet. Above the salmon place a couple thin slices of mango across the nori sheet. Then place slices of cucumber above the mango. If you are using them, then place above the cucumber a half-spear of the asparagus and a length of the scallions.

Starting from the bottom, fold the nori over all the ingredients, then roll tightly until you have a compact sushi roll. With a very sharp knife, cut the roll into about 8 pieces. Set them aside and repeat the steps with the remaining ingredients to create more rolls.

Serve the sushi on its own or with a bowl of coconut aminos or Ume Plum Vinaigrette (page 236) for dipping.

Crispy Coconut Shrimp

SERVES 4

Yum! The unsweetened coconut flakes give this shrimp a sweet, nutty crunch!

24 jumbo wild-caught shrimp, peeled and deveined
¼ cup coconut flour
2 to 4 tablespoons coconut oil

3 garlic cloves, minced

⅓ cup unsweetened coconut flakes

In a large bowl, toss the shrimp in the coconut flour to coat each piece well. Set them aside.

Heat the coconut oil in a large pan set over medium heat. Sauté the garlic in the oil until it is slightly browned, then add the shrimp. Cook, flipping each piece, until the shrimp is pink on both sides, then sprinkle them with coconut flakes. Stir to coat well and serve.

Lemon and Mushroom Baked Trout

Serves 4

4 8-ounce wild-caught trout fillets

½ teaspoon sea salt

Pinch of ground black pepper

4 tablespoons coconut oil, plus more for greasing the baking dish

2 shallots, sliced

2 garlic cloves, minced

1-inch piece ginger root, minced

1½ cups sliced mushrooms (eliminate on Yeast Overgrowth / SIBO Dietary Protocol)

Juice of large lemon

4 scallions, sliced

4 teaspoons chopped fresh parsley or cilantro

Place the trout fillets in an oiled glass baking dish. Sprinkle each fillet with salt and pepper, then set them aside.

Preheat the oven to 325°F.

Heat the coconut oil in a pan set over medium heat. Sauté the shallot in the oil for about 30 seconds, then add the garlic and ginger. Cook for another 30 seconds, then add the mushrooms, lemon juice, scallions, and parsley or cilantro. Simmer the mixture until the mushrooms are soft.

Spread the mushroom mixture over each fillet. Bake the trout uncovered for about 20 minutes, or until the fillets are flaky.

Spicy Fish Tacos

Serves 4

We love fish tacos in Austin, Texas! If you like, you can substitute the red onion, avocado, and cilantro with the Tangy Mango Salsa (page 237).

3 wild-caught whitefish fillets
Pinch of sea salt
Pinch of ground black pepper
Juice of 2 limes
1 to 2 tablespoons extra-virgin olive oil
1 garlic clove, minced
¼ teaspoon ground turmeric
8 lettuce or cabbage leaves
½ head red cabbage, cored and thinly sliced
½ red onion, minced
2 avocados, sliced
¼ cup chopped fresh cilantro
1 large lime, cut into wedges, as a garnish

Preheat the oven to 325°F or prepare a grill to cook the fish.

Place the whitefish fillets in a glass baking dish. Sprinkle each with salt and pepper, and drizzle them with the lime juice and olive oil, coating both sides. Top each fillet with garlic and turmeric. Bake or grill the fish for about 20 minutes, or until the fillets are flaky.

To serve, place the lettuce or cabbage leaves on four serving plates and top them with flaked fish, as well as the sliced cabbage, onion, avocado, and cilantro (or Tangy Mango Salsa, if you prefer). Drizzle each plate with extra lime juice and garnish with a lime wedge.

POULTRY, BEEF, PORK, and LAMB

Lemon Garlic Oven-Roasted Chicken

SERVES 6 TO 8

This dish is so simple and definitely a staple on The Myers Way. It's a great recipe to enjoy chicken throughout the week and to make Gut Healing Broth with the leftovers.

1 whole organic, pasture-raised chicken (approximately 5 to 6 pounds), giblets removed
1 to 2 garlic cloves, minced
1 tablespoon extra-virgin olive oil
⅛ teaspoon sea salt
⅛ teaspoon ground black pepper
1 lemon, sliced
2 tablespoons broth (optional)
1 tablespoon apple cider vinegar (optional)

Preheat the oven to 375°F.

Place your chicken on a clean surface and cut slits in the skin, then press into each slit some of the garlic. Drizzle the chicken with olive oil, sprinkle it with salt and pepper, and rub the seasonings in. Insert the lemon slices inside the chicken cavity.

Set the chicken into a baking dish. If desired, pour the broth and vinegar in the bottom of the dish. Roast it for about 1 hour and 30 minutes, or until the chicken is cooked through and has reached 165°F.

Let the chicken cool before removing the meat from the bones. Save the bones to make Gut Healing Broth (page 226).

Chicken Coconut Curry

SERVES 4

This recipe is a favorite among patients, family, and friends. It is a wonderful mix of nutritional vegetables, savory spices, and creamy coconut. For those of you who like to cook in bulk, this is a great recipe to make a lot of and enjoy later.

1 tablespoon extra-virgin olive oil

2 garlic cloves, chopped

1 medium onion, diced

½ tablespoon ground turmeric

½ tablespoon ground cumin

1 tablespoon ground coriander

½ teaspoon onion powder

1 sweet potato, peeled and chopped into ½-inch cubes

2 celery stalks, chopped

½ cup chopped scallions

1 cup water

1 teaspoon sea salt

1 organic, pasture-raised chicken breast, cooked and cut into bite-size
   pieces

1 13.5-ounce can full-fat coconut milk

1 avocado, sliced

Heat a large skillet over medium heat. Coat the pan with the olive oil. When the pan is hot, sauté the garlic until it is slightly browned. Add the onion, and more oil if needed, then cover the pan and let the mixture simmer until the onions are translucent. Stir in the turmeric, cumin, coriander, and onion powder, coating the onions, then add the sweet potato, celery, scallions, water, and salt. Simmer the vegetables until the sweet potatoes are soft. Add the cooked chicken and coconut milk, and continue to simmer to mix the flavors.

Serve topped with slices of avocado.

Sweet Organic Chicken and Spiced Apples

SERVES 2

A great option as you rethink breakfast, but you can still enjoy the sweetness of cinnamon apples in the morning.

2 teaspoons coconut oil
2 cups cooked organic, pasture-raised chicken, cut into bite-size pieces
(you can use leftover Lemon Garlic Oven-Roasted Chicken, page 247)
1 large apple, chopped
¼ teaspoon ground cinnamon
Pinch of ground nutmeg
Pinch of sea salt

Heat the coconut oil in a pan set over medium heat. Add the chicken, apple, cinnamon, nutmeg, and salt. Cook covered for about 5 to 7 minutes until food is warm and apples are soft. Add water if needed to prevent burning.

Organic Herb Roasted Chicken Tenders

SERVES 2 TO 4

These tenders are great for salads the next day. Pop them in the oven while you are making dinner and pack them up for your lunch.

1 pound boneless, skinless organic chicken tenders
1 tablespoon olive oil
Pinch sea salt
Pinch ground black pepper
1 to 2 cloves garlic, minced
1 tablespoon apple cider vinegar

Preheat oven to 350°F. Put chicken tenders in oven safe baking dish and drizzle with olive oil. Sprinkle with salt, pepper, and garlic. Turn to coat all sides of chicken with oil and seasonings. Add apple cider vinegar to bottom of dish and bake in oven for 20 to 25 minutes until chicken reaches 165°F.

Free-Range Organic Chicken and Veggie Scramble

SERVES 4

- 1 pound free-range organic cooked chicken, shredded
- 1 tablespoon coconut oil
- 1 small sweet onion, diced
- 1 zucchini, cut into thin half moons
- 1 yellow squash, cut into thin half moons
- Pinch of sea salt
- Pinch of ground black pepper
- 1 large avocado, halved

Heat large pan over medium heat with coconut oil. Add onions and let cook for 3 minutes. Add zucchini, squash, and chicken and sauté for about 5 minutes until veggies are tender. Add salt and pepper. Mix well and serve hot with a side of avocado.

Loaded Sweet Potatoes

SERVES 4

- 2 medium sweet potatoes
- 1 pound organic, grass-fed ground beef
- ½ sweet onion, chopped
- Sea salt to taste
- 2 garlic cloves, minced
- ½ medium avocado, chopped
- Fresh chopped chives or cilantro leaves

Preheat the oven to 400°F.

Wash the sweet potatoes well with a vegetable brush, then pat them dry. Pierce each potato several times with a fork. Place them on a baking sheet and bake them for 45 minutes. Remove the potatoes from the oven and lower the oven heat to 375°F.

While the potatoes cool, brown the ground beef in a skillet. Add the onion, sautéing it until it's translucent, and add salt to taste. Sprinkle the minced garlic over the meat and onion mixture and continue cooking a few more minutes.

When the sweet potatoes are cool enough to touch, cut them in half lengthwise. Set each sweet potato half faceup in an oiled 10 × 13-inch baking dish.

Scoop the meat mixture on top of each sweet potato half. Bake them for 20 minutes.

To serve, top each sweet potato with chopped avocado and sprinkle with chives or cilantro.

Spicy Turkey Cabbage Wraps

SERVES 2 TO 4

These wraps have a really great flavor. The filling would also be great on a salad or by itself!

8 intact leaves from a head of green cabbage (or substitute any leafy
    greens of your choice)
1 tablespoon coconut oil
1 to 2 garlic cloves, minced
1 teaspoon grated or minced fresh ginger root
1 yellow onion, diced
10 stalks asparagus, cut into bite-size segments
½ pound ground organic, pasture-raised turkey
⅛ teaspoon ground turmeric
Juice of 1 large orange wedge (about 2 tablespoons)
Juice of ½ lime
1 tablespoon chopped fresh basil
1 tablespoon chopped scallions

Try to keep each cabbage leaf intact as you separate them from the head (it is okay if there are some cracks). Wash them and set them aside.

Fill a large pot halfway with water. Begin heating the water over low heat while you prepare the turkey filling.

In a large skillet, heat the coconut oil, then sauté the garlic, ginger, and onion for a few minutes. Add the asparagus and continue to cook for about 3 more minutes, then add the turkey, turmeric, orange juice, and lime juice. When the turkey is almost cooked through, add the basil and scallions. Cook the mixture until the turkey is done, then remove the skillet from the heat.

When the pot of water begins to boil, add a few cabbage leaves using tongs. After about 30 seconds, remove the leaves and arrange them on a serving plate. Fill each cabbage leaf with turkey mixture, roll tightly to enclose filling, and enjoy!

Spicy Chicken and Sausage Gumbo

SERVES 4 TO 6

This is a spin on a classic. It can be made so many different ways. Get creative and feel free to change it up.

1½ pounds organic, pasture-raised chicken or duck, cut into 1- to 2-inch pieces

2½ tablespoons Creole Spice Blend (page 260)

¾ cup coconut flour

5 tablespoons coconut oil

1 sweet onion, diced

5 celery stalks, diced

5 carrots, peeled and diced

6 cups Gut Healing Broth (page 226)

½ pound organic sausage, sliced into ¼-inch slices

1 tablespoon garlic, minced

Sprinkle and rub the chicken with 1½ tablespoons of the Creole Spice Blend.

In a large bowl, stir together the remaining 1 tablespoon of Creole Spice Blend and the coconut flour. Remove about 1 tablespoon of the flour mixture and set it aside for use later. Add the chicken pieces to the remaining flour mixture and shake or stir to coat each chicken piece evenly.

Heat 3 tablespoons of the coconut oil in a large pan. When the oil is hot, carefully place the chicken in the oil and brown the pieces on all sides. As you work, scrape the bottom of the pan to prevent the flour from burning. Add more oil as needed. You may need to cook the chicken in two batches to cook all of it effectively. When it's ready, transfer the cooked chicken to a plate.

Drain the oil from the pan and clean the pan with a paper towel. Heat 2 more tablespoons of the coconut oil in the same pan, then add the onion, celery, and carrots. Sauté the vegetables for 3 to 5 minutes. Add the tablespoon of reserved seasoned flour and cook the vegetables for another 2 to 3 minutes, then add the broth. Bring the mixture to a boil. Add the cooked chicken, sausage, and garlic, and continue to simmer for another 20 minutes, or until the chicken is cooked through.

Slow-Cooked Moroccan Lamb Curry

SERVES 4 TO 6

This dish cooks for 4 to 8 hours in the slow cooker, so prepare in the morning to enjoy for dinner.

- 1½ to 2 pounds organic, grass-fed lamb, cut into 1-inch pieces, or stew meat
- 1 teaspoon sea salt
- 2 to 3 tablespoons coconut oil
- 2 sweet onions, chopped
- 2 garlic cloves, minced
- ½-inch piece ginger root, minced
- 2 teaspoons ground cumin
- 2 teaspoons ground turmeric
- 1 teaspoon ground cinnamon
- 1 bay leaf
- 8 ounces (1 cup) Gut Healing Broth (page 226)
- 1 13.5-ounce can coconut milk
- 6 cups chopped fresh greens (kale, spinach, etc.)
- 2 tablespoons chopped fresh mint, as a garnish

Sprinkle the lamb with salt and place the pieces in a slow cooker.

Heat the coconut oil in a medium pan. Add the onions and garlic, and sauté the mixture for a few minutes. Add the ginger, cumin, turmeric, cinnamon, and bay leaf, and sauté for another 5 minutes, or until some caramelizing appears on the bottom of the pan. Add the broth and coconut milk, and scrape the bottom of the pan with a wooden utensil to deglaze it. Bring the mixture to a boil, then pour it over the lamb in the slow cooker. Cook the lamb on a low setting for about 8 hours or on a high setting for about 4 hours. Stir in the greens about 30 minutes before the lamb is done and cook them until they are soft. Serve the curry garnished with fresh mint.

Creamy Basil Pesto Sauce over Spaghetti Squash

SERVES 4

Spaghetti squash is so easy to make, and you won't even miss your plain old spaghetti! This recipe is great with grass-fed ground beef or organic chicken.

- 1 spaghetti squash, cut in half lengthwise, seeds discarded
- 1 tablespoon coconut oil, plus extra for greasing baking sheet
- 1 pound grass-fed ground beef or 1 pound organic chicken breasts (can use leftover Lemon Garlic Oven-Roasted Chicken, page 247)
- 1 zucchini, grated
- 4 cups fresh spinach
- Creamy Basil Pesto Sauce (page 235)

Preheat the oven to 375°F.

Grease a baking sheet and place each squash half facedown on the sheet. Bake them for about 35 minutes, or until they are soft. Remove the sheet from the oven and turn the squash faceup with tongs or hot pads. Let cool for 10 minutes.

While squash is cooking brown the beef in a medium sized sauce pan or sauté chicken breasts with additional coconut oil until cooked through.

When squash is done, heat the coconut oil in a large pan set over medium heat. Scoop out the flesh of the spaghetti squash with a spoon and add to pan along with the zucchini, the spinach, and the Creamy Basil Pesto Sauce. Stir to combine, heating the mixture for a couple minutes until it is hot. Mix in cooked beef or chicken, then serve.

Variation: Use Olive Tapenade (page 235) instead of Creamy Basil Pesto Sauce.

Seared Grass-Fed Steak and Sweet Potatoes

SERVES 4

This is a spin on the classic meat and potatoes.

- 2 8- to 10-ounce organic, grass-fed steaks
- 2 teaspoons sea salt
- ½ teaspoon ground black pepper
- 2 teaspoons extra-virgin olive oil
- Simply Delicious Baked Sweet Potatoes, double recipe to make 4 full potatoes (1 potato per serving) (page 221)

Let the steaks sit at room temperature for about 30 minutes before cooking them.

Set a medium pan over high heat. Sprinkle the steaks with salt and pepper, and drizzle them with olive oil. Carefully place the steaks into the hot pan and sear them on one side. Wait until the steaks are not sticking to the pan before flipping them to the opposite side, about 3 to 4 minutes. Sear their other sides until they are cooked through to a desired doneness. Remove them from the pan and let them rest a few minutes before serving them with the baked sweet potatoes. Enjoy!

Easy Chicken Lettuce Wraps

SERVES 4 TO 6

There are so many ways to make a good wrap. I recommend taking a container of these sliced ingredients to work and prepping your portion in less than 5 minutes at lunchtime.

> 10 to 12 leaves green or red leaf lettuce, rinsed
> 2 avocados, thinly sliced, or use leftover Zucchini "Noodle" Salad (page 232)
> Lemon Garlic Oven-Roasted Chicken (page 247), boned and shredded
> ½ cup sliced black olives
> 3 cups baby spinach leaves
> ½ red onion, sliced
> ¾ cup matchstick carrots, freshly chopped or purchased precut
> ½ cup broccoli sprouts
> Handful of fresh cilantro or basil leaves
> Squeeze of fresh lemon juice

Lay out the lettuce leaves on a work surface and divide the avocado slices (or the Zucchini "Noodle" Salad) evenly between them. Next, evenly distribute the shredded chicken, olives, spinach, onion, carrots, and broccoli sprouts between each leaf. Top with cilantro or basil, and squeeze a bit of lemon juice on each. Roll tightly to enclose filling and enjoy!

Savory Breakfast Sausage

SERVES 4 (MAKES 8 SAUSAGE PATTIES)

This recipe is a wonderful staple for the program and so easy to make ahead of time so breakfast can be quick!

    1 pound free-range organic ground turkey or chicken
    1 teaspoon garlic, minced
    2 tablespoons red onion, finely chopped
    ¼ teaspoon salt
    ⅛ teaspoon ground mustard
    ⅛ teaspoon cumin
    ¼ teaspoon ground black or white pepper
    2 tablespoons coconut oil
    ¼ cup bone broth or water (optional)

Put meat, garlic, onions, and spices in large mixing bowl. Using your hands, mash ingredients together to incorporate spices well into meat. Form meat into 8 sausage patties.

Heat coconut oil in large pan. Add sausage patties to hot oil and cook for about 5 minutes, flipping to brown all dies. Add broth or water and cook covered for another 3 to 5 minutes until cooked through.

Enjoy fresh or store in fridge or freezer to enjoy later.

Variation: Top with fresh avocado.

Sweet Apple Breakfast Sausage

SERVES 4 (MAKES 8 SAUSAGE PATTIES)

Yum! What a sweet start to your day. Remember, if you want to save time in the morning, these are easy to make beforehand.

    1 pound free-range organic ground turkey or chicken
    ½ teaspoon cinnamon
    ¼ teaspoon nutmeg
    ¼ teaspoon salt
    ½ green apple, finely chopped (optional)
    2 tablespoons coconut oil
    ¼ cup bone broth or water (optional)

Put meat, spices, and apple in large mixing bowl. Using your hands, mash ingredients together to incorporate spices well into meat. Form meat into 8 sausage patties.

Heat coconut oil in large pan. Add sausage patties to hot oil and cook for about 5 minutes, flipping to brown all dies. Add broth or water and cook covered for another 3 to 5 minutes until cooked through.

Enjoy fresh or store in fridge or freezer to enjoy later.

Variation: Top with fresh avocado.

Rosemary and Basil Grass-Fed Burgers/Meatballs

SERVES 4

1 pound organic, grass-fed
ground beef (or use organic, pasture-raised
turkey, chicken, lamb, etc.)
1 teaspoon minced garlic
2 tablespoons finely chopped yellow onion
1½ teaspoons dried rosemary
1½ teaspoons dried basil
¼ teaspoon sea salt
¼ teaspoon ground black pepper
2 tablespoons coconut oil
¼ cup Gut Healing Broth (page 226) or water (optional)

In a large bowl, combine the meat, garlic, onion, rosemary, basil, salt, and pepper. Using your hands, mash the ingredients together to incorporate the spices well into the meat. Form the mixture into 8 patties or 24 meatballs.

Heat the coconut oil in a large pan. Add the patties or meatballs to the hot oil and cook them for about 5 minutes, flipping them to brown all sides. Add the broth or water and simmer them, covered, for another 3 to 5 minutes, or until the patties or meatballs are cooked through.

Enjoy them warm, or store them in the fridge or freezer to enjoy later.

Chinese Spice Slow-Cooked Pork

SERVES 4 TO 6

This dish has really bold flavors that make you want to keep coming back for more. If you are making this dish for dinner, start cooking in your slow cooker earlier in the day.

1½ to 2 pounds boneless organic, grass-fed pork shoulder
Sea salt to taste
Ground black pepper to taste
2 yellow onions, sliced
½ cup coconut aminos (eliminate on Yeast Overgrowth / SIBO Dietary Protocol)
3 garlic cloves, minced
2 teaspoons grated fresh ginger root
4 to 5 teaspoons Chinese Spice (page 260)
4 stalks collard greens, chopped

Season the pork with salt and pepper and place it in a slow cooker on top of the onion slices.

In a small bowl, combine the coconut aminos, garlic, ginger, and Chinese Spice. Pour the mixture over the pork in the slow cooker, then cook the pork for 4 hours on a high setting or 6 hours on a low setting, or until the meat is tender. In the last half hour, add the collard greens to cook until they are soft.

BEVERAGES

Spring Green Veggie Juice

SERVES 2

> 2 cucumbers
> 1 green apple
> 1 lemon or lime
> ½- to 1-inch piece ginger root
> 2 leaves kale
> Fresh herbs: basil, mint, parsley, cilantro, fennel (optional)
> ¼ cup aloe juice (optional)

Juice the cucumbers, apple, lemon or lime, ginger, kale, and optional herbs in a juicer or blend them together in a high-speed blender with some water. If you are using a blender, strain the pulp out with cheesecloth. Stir in the aloe juice before drinking.

Chai Tea Latte

SERVES 1

> 1 tea bag chai tea (Numi Organic Rooibos Chai is one of many options)
> Full-fat coconut milk to taste
> Dash of ground cinnamon

In a mug of your choice, steep the tea bag in boiling water, but leave enough room for the coconut milk. After about 5 minutes, remove the tea bag and add the coconut milk to taste. Top with cinnamon.

SPICES

Creole Spice Blend

MAKES APPROXIMATELY 3 ½ TABLESPOONS

2 teaspoons onion powder

2 teaspoons garlic powder

2 teaspoons dried oregano

2 teaspoons dried basil

¼ teaspoon dried thyme

¼ teaspoon ground black pepper

¼ teaspoon ground white pepper

2 teaspoons sea salt

Mix the herbs and spices together in a small bowl and store in a small glass mason jar.

Chinese Spice

MAKES APPROXIMATELY 4 ½ TEASPOONS

1 teaspoon ground star anise

1 teaspoon ground cinnamon

½ teaspoon ground clove

1¼ teaspoons ground fennel seeds

½ teaspoon sea salt

¼ teaspoon ground black pepper

Mix the spices together in a small bowl and store in a small glass mason jar.

CREATE YOUR OWN RECIPES

Create Your Own Organic Mixed Salad

Salads can be so much more than iceberg lettuce and ranch dressing. Get creative with vibrant colors and enjoy how delicious a salad can be!

Choose Your Greens
- Kale (baby, dinosaur, curly)
- Spinach
- Bok choy
- Mustard greens
- Arugula
- Cabbage
- Romaine lettuce

Choose Your Vegetables
- Cucumber
- Carrots
- Broccoli
- Cauliflower
- Asparagus
- Zucchini
- Yellow squash
- Roasted or grated fresh beets
- Onion
- Scallions
- Avocado (though this one is technically a fruit)
- Celery

Choose Your Protein
- Sliced organic, pasture-raised chicken
- Ground organic, pasture-raised turkey
- Organic, grass-fed ground beef
- Pulled organic, grass-fed pork
- Grilled wild-caught salmon
- Wild-caught sardines

Choose Your Sweetness (Minimal and Optional)
 Apples
 Pears
 Oranges
 Dried unsweetened cranberries
 Dried unsweetened cherries
 Unsweetened coconut flakes

Top with Herbs/Spices
 Cilantro
 Mint
 Parsley
 Basil
 Freshly grated ginger root

Choose Your Dressing
 Ume Plum Vinaigrette (page 236)
 Whipped Avocado and Lemon Dressing (page 237)
 Create Your Own Salad Dressing (below)

Create Your Own Salad Dressing

A note about salad dressings: Use the ratio of three parts oil to one part vinegar.

Choose Your Oil
 Extra-virgin olive oil
 Grapeseed oil
 Avocado oil

Choose Your Vinegar
 Apple cider vinegar
 Ume plum vinegar (eliminate on Yeast Overgrowth / SIBO Dietary
  Protocol)
 Balsamic vinegar (eliminate on Yeast Overgrowth / SIBO Dietary
  Protocol)

Choose Your Juice (Optional)
 Lemon juice
 Lime juice
 Orange juice

Choose Your Seasoning
    Sea salt
    Ground black pepper
    Minced garlic
    Minced onion or shallot
    Fresh herbs (basil, cilantro, mint, parsley)
    Spices (cinnamon, turmeric)

Create Your Own Meal

I know you are busy and sometimes following a recipe doesn't fit into your schedule. Use this guide to create your own meal with lots of nutrition and some of your favorite ingredients!

Choose Your Protein
    Organic, grass-fed beef, lamb, or pork
    Organic, pasture-raised poultry (chicken, turkey, duck)
    Wild-caught seafood (fish, shellfish)
    Wild game

Choose Your Vegetables
    Leafy greens (kale, spinach, collards, etc.)
    Green veggies (asparagus, broccoli, etc.)
    Colorful veggies (red cabbage, carrots, beets, etc.)
    See comprehensive approved vegetable list for more ideas
        (pages 180–81)

Choose Your Starch
    Sweet potatoes
    Butternut squash
    Acorn squash
    Kabocha squash
    Spaghetti squash

Choose Your Fat
    Coconut oil
    Olive oil
    Avocado
    Olives

SNACK IDEAS

Smoked salmon served with avocado

A cup of leftover soup

Crispy Kale Chips (page 225)

Spring Green Veggie Juice (page 259)

Veggies and Super Guacamole (page 236)

Chicken and Super Guacamole (page 236)

Leftover Roasted Wild-Caught Salmon with Tangy Mango Salsa (page 238)

Roasted Veggies (page 224)

Crispy Sweet Potato Fries (page 222)

DESSERTS

Coconut Cream Mousse

SERVES 2

1 13.5-ounce can coconut milk, chilled in the fridge overnight

Pinch of ground cinnamon, or more to taste

Pinch of sea salt

Stevia to taste (optional)

Skim off the top layer that has thickened into coconut cream from the chilled can of milk and place into a medium bowl, leaving behind the watery layer in the bottom of the can. Using a hand whisk or an electric mixer, beat the coconut cream into a desired texture.

With a spoon, fold into the whipped coconut cream the cinnamon, salt, and stevia. Divide the mousse between two serving bowls. Enjoy!

Variation: To make Coconut Cream Chocolate Mousse fold 1 tablespoon unsweetened cacao powder, or more to taste, to coconut cream with cinnamon, salt, and optional stevia.

Coconut Cream Berry Parfait

SERVES 2

You'll love starting your day with this refreshing and satisfying parfait. To save time in the morning make the Coconut Cream Mousse beforehand and store in the fridge.

Coconut Cream Mousse (page 264)
½ cup organic mixed berries (raspberries, blueberries, blackberries, strawberries)
1 tablespoon unsweetened coconut flakes

Top Coconut Cream Mousse with berries and coconut flakes.

Cinnamon Apple Crisp

SERVES 4 TO 6

2 tablespoons coconut oil, melted or very soft, plus more for greasing the baking dish
4 to 5 apples, peeled and sliced into thin wedges
Juice of 1 lemon
¾ teaspoon ground cinnamon, divided
¼ teaspoon sea salt, divided
½ cup coconut flour
¼ cup unsweetened coconut flakes
4 dried dates, pitted and chopped

Preheat the oven to 350°F.

Grease an 8 × 8-inch baking dish with coconut oil. In a medium bowl, stir together the apples, lemon juice, ¼ teaspoon of the cinnamon, and ⅛ teaspoon of the salt. Spread the apple mixture in the baking dish.

In a food processor or a high-speed blender, combine the coconut flour, coconut flakes, remaining ½ teaspoon of cinnamon, remaining ⅛ teaspoon of salt, dates, and the 2 tablespoons of coconut oil. Sprinkle the mixture over the apple mixture in the baking dish. Cover the dish with foil and bake for about 45 minutes, or until the apples are soft, then uncover the dish and bake it for another 10 minutes, or until the topping is crispy.

Variation: Top each serving of the Cinnamon Apple Crisp with Coconut Cream Mousse (page 264).

Banana Cream Mini Cake Bites

MAKES ABOUT 12 MINI CAKES

Sometimes you need something sweet and want to sink into a soft, chewy treat. These cake bites are sweetened with banana, coconut, and cinnamon. Enjoy one or two with a hot Chai Tea Latte (page 259).

1 ripe banana, mashed

2 teaspoons coconut oil, plus extra to grease the baking sheet

¾ cup canned coconut milk

2 teaspoons water

1 tablespoon coconut butter or manna

⅓ cup coconut flour

1 teaspoon vanilla extract

1 teaspoon ground cinnamon

Pinch of sea salt

Preheat the oven to 350°F.

Mix all the ingredients in a large bowl. Spoon 1-inch drops of the dough onto a greased baking sheet and bake them for about 12 minutes.

KITCHEN EQUIPMENT

Recommended

- meat thermometer
- high-speed blender
- food processer
- spiral slicer or julienne peeler

Optional

- juicer (citrus and vegetable juicers)
- steamer basket
- sushi mat

THE MYERS WAY AUTOIMMUNE SOLUTION
THIRTY-DAY MEAL PLAN FOR TWO

Remember that this meal plan is based on the idea that you will be cooking for two people, so each meal accounts for two servings to be enjoyed. Feel free to adjust to fit your family's needs. If you are cooking for one, simply cut in half the number of servings you are instructed to make. That still leaves you plenty of leftovers. I recommend doing your Prep Day on a Saturday, and having Sunday be your Day 1, since there is somewhat more cooking involved on Day 1 than on the other days of the week. That way, you get plenty of leftovers on Day 1 to cut down on cooking time during your workweek.

THE MYERS WAY RECIPE	Enjoy Leftovers	Number of Servings to Make	Number of Servings to Save in the Fridge
PREP DAY			
Lemon Garlic Oven-Roasted Chicken		6 to 8	4 to 6
Gut Healing Broth		16	16
Sweet Apple Breakfast Sausage		4	4
DAY 1			
Breakfast			
Sweet Apple Breakfast Sausage	✓		
Hearty Sweet Potato Hash		4	2
Spring Green Veggie Juice		2	
Lunch			
Organic Citrus Kale Salad with Cranberries		2	
Organic Farm Five-Veggie Soup		4	2
Dinner			
Creamy Basil Pesto Sauce over Spaghetti Squash		4	2
½ cup organic mixed berries		2	
DAY 2			
Breakfast			
Sweet Apple Breakfast Sausage	✓		
Hearty Sweet Potato Hash	✓		
Gut Healing Broth	✓		
Chai Tea Latte or decaf green tea		2	

THE MYERS WAY RECIPE	Enjoy Left-overs	Number of Servings to Make	Number of Servings to Save in the Fridge
Lunch			
Creamy Basil Pesto Sauce over Spaghetti Squash	✓		
Dinner			
Roasted Wild-Caught Salmon with Tangy Mango Salsa		4	2
Sautéed Organic Mixed Greens with Garlic		2	
Simple Organic Roasted Asparagus		2	
DAY 3			
Breakfast			
Roasted Wild-Caught Salmon with Tangy Mango Salsa	✓		
Spring Green Veggie Juice		2	
Gut Healing Broth	✓		
Lunch			
Tropical Nicaraguan Salad		2	
Organic Farm Five-Veggie Soup	✓		
Dinner			
Organic Baby Kale and Spinach Salad with Rosemary and Basil Grass-Fed Burgers		4	2
Creamy Acorn Squash		4	2
½ cup organic mixed berries		2	
DAY 4			
Breakfast			
Savory Breakfast Sausage		4	2
Coconut Cream Berry Parfait		2	
Gut Healing Broth	✓		
Lunch			
Organic Baby Kale and Spinach Salad with Rosemary and Basil Grass-Fed Burgers	✓		
Creamy Acorn Squash	✓		
Dinner			
Spicy Fish Tacos		4	2
Brussels Sprouts with Dark Organic Cherries		2	
DAY 5			
Breakfast			
Wild-Caught Seafood, Kale, and Zucchini Scramble		2	
Gut Healing Broth	✓		

THE MYERS WAY RECIPE	Enjoy Left-overs	Number of Servings to Make	Number of Servings to Save in the Fridge
Lunch			
Arugula, Blood Orange, and Fennel Salad		2	
Dinner			
Chicken Coconut Curry		4	2
Cauliflower "Pilaf"		4	2
½ cup organic mixed berries		2	
Food Preparation			
Freeze any remaining Gut Healing Broth			
DAY 6			
Breakfast			
Savory Breakfast Sausage	✓		
Hearty Sweet Potato Hash		4	2
Lunch			
Chicken Coconut Curry	✓		
Cauliflower "Pilaf"	✓		
Dinner			
Wild-Caught Halibut with Caramelized Sweet Onions		2	
Organic Broccolini with Garlic and Lemon		2	
Sautéed Organic Mixed Greens with Garlic		2	
DAY 7			
Breakfast			
Sweet Apple Breakfast Sausage		4	2
Hearty Sweet Potato Hash	✓		
Spring Green Veggie Juice		2	
Chai Tea Latte or decaf green tea		2	
Lunch			
Clean Cobb Salad		2	
Simple Organic Roasted Asparagus		2	
Dinner			
Creamy Basil Pesto Sauce over Spaghetti Squash		4	2
Gut Healing Broth		16	16
½ cup organic mixed berries		2	
Food Preparation			
Put Gut Healing Broth in the slow cooker to make overnight.			

THE MYERS WAY RECIPE	Enjoy Left-overs	Number of Servings to Make	Number of Servings to Save in the Fridge
DAY 8			
Breakfast			
Sweet Apple Breakfast Sausage	✓		
Coconut Cream Berry Parfait		2	
Gut Healing Broth	✓		
Chai Tea Latte or decaf green tea		2	
Lunch			
Creamy Basil Pesto Sauce over Spaghetti Squash	✓		
Dinner			
Thai Green Curry with Shrimp		4	2
Organic Broccolini with Garlic and Lemon		2	
DAY 9			
Breakfast			
Savory Breakfast Sausage		4	2
Hearty Sweet Potato Hash		4	2
Gut Healing Broth	✓		
Chai Tea Latte or decaf green tea		2	
Lunch			
Thai Green Curry with Shrimp	✓		
Dinner			
Chinese Spice Slow-Cooked Pork		4	2
Cauliflower "Pilaf"		4	2
Food Preparation			
Put Chinese Spice Slow-Cooked Pork in slow cooker in the morning for dinner.			
DAY 10			
Breakfast			
Savory Breakfast Sausage	✓		
Coconut Cream Berry Parfait		2	
Gut Healing Broth	✓		
Lunch			
Chinese Spice Slow-Cooked Pork	✓		
Cauliflower "Pilaf"	✓		
Dinner			
Spicy Turkey Cabbage Wraps		4	2
Zucchini "Noodle" Salad		2	

THE MYERS WAY RECIPE	Enjoy Left-overs	Number of Servings to Make	Number of Servings to Save in the Fridge
DAY 11			
Breakfast			
Sweet Apple Breakfast Sausage		4	2
Hearty Sweet Potato Hash	✓		
Gut Healing Broth	✓		
Lunch			
Spicy Turkey Cabbage Wraps	✓		
Zucchini "Noodle" Salad or Create Your Own Organic Mixed Salad		2	
Dinner			
Sweet Citrus Salmon Salad		2	
Brussels Sprouts with Dark Organic Cherries		2	
Food Preparation			
Freeze any remaining Gut Healing Broth			
DAY 12			
Breakfast			
Wild-Caught Seafood, Kale, and Zucchini Scramble		2	
Lunch			
Organic Citrus Kale Salad with Cranberries		2	
Dinner			
Garlic Oven-Roasted Cabbage		4	2
DAY 13			
Breakfast			
Sweet Apple Breakfast Sausage	✓		
Coconut Cream Berry Parfait		2	
Lunch			
Tropical Nicaraguan Salad		2	
Dinner			
Organic Baby Kale and Spinach Salad with Rosemary and Basil Grass-Fed Burgers		2	
Crispy Sweet Potato Fries		2	
DAY 14			
Breakfast			
Free-Range Organic Chicken and Veggie Scramble		2	
Chai Tea Latte or decaf green tea		2	

THE MYERS WAY RECIPE	Enjoy Left-overs	Number of Servings to Make	Number of Servings to Save in the Fridge
Lunch			
Creamy Pesto "Pasta" with Shrimp		4	2
Simple Organic Roasted Asparagus		2	
Dinner			
Slow-Cooked Moroccan Lamb Curry		4	2
Roasted Kabocha Squash with Cinnamon		4	2
½ cup organic mixed berries		2	
Food Preparation			
Put Slow-Cooked Moroccan Lamb Curry in slow cooker in the morning for dinner.			
DAY 15			
Breakfast			
Free-Range Organic Chicken and Veggie Scramble	✓		
Roasted Kabocha Squash with Cinnamon	✓		
Lunch			
Spicy Fish Tacos		4	2
Cucumber Seaweed Salad		2	
Dinner			
Creamy Pesto "Pasta" with Shrimp	✓		
Simple Organic Roasted Asparagus		2	
DAY 16			
Breakfast			
Slow-Cooked Moroccan Lamb Curry	✓		
Lunch			
Spicy Fish Tacos	✓		
Cucumber Seaweed Salad or Create Your Own Organic Mixed Salad		2	
Dinner			
Lemon Garlic Oven-Roasted Chicken		6 to 8	
Grandma's Hearty Chicken "Noodle" Soup		4	2
Gut Healing Broth		16	16
Food Preparation			
Use Lemon Garlic Oven-Roasted Chicken for Grandma's Hearty Chicken "Noodle" Soup.			

THE MYERS WAY RECIPE	Enjoy Left-overs	Number of Servings to Make	Number of Servings to Save in the Fridge
DAY 17			
Breakfast			
Grandma's Hearty Chicken "Noodle" Soup	✓		
Chai Tea Latte or decaf green tea		2	
Lunch			
Cilantro Salmon Stuffed Avocado		2	
Arugula, Blood Orange, and Fennel Salad		2	
Dinner			
Creamy Basil Pesto Sauce over Spaghetti Squash		4	2
Crispy Kale Chips		2	
½ cup organic mixed berries		2	
DAY 18			
Breakfast			
Savory Breakfast Sausage		4	2
Coconut Cream Berry Parfait		2	
Gut Healing Broth	✓		
Lunch			
Clean Cobb Salad		2	
Dinner			
Spicy Chicken and Sausage Gumbo		4	2
Organic Broccolini with Garlic and Lemon		2	
DAY 19			
Breakfast			
Savory Breakfast Sausage	✓		
Coconut Cream Berry Parfait		2	
Gut Healing Broth	✓		
Lunch			
Spicy Chicken and Sausage Gumbo	✓		
Organic Broccolini with Garlic and Lemon		2	
Dinner			
Wild-Caught Halibut with Caramelized Sweet Onions		4	2
Creamy Butternut Squash Soup with Cinnamon		4	2

THE MYERS WAY RECIPE	Enjoy Left-overs	Number of Servings to Make	Number of Servings to Save in the Fridge
DAY 20			
Breakfast			
Sweet Apple Breakfast Sausage		4	2
Creamy Butternut Squash Soup with Cinnamon	✓		
Gut Healing Broth	✓		
Chai Tea Latte or decaf green tea		2	
Lunch			
Wild-Caught Halibut with Caramelized Sweet Onions	✓		
Organic Citrus Kale Salad with Cranberries		2	
Dinner			
Tropical Nicaraguan Salad		2	
Brussels Sprouts with Dark Organic Cherries		2	
Cinnamon Apple Crisp		4	2
DAY 21			
Breakfast			
Sweet Apple Breakfast Sausage	✓		
Hearty Sweet Potato Hash		4	2
Spring Green Veggie Juice		2	
Gut Healing Broth	✓		
Lunch			
Lemon Garlic Oven-Roasted Chicken		6 to 8	4 to 6
Clean Cobb Salad		2	
Organic Farm Five-Veggie Soup		4	2
Gut Healing Broth		16	16
Dinner			
Saturday Night Sushi		2	
Crispy Coconut Shrimp		4	2
Roasted Veggies		4	2
Food Preparation			
Use last weeks remaining Gut Healing Broth for Organic Farm Five-Veggie Soup.			
DAY 22			
Breakfast			
Cinnamon Apple Crisp	✓		
Spring Green Veggie Juice		2	
Gut Healing Broth	✓		

THE MYERS WAY RECIPE	Enjoy Left-overs	Number of Servings to Make	Number of Servings to Save in the Fridge
Lunch			
Artichokes with Ume Plum Vinaigrette		4	2
Arugula, Blood Orange, and Fennel Salad		2	
Dinner			
Chicken Coconut Curry		4	2
Artichokes with Ume Plum Vinaigrette	✓		
DAY 23			
Breakfast			
Savory Breakfast Sausage		4	2
Coconut Summer Squash		2	
Gut Healing Broth	✓		
Chai Tea Latte or decaf green tea		2	
Lunch			
Chicken Coconut Curry	✓		
Organic Citrus Kale Salad with Cranberries or Create Your Own Organic Mixed Salad		2	
Dinner			
Loaded Sweet Potatoes		4	2
Organic Farm Five-Veggie Soup	✓		
DAY 24			
Breakfast			
Savory Breakfast Sausage	✓		
Coconut Cream Berry Parfait		2	
Gut Healing Broth	✓		
Lunch			
Loaded Sweet Potatoes	✓		
Zucchini "Noodle" Salad or Create Your Own Organic Mixed Salad		2	
Dinner			
Cilantro Salmon Stuffed Avocado		2	
Simple Organic Roasted Asparagus		2	
DAY 25			
Breakfast			
Sweet Apple Breakfast Sausage		4	2
Hearty Sweet Potato Hash		4	2
Gut Healing Broth	✓		

THE MYERS WAY RECIPE	Enjoy Left-overs	Number of Servings to Make	Number of Servings to Save in the Fridge
Lunch			
Tropical Nicaraguan Salad		2	
Dinner			
Chinese Spice Slow-Cooked Pork		4	2
Cauliflower "Pilaf"		4	2
Food Preparation			
Put Chinese Spice Slow-Cooked Pork in slow cooker in the morning for dinner.			
DAY 26			
Breakfast			
Sweet Apple Breakfast Sausage	✓		
Hearty Sweet Potato Hash	✓		
Spring Green Veggie Juice		2	
Lunch			
Chinese Spice Slow-Cooked Pork	✓		
Cauliflower "Pilaf"	✓		
Dinner			
Spicy Fish Tacos		4	2
Cucumber Seaweed Salad		2	
½ cup organic mixed berries		2	
DAY 27			
Breakfast			
Savory Breakfast Sausage		4	2
Coconut Cream Berry Parfait		2	
Chai Tea Latte or decaf green tea		2	
Lunch			
Spicy Fish Tacos	✓		
Cucumber Seaweed Salad or Create Your Own Organic Mixed Salad		2	
Dinner			
Seared Grass-Fed Steak and Sweet Potatoes		4	2
Sautéed Organic Mixed Greens with Garlic		2	
Banana Cream Mini Cake Bites		12	8
Food Preparation			
Enjoy Banana Cream Mini Cake Bites over the next couple days.			

THE MYERS WAY RECIPE	Enjoy Left-overs	Number of Servings to Make	Number of Servings to Save in the Fridge
DAY 28			
Breakfast			
Seared Grass-Fed Steak and Sweet Potatoes	✓		
Spring Green Veggie Juice		2	
Lunch			
Lemon Garlic Oven-Roasted Chicken		6 to 8	4 to 6
Easy Chicken Lettuce Wraps		4	2
Organic Broccolini with Garlic and Lemon		2	
Gut Healing Broth		16	16
Dinner			
Saturday Night Sushi		2	
Oven-Roasted Cod in Coconut Oil with Spinach		4	2
Cucumber Seaweed Salad		2	
DAY 29			
Breakfast			
Wild-Caught Seafood, Kale, and Zucchini Scramble		2	
Spring Green Veggie Juice		2	
Gut Healing Broth	✓		
Lunch			
Easy Chicken Lettuce Wraps	✓		
Dinner			
Organic Baby Kale and Spinach Salad with Rosemary and Basil Grass-Fed Burgers		2	
DAY 30			
Breakfast			
Savory Breakfast Sausage	✓		
Hearty Sweet Potato Hash		4	2
Gut Healing Broth	✓		
Chai Tea Latte or decaf green tea		2	
Lunch			
Arugula, Blood Orange, and Fennel Salad		2	
Dinner			
Creamy Basil Pesto Sauce over Spaghetti Squash		4	2
Brussels Sprouts with Dark Organic Cherries		2	

THE MYERS WAY AUTOIMMUNE SOLUTION SEVEN-DAY SEAFOOD MEAL PLAN FOR TWO

This meal plan was created for those of you who are not currently eating meat and is loosely designed for two people; thus two servings per meal are accounted for here. If you are doing the program by yourself make half the number of servings instructed in this chart. Enjoy flexibility to make it your own! I recommend prepping on a Saturday and beginning the first day on a Sunday.

THE MYERS WAY RECIPE	Enjoy Left-overs	Number of Servings to Make	Number of Servings to Save in the Fridge
PREP DAY			
Creamy Butternut Squash Soup with Cinnamon		4 to 6	4
Chicken Coconut Curry without chicken		4	4
DAY 1			
Breakfast			
Coconut Cream Berry Parfait		2	
Spring Green Veggie Juice		2	
Chai Tea Latte or decaf green tea		2	
Lunch			
Organic Citrus Kale Salad with Cranberries		2	
Chicken Coconut Curry without chicken	✓		2
Dinner			
Lemon and Mushroom Baked Trout		4	2
Organic Broccolini with Garlic and Lemon		2	
DAY 2			
Breakfast			
Wild-Caught Seafood, Kale, and Zucchini Scramble		2	
Creamy Butternut Squash Soup with Cinnamon	✓		2
Lunch			
Lemon and Mushroom Baked Trout	✓		
Organic Citrus Kale Salad with Cranberries		2	

THE MYERS WAY RECIPE	Enjoy Left-overs	Number of Servings to Make	Number of Servings to Save in the Fridge
Dinner			
Wild-Caught Halibut with Caramelized Sweet Onions		4	2
Sautéed Organic Mixed Greens with Garlic		4	2
Spiced Butternut Squash with Turmeric		2	
DAY 3			
Breakfast			
Chicken Coconut Curry without chicken	✓		
Lunch			
Wild-Caught Halibut with Caramelized Sweet Onions	✓		
Creamy Butternut Squash Soup with Cinnamon	✓		
Sautéed Organic Mixed Greens with Garlic	✓		
Dinner			
Creamy Pesto "Pasta" with Shrimp		4	2
½ cup organic mixed berries		2	
DAY 4			
Breakfast			
Coconut Cream Berry Parfait		2	
Spring Green Veggie Juice		2	
Lunch			
Creamy Pesto "Pasta" with Shrimp	✓		
Dinner			
Roasted Wild-Caught Salmon with Tangy Mango Salsa		4	2
Twice-Baked Perfect Sweet Potatoes with Cinnamon and Nutmeg		2	
Simple Organic Roasted Asparagus		2	
DAY 5			
Breakfast			
Coconut Cream Berry Parfait		2	
Spring Green Veggie Juice		2	
Lunch			
Roasted Wild-Caught Salmon with Tangy Mango Salsa	✓		
Tropical Nicaraguan Salad		2	

THE MYERS WAY RECIPE	Enjoy Left-overs	Number of Servings to Make	Number of Servings to Save in the Fridge
Dinner			
Oven-Roasted Cod in Coconut Oil with Spinach		4	2
Cauliflower "Pilaf"		4	2
DAY 6			
Breakfast			
Wild-Caught Seafood, Kale, and Zucchini Scramble		2	
Lunch			
Oven-Roasted Cod in Coconut Oil with Spinach	✓		
Cauliflower "Pilaf"	✓		
Dinner			
Crispy Coconut Shrimp		4	2
Arugula, Blood Orange, and Fennel Salad		2	
Cinnamon Apple Crisp		4	2
DAY 7			
Breakfast			
Coconut Cream Berry Parfait		2	
Spring Green Veggie Juice		2	
Chai Tea Latte or decaf green tea		2	
Lunch			
Spicy Fish Tacos		4	2
Artichokes with Ume Plum Vinaigrette		2	
Dinner			
Saturday Night Sushi		2	
Cucumber Seaweed Salad		2	

Part Four

Live the Solution

CHAPTER 10

The Myers Way as a Way of Life

YOU'RE EXCITED ABOUT all the great results from your new diet, which has left you feeling better than you have in years. Yet Thanksgiving is coming up, and you just know the table will be loaded with gluten, grains, and legumes, not to mention sugar and alcohol. At this point you're not even tempted by the foods you know would derail you. But how do you handle all those relatives who will want you to taste their treats?

One of the things you enjoy most is going out with your colleagues on Friday after work and blowing off steam about everything that went on that week. You don't want to give up this social time, and you also don't want to draw attention to yourself, your health, and your special diet. What should you do?

You've been doing great on The Myers Way so far—you've cleaned up your kitchen, prepared lots of great lunches to bring to work, and even found a few favorite restaurants where you know what to order. But now you're about to go on a business trip or a vacation with your family, and you can't be sure what will be available. How do you travel on The Myers Way?

LIVE THE SOLUTION

Here's the great news about The Myers Way: Once you start following this way of life, you feel so terrific, you have tons of motivation to keep going. Your symptoms fade and, in many cases, they disappear entirely. Your energy returns. You feel vibrant and healthy. You look radiant—getting rid of inflammation makes your skin glow, makes your hair grow thicker, and often helps you lose weight. Many of my patients tell me they feel better than they have in years—maybe in their whole lives. They're thrilled about getting off their medications. And they soon get used to hearing—sometimes frequently—"What have you been doing? You look terrific!"

One of the first things you'll notice is that it isn't willpower keeping you on The Myers Way; it's simple cause and effect. Once you see how great you feel and how good you look, those inflammatory foods simply lose their appeal. Many of my patients tell me they don't even "see" inflammatory foods anymore—they register immediately that the food has gluten or dairy or something else they know will bring their symptoms back, and it's as though the food disappears from their line of vision. It's simply not on their list of possibilities now, the way putting ketchup on ice cream wasn't on their list of possibilities before—not something they try to resist but something they don't even want.

I had that experience myself the other day. I was out for lunch with a group of friends, and a few of them decided to get a chocolate dessert—one of those molten cakes, topped with a big mound of whipped cream. I'll be honest with you. Before The Myers Way, this would have been my downfall, because I love chocolate, and I used to love cake. Who doesn't?

After the dessert arrived, my friends dug in, exclaiming with joy over the luscious treat. Then they stopped suddenly and looked at me.

"Oh, Amy, we're so sorry," one of them said. "We just weren't thinking."

It actually took me a few moments to realize what they were talking about. I had glanced at the food, registered "gluten, sugar, dairy," and just stopped thinking about it. I didn't have to resist temptation; I really wasn't tempted. If I had thought about the cake at all, I would have had an immediate flash of what it would feel like for my symptoms to return, and then I *really* wouldn't have been tempted.

Honestly, I didn't even get that far. If I want a chocolate treat, I can have a square or two of an 90 percent dark chocolate bar (which you too can consider after you have progressed on The Myers Way), or I can make my special mousse of whipped coconut milk, cinnamon, and cacao—mmmm! (Of course I've included the recipe on page 264 for you to enjoy as well!) But I really wasn't tempted by my friends' inflammatory dessert, any more than I'd have been tempted by . . . well, ketchup on ice cream. It simply didn't appeal to me.

If you're reading these pages in your early days on The Myers Way, these words may seem hard to believe, but trust me, they're true. The rewards of losing your symptoms and feeling terrific are the best motivation ever. And once you're eating in a way that supports your body instead of punishing it, you won't even need "motivation." Eating healthily will simply be what you naturally feel like doing.

WHEN TEMPTATION STRIKES . . .

Now, having said all that, I'm going to turn around and admit that I too sometimes want foods that are not perfectly healthy. Maybe I'm not tempted to order a sugary, gluten- and dairy-filled dessert, but there are times I want something sweet or salty or crunchy or starchy. After all, I'm only human!

So here's my secret for handling those times: *Find something to eat that satisfies you but does not completely derail you.*

Let me be perfectly clear: I'm not talking about your first thirty days on The Myers Way. For that first month you really do need to follow the eating plan 100 percent, because even a tiny deviation could cause your immune system to go off the rails again. If you have an autoimmune condition or are high on the spectrum, your body is by definition highly inflamed. Your number-one priority is to bring that inflammation down, and because of the way your body's chemistry works, even small amounts of inflammatory food can completely derail the process.

For many of you, thirty days may be enough to right the balance and give you a little leeway: some sugar, some gluten-free grains, maybe a little caffeine. For many others, you might need longer than thirty days, especially if your symptoms have been severe, you suffer from multiple conditions, or you've had your autoimmune condition for a few years. When your symptoms have been gone for a few months, if you want to experiment a little, then you might try adding some foods back in. Check out the bonus chapter on my website to find out how, because there's a healthy way and a dangerous way to go about reintroducing foods, and I want you to stay safe and healthy.

Just to be clear, no matter how healthy you feel, I never want you eating gluten or dairy, and I never want you consuming high amounts of caffeine, sugar, alcohol, salt, grains, or legumes. The resulting inflammation is likely to start your symptoms right back up again and might even bring on a second or third autoimmune condition.

The challenge is that you won't necessarily feel the difference right away. I had a patient whose thyroid antibodies had shot up, and neither of us could figure out why. Then she said, "Oh, wait a minute, I had a vegan cookie the other day. Would that be the reason?" Well, yeah. Unless it was labeled "gluten-free," that cookie was surely made with wheat or some other gluten-bearing grain. My patient couldn't *feel* that her thyroid antibodies had just risen to a significantly higher level, but I could measure that change in her blood, and I knew those gluten-triggered antibodies were at that very moment instructing her immune system to destroy her thyroid, not to mention putting her at risk for developing other autoimmune conditions.

Most of the time this patient was perfectly satisfied on The Myers Way. Every so often she craved something else. So I told her what I just told you: Find something to eat that satisfies you but does not completely derail you. Unfortunately, that little bit of wheat in the vegan cookie was enough to derail her. If she occasionally had a gluten-free cookie, she probably would have been fine.

JOIN THE MYERS WAY FAMILY!

I'm excited to continue building The Myers Way family and to have my patients and readers share information with each other while continuing to stay in touch with me. If you'd like to be part of a supportive community where you can share stories, ask questions, get advice, and hear big cheers for all your progress, please join us at AmyMyersMD.com.

MAKE IT A FAMILY AFFAIR

I love the name "The Myers Way," because I really do see this approach to eating as a way of life. If you can make The Myers Way a way of life not only for yourself but also for the people you live with, you'll find it easier to stay on your eating plan—and your loved ones will all get a lot healthier. The Myers Way can help with all sorts of symptoms: brain fog, anxiety, depression, acne, headaches, migraines, indigestion, acid reflux, irritable bowel syndrome, PMS, menopausal issues, joint pain, and seasonal allergies, as well as a host of other low-grade miseries that most people have simply learned to live with. They don't have to, though. Just turn down that inflammatory heat, and watch your body respond with gratitude, energy, and vibrant, glowing health.

The Myers Way is also a terrific way to lose weight and keep the weight off once you've lost it. As you saw earlier, inflammation induces weight gain, and excess body fat is inflammatory. The Myers Way can help break that vicious cycle, rewarding your discipline with the healthy body and the healthy weight you've always wanted.

So, if possible, get the other people in your household to do The Myers Way with you. Make it a family affair, so you can all support each other. If one of your children needs the support of The Myers Way and the others don't, putting them all on the same diet eliminates a lot of bickering, and it's definitely easier for you to prepare just one set of meals. You eliminate the chance for one kid to say, "How come *he* gets to have that ice cream and I don't?" You also eliminate the possibility of cross-contamination, where you pick up some gluten from the pot someone else made pasta in or get exposed to some dairy from another person's butter knife. If The Myers Way becomes a family project, the whole family gets both healthier and closer. Added benefits: Both you and your children will enjoy increased athletic performance, better brain function, healthy weights, and way less acne!

Of course if your family doesn't want to come along for the ride, let them get there in their own time. You need to do this for *you*, which means you need to let other people do what's right for them. A lot of the time, though, spouses, girlfriends, and boyfriends want to support their partners and parents want to support their children. If you all do The Myers Way together, you have a great home base.

KNOW YOUR OWN BOUNDARIES

I'm betting that you'll get a lot of positive reinforcement from your loved ones, and most of the time what you'll hear is "You look terrific! What have you been doing?"

Sometimes, though, you might hear statements like the following:

"Oh, come on. One little bite of ice cream isn't going to hurt you!"

"Why can't I make your child a sandwich? He loves my sandwiches!"

"You have to at least *taste* Aunt Sarah's stuffing or her feelings will be hurt."

"Ever since you started doing this new diet, there's nowhere we can go to eat without you making a whole big deal about it."

Sound familiar? For your sake, I hope not, but most of us meet at least some resistance along the way. I get it, believe me. Nobody wants to feel like a picky eater.

However, this is a health issue for you—or, if you're reading this book as a parent, it's a health issue for your child. And in my book, health comes first. You've seen firsthand the misery autoimmune symptoms can bring, and now you also know that you're three times more likely to develop a second autoimmune condition after you have the first. If other people don't want to believe you, that's their right, but you still need to stand strong and stick to the choices you know are healthiest for you.

One of the things that makes me saddest is hearing about parents of autoimmune kids whose own parents don't support them. My patients tell me stories about grandparents who insist on bringing cookies or making sandwiches or giving yogurt to their autoimmune grandchild, or who say in front of the child, "I don't see why you're being so strict. Every child deserves a treat once in a while."

This isn't an easy situation, but giving in is *not* the solution. Figure out how to set your boundaries and stick to them, knowing that you, as the parent, have to decide what's best for your child.

What if you're the one with the autoimmune condition and someone in your life is just not sensitive to your decision to follow The Myers Way? What if they're always saying "Hey, let's go out for pizza!" when they know you can't join them or leaving tempting gluten-filled treats around the house or teasing you about your diet, especially when other people are around?

That's also a tough situation. If you can just say no, good for you. If you need some help setting boundaries, maybe you'd like to find a life coach, counselor, or therapist who can support you in standing up for yourself, your health, and your right to respect. You might find a way to set boundaries and still maintain a close relationship with the "challenging" person. Or maybe you'll decide that it's a toxic relationship you choose to let go of along with the gluten and the sugar.

Let me just remind you that stress and painful situations raise your inflammation just as much as dairy and alcohol (see chapter 7 for reinforcement!), and your first responsibility is to protect your own health. If someone chooses not to follow The Myers Way with you, that's one thing. If they're repeatedly sabotaging your efforts, that's something else entirely.

KEEP YOUR EYES ON THE PRIZE

"Why can't you just follow your regular doctor's advice?"

That's one my patients hear a lot, and believe me, I understand that one too. Even though I'm a physician myself, my relatives don't always understand why I've taken such a "contrary" view. With conventional medicine dismissing the impact of diet and elevating the value of medication, sometimes you feel like that little boy in the crowd full of cheering citizens, a lone voice shouting, "But the emperor has no clothes!"

Well, you already know my opinion about that. I'm willing to be a minority voice, especially because I believe that someday soon this approach will become standard, even in conventional medicine. Meanwhile, I believe that health decisions are very personal, and none of us can ever say what another person should do. Even I can only tell my patients what I think is best for them; what they actually do is up to them.

So if this book resonates with you and you want to give this approach a try, no one has any business getting in your way. Let them raise their objections and ask their questions one time. Then they need to keep quiet and respect your decision. If they can't—if you experience their questions or concerns as sabotaging your commitment to your health—then you have some more decisions to make. After all, you deserve a healthy, fulfilling life. The people who care about you should want that for you also.

JOIN A COMMUNITY OF SUPPORT

I know that one of the key things that helps us all make changes is getting support—joining forces with like-minded people to share triumphs, exchange advice, and come up with new ideas for moving forward. That's why I'm thrilled to offer you the support of The Myers Way family, which you can join by visiting my website, AmyMyers MD.com.

You might already have been pointed to some support groups by your conventional medical specialist or perhaps you've found some groups online. Here's where it can get tricky, because you probably will not find it so supportive to be told that diet doesn't matter or that you have to be on your medication for the rest of your life—and that conventional medicine perspective is shared by many autoimmune support groups.

What you're really looking for is a community of people who are also letting go of gluten, grains, and legumes; people who are also trying to detoxify their lives; and people who share your concern with inflammation, food sensitivities, and environmental toxins. Try Googling "Paleo," "celiac," "gluten-free," or "allergy-free." Many of my patients have found more helpful resources on those types of websites, rather than the conventional autoimmune ones.

Be careful of the Internet generally, because you can find an awful lot of gloom and doom that can really shake your confidence or, if you're easily suggestible, frighten you to death! You can end up reading story after story of people whose symptoms don't get better or whose medications don't work. Why expose yourself to all that negativity? Whether online or live, make sure your support group is full of positive, determined people who, like you, want to change their diet, detox their environment, and de-stress their lives—people who believe that health is their birthright and they *can* attain it. Surround yourself with positive energy and let the doomsayers be gloomy somewhere else.

ENJOY RESTAURANT DINING

"What about restaurants and dining out?"

That's something a lot of my patients want to know. I'm happy to tell you that there will be lots of things you can eat at just about any restaurant as long as you're willing to ask some questions and work with the restaurant staff.

For your first thirty days on The Myers Way, I'm hoping you'll eat at home because of the chances of cross-contamination—the possibility that something that *is* safe for you to eat has come in contact with something that *isn't*. I would hate for you to spend thirty days on The Myers Way and think the program isn't working for you simply because your restaurant food kept exposing you to problem foods.

Even during the first thirty days, however, you can enjoy an occasional restaurant meal, and after the thirty days are up, you might find yourself eating out quite often. I personally like to do a little advance work if I'm visiting a new restaurant, especially if I'm going there with friends who are *not* following The Myers Way or a similar diet. I don't like to call attention to myself, so I usually check out the restaurant menu online and figure out what I'm going to be able to eat. If I'm not 100 percent sure, I call the restaurant to explain what I'm trying to avoid and work with them to put together a meal.

"I eat meat, chicken, fish, fruits, and vegetables," I tell them. "What do you suggest?" Then when I sit down to order, I can tell the waiter, "I'd like the chicken breast with steamed broccoli, but please hold the sauce—I understand it has butter." Easy breezy, and I'm back to talking with my friends. Lots of people don't even notice that I've asked for anything special.

Of course you can also have that conversation with the waiter. These days a lot of people are avoiding gluten, and the restaurant might even have a special gluten-free menu. They're likely to be familiar with other special requests too, since these are becoming increasingly common.

TIPS FOR EATING OUT

- Remember you are a customer at the restaurant and they are there to serve you. A smile, "please," and "thank you" help too.

- Make your own salad dressing with olive oil, lemon or vinegar, and maybe an avocado.

- Substitute vegetables for the potato- or grain-based side dish.

- Avoid all sauces. That's where butter, flour, sugar, and gluten-bearing soy sauce often hide. Ask for plain broiled fish, chicken, or steak, with olive oil instead of butter. Remind them to leave out the soy sauce too, since that usually contains gluten.

- Ask how meats are marinated. Many times marinades include soy sauce, and rarely is that soy sauce gluten-free.

- Sautéed food is fine; just ask them to use olive oil instead of butter and leave out the flour.

- During your first thirty days, deep-fried food is best avoided, because of the risk of cross-contamination. Later on you can occasionally enjoy a treat such as sweet potato fries as long as the restaurant makes only French fries and not gluten-bearing foods (like fried fish or chicken) in the fryer.

- Last but not least, be creative! Most restaurants will be happy to make you a plain grilled piece of fish or chicken or a small steak and bring you steamed, grilled, or sautéed vegetables on the side.

BRING YOUR OWN DISH WHEN YOU VISIT FRIENDS

Recently, I was invited to a buffet lunch thrown by a friend to celebrate her new baby. Of course I wanted to meet the baby, but I was pretty sure that the spread would feature casseroles full of dairy, gluten, and other things I can't eat. I'd never inconvenience a mother with a new baby by asking her to cook something special. Instead I said, "I'd like to bring some food. What do you need?"

"Oh," she said, "I would love a salad!"

Okay, but I knew a salad wouldn't hold me through the whole party. So while I was at the grocery store, I picked up a rotisserie chicken.

"I thought you might enjoy some chicken too," I said when I arrived with my two dishes. Problem solved! I hadn't had to say "I can't eat anything you're serving" or "Can you make me something special?" I had managed to bring my own food without making a big deal about it.

What I usually do when someone invites me to a dinner party is offer to bring something and maybe also find out what they're planning to serve. These days lots of people are aware of food allergies and sensitivities, so your host might welcome being told about your diet ahead of time. Alternately, bring a gift of food and eat something ahead of time. You're going for the company, not the food, right?

If I know a party is going to be all finger food, I definitely eat beforehand. That way I can focus on the people. If I happen to find something I can eat, awesome! If not, no worries.

"Be prepared" works in this situation too. I usually have some food with me—in my bag or in my car—so I always have something to eat in any situation. My standbys are canned salmon, some veggies, and Epic protein bars (see "Resources"). I feel empowered knowing that I can go anywhere, do anything, and still eat the foods that will make me healthy.

ENJOY "HAPPY AND HEALTHY" HOUR

I'd like you not to drink any type of alcohol during your first thirty days on The Myers Way because the alcohol and sugar suppress your immune system, feed unhealthy bacteria, promote yeast overgrowth and SIBO, and make it more difficult to heal from any infections you might be trying to get rid of. What I do is order a Pellegrino with a splash of cranberry and lime, so that I feel I'm having something special. My focus at social gatherings is hanging out with friends, so I don't usually miss the alcohol.

As you get better, you can have some vodka or tequila every so often, like once or twice a month. Wine has lots of sugar, plus it's fermented, which makes it basically a form of liquid yeast. Since many people with autoimmunity or on the spectrum have yeast infections, I'd like you to avoid it for at least thirty days. You might be able to go back to it later. Beer is also fermented and in addition has gluten, so you'll be avoiding that permanently. "Colored" liquors such as whiskey or bourbon tend to have more problematic ingredients than clear liquors, so keep it to a minimum. Definitely choose club soda or sparkling water for your mixer, rather than some sugar or fruit concoction. Avoid the innocent-seeming tonic, which is actually full of sugar or, worse, high-fructose corn syrup. And remember, alcohol depresses your immune system, so stick to just one drink or, at most, two.

PLAN AHEAD FOR TRAVELING

I travel all the time, to all sorts of places, and I've always been able to stick to The Myers Way. If I can do it, so can you. Once again, the secret is being prepared. Here are my top four Myers Way Travel Tips:

❶ **Do some advance research.** Check out the menus at the hotel where you'll be staying, and Google "gluten-free + [city name]" to find out some restaurant options in the area. You can also Google "restaurants near [hotel name or address]" to find some nearby eating options, and then check them out online as well. Your advance planning will pay off when you arrive in a new city and know exactly where to get some broiled fish and a salad or which Italian restaurant will sauté you a nice chicken breast in lemon and olive oil.

❷ **Pack your own food.** Lots of healthy foods don't require refrigeration. Bring them along so you always have something satisfying to eat: unsweetened organic applesauce cups, clean nutrition bars, gluten-free beef jerky, and canned salmon. (See "Resources" for many of these.)

❸ **Bring ice packs and insulated bags.** You can stick the ice packs in the hotel fridge or freezer. Then pack them and some veggies, fruits, or leftovers from last night's dinner in an insulated bag.

❹ **Ask for a fridge or buy a cooler.** Often you can clear out the minibar and use it as a fridge—just make sure it isn't set to charge you every time you open the door or remove an item, as some minibars are. Alternately, most hotels will put a small refrigerator in your room at no charge if you request it ahead of time and tell them you need it for medical reasons. If you can't score a fridge, buy an inexpensive cooler at your destination to store approved foods from a local health food store or, in a pinch, from any grocery store.

If you'd like to see the products I rely on when I travel, go to my website: http://store.amymyersmd.com/product-category/more/food/.

FOCUS ON LOVED ONES DURING THE HOLIDAYS

Most of my patients tell me that, for them, holidays are the most challenging times. There are lots of tempting foods, people are in an indulgent mood, and can't we have a little fun before settling down to keep our New Year's resolutions?

For me, the holidays are a time to get together with the people I love. I still have such vivid memories of what happened to my body *before* The Myers Way, and I like feeling healthy, vital, and energized. Why jeopardize that for a cookie or a piece of cake? It's just not worth it.

The suggestions I've made throughout this chapter should stand you in good stead: Bring your own dishes to parties; eat ahead of time if you have to; and keep your eyes on the prize, which is how terrific you feel and look on this new approach to eating. Often if you don't make a point of focusing on your diet, no one else will either. They'll just tell you how great you look and how good it is to see you so full of energy and joy.

I personally love the holidays because they're a chance for me to reach more people. A couple of years ago a relative from Alabama started telling me about his joint pain. Of course he knew I was a doctor, but I soon saw that he didn't know anything about the kind of medicine I practice. To be honest, I didn't expect him to be receptive, but I did give him a quick-and-dirty explanation of how gluten was probably responsible. He nodded politely, and I figured that was the end of it.

Imagine my surprise the following year when this same man came bounding up to me, a big grin on his face! "I just can't thank you enough," he said, beaming. "You have changed my life! I stopped eating gluten, just like you told me to, and guess what. All my joint pain disappeared!" I was so happy that I had not given in to the temptation to underestimate him. The holidays had brought my family and me together in a whole new way.

A MYERS FAMILY HOLIDAY

Okay, I have to share with you just one more holiday story. This one exemplifies for me The Myers Way's promise of hope. Sure, there are times when it seems challenging to handle a rigorous diet and deal with all the family negotiations. But there are also those rewarding times when it all seems worthwhile.

For me, last Christmas was one of those times. Before, in my family, we each always had our own separate meals. My stepmother had been a vegetarian for thirty-five years. I had been a vegetarian for a while, then I went gluten-free, then I started following The Myers Way. And my father had always followed a conventional diet, plus he had an enormous sweet tooth. We'd sit around the table, figuring out which dishes each of us could and could not have—and I don't even want to get into what cooking and planning that meal was like.

Last year, though, my father started following The Myers Way. He suffers from an autoimmune condition known as polymyositis, and although he had held out for many years, his condition had taken a turn for the worse. At age seventy-five, he took the leap and decided to listen to his daughter. To support him, my stepmother actually started eating meat so she could follow The Myers Way with him.

So for the first time I could ever remember, all of us were cooking together and eating together. By Christmas, my father had lost fifteen pounds and his condition was much improved. He told me he didn't even miss the sweet things, and I could see how much better he looked. My stepmother was thrilled to see her husband doing so well.

And I loved sharing every step of the holiday dinner with them: shopping, cooking, and sitting down together to eat.

I can't tell you how much it meant to me that all of us were sharing a single meal. It meant even more to see my father so happy and to know that The Myers Way had given him this new opportunity to feel energized and alive.

So if you are the only one in your family following The Myers Way, take heart. You never know when someone will be ready to hear your message of health or when they will be ready to support you—or even join you—on your healing journey.

CHAPTER 11

Navigating the Medical Maze

WHEN I HEAR HOW MANY DOCTORS my patients have seen before they get to me, and consider how hard it is even to find autoimmune specialists in many small or rural communities, I often think the medical maze is almost as challenging as the actual autoimmune disorder. I went through it myself as a patient, and now I hear these stories from so many of my own patients. So in this chapter I offer my services as navigator and guide.

Of course my hope is that most of the help you need will be right here in this book. You can go a long way—ideally even all the way—in resolving symptoms, preventing new flares, and even reversing the course of your disease just by changing your diet, healing your gut, lightening your toxic burden, managing your infections, and relieving your stress.

Still, I sometimes spend months working with patients whose cases are more challenging: the ones with multiple autoimmune disorders or the ones who have been suffering for many years with the conventional approach before they came to me. If you are in this situation, you will definitely see some improvements in your thirty days on The Myers Way, but it may take you another few months before you enjoy a full reversal of your condition or can consider going off your medications. As I tell my patients, it took more than thirty days to get you into this situation, so it's going to take more than thirty days to get you out. In that case, you will probably want to find a functional medicine practitioner or continue working with your current practitioner. And of course whatever the status of your symptoms, you will certainly need some kind of ongoing relationship with a health-care provider.

The medical maze can be challenging—but it *can* work for you. Here are my suggestions for giving yourself the best chances at success on your own medical journey.

BE PREPARED

Before you go for your appointment, write down all the questions you have. Check them off as the doctor answers them, and of course write down the answers too. You might even ask the doctor if you can record the conversation so you can listen to it afterward, perhaps with a friend or family member. Doctor visits can be very overwhelming, so make the whole experience as easy on yourself as possible. Make an audio recording using that app on your iPhone or bring in a small tape recorder. I am always happy to have my patients record their appointments with me if they simply ask.

KEEP GOOD RECORDS

Keeping records might be the last thing on your mind when you show up to visit the doctor, especially if you're feeling anxious, confused, or overwhelmed by your condition. The best thing you can do, though, is stay organized and keep good records.

In my office, we actually give you a binder so you can keep track of all the information we give you, with tabs for The Myers Way diet, my recommended course of action, any labs you need, your lab results, and labs that are pending, as well as our Medical Symptoms Questionnaire, which each patient fills out, and the food diary we ask each patient to keep. You have seen The Myers Way Symptom Tracker on pages 22–25. You can find another copy in appendix G. As I said in chapter 1, I encourage you to make several photocopies and fill it out each week while following The Myers Way. It's a great way to track your progress and share your results with your physician.

Make sure to request a copy of your lab reports before you leave the doctor's office. Getting your labs after the fact can be like trying to smuggle gold out of Fort Knox. Doctors have to release your lab reports, but if you don't get a copy on the spot, it can take weeks and even months for most conventional doctors to get them to you. Most functional medicine practitioners, by contrast, give you a copy at the time of your appointment. If the doctor doesn't offer, just ask the staff, "Would you be willing to make a photocopy of those reports so I can take them with me when I go?" and don't leave until you get them. Then store them safely in your binder or scan them into your computer so you have an ongoing record of your progress.

Some people even make a spreadsheet to keep track of each set of lab results.

BRING A FRIEND OR LOVED ONE

It's helpful to have your own personal health advocate with you, a friend or loved one who can take notes, remind you of questions you forgot to ask, and help you remember afterward exactly what the doctor said. You also might appreciate the emotional support, since it can be challenging to deal with an autoimmune diagnosis.

BE ASSERTIVE

Make sure you get all your questions answered. If the doctor doesn't have time to tell you everything you want to know, make a second appointment. This is your health. You have a right to be informed.

Be aware, too, that "standard of care" isn't necessarily the best care. For example, if you're having routine surgery, standard of care involves loading you up with antibiotics to prevent the risk of infection. You probably won't be told that you need to take extra probiotics to make up for the damage the antibiotics do to your friendly bacteria, but now that you've read this book, you can take that step. To do so, though, you need to find out exactly what is involved in the procedure, so you know about the antibiotics in the first place. You may not even really need them.

I know that, for many of us, being assertive with a doctor can be a challenging suggestion. Doctors have a kind of aura in our culture—a kind of "doctor knows best" authority that both doctors and patients tend to believe in. So I get it: Asserting yourself with a doctor can seem to go against the grain. You might worry that if you start asking too many questions or insisting upon answers, your doctor will become impatient with you or disapprove or even become offended. You might simply feel uncomfortable challenging an authority figure.

The thing to remember is that this is *your* health. It's both your responsibility and your right to be informed, proactive, and able to make the best possible decisions for yourself. Some doctors might become impatient or offended. Others might be more open and willing to engage in dialogue or respond to their patients' concerns. Either way, at the end of the day, stand up for yourself by keeping your eyes on the prize. Remember that what's at stake is your ability to lead a long and healthy life. Figuring out how to get the answers you need isn't always easy—but isn't it worth it?

If being assertive with a doctor is tough for you, you might bring with you a more assertive spouse, partner, family member, or friend to act as your health advocate. Especially if you're feeling sick and vulnerable, having someone else stand up for you can be an amazing, energizing experience.

You might also bring this book with you, perhaps with a couple of specific passages marked, so you can show your doctor exactly what you are concerned about. While expressing respect for your doctor's authority, you might ask if he or she would like a copy of this book.

Another option, of course, is to find another doctor who is better at sharing information. In many cases, simply knowing in your own mind that you intend to look elsewhere if you don't get the answers you need will free you to become more assertive.

TREAT THE OFFICE STAFF WELL

This is one of those things that should go without saying, but sadly it must be said. In my view, you have a whole team helping you to get well. The physician is an important part of that team, but she is only a part. The rest of the team includes the nurse, the person who takes your blood, the person who answers the phone and keeps the schedule, and the person sitting at the reception desk when you arrive. The more you recognize these people as part of the team—the more you see them as health-care workers who are all trying to help you and get you well—the more readily they will help you. They'll appreciate the respect and appreciation you show them, and they'll repay it in kind.

To me, this comes under the heading of basic human decency. However, if you are asking for any "extras"—anything that most patients don't ask for—you will be far more likely to get them if you have developed a good relationship with the staff. Many people don't ask for copies of their lab reports, for example, as I am advising you to do. If you have been friendly, polite, and appreciative to the office staff, they'll be a lot more willing to grant your request.

TREAT YOUR DOCTOR WELL TOO!

I know I've spent a lot of time telling you the flaws of conventional medicine, and I stand by what I've said. But I also have a lot of sympathy for conventional doctors, especially those who spend most of their time treating autoimmune patients. While I have the satisfaction of seeing my patients recover in a few weeks or months, most conventional physicians have to live with the fact that *their* patients are not really getting well. These doctors probably got into medicine because they wanted to help people, and yet, given conventional protocols, they have to live with a lot of discouraging cases and patients whose symptoms are growing steadily worse. Even when patients are improving, they're probably taking lots of high-risk drugs, whose side effects the doctors then have to treat. I don't think I could handle that, and I feel a lot of compassion for the physicians who do.

On a side note, I should remind you that how you come into the office will affect your doctor's response, just the way your attitude would affect any other person you're working with. After all, doctors are people too. If you show up friendly, positive, and willing to engage with your doctor, he or she will be far more likely to respond in kind.

RESEARCH YOUR INSURANCE THOROUGHLY

Okay, here's some bad news: Many functional medicine practitioners don't take insurance. That's because by the very nature of how we practice medicine, we spend far more time with our patients than the fifteen minutes most insurance companies reimburse for, and we often call for tests that aren't always covered by conventional insurance.

This requires patients to get a bit creative. You might get a policy with a very high deductible or even a "catastrophe only" policy so that you're covered for emergencies. The money you save in premiums you can use toward seeing a functional medical practitioner. The good news is that once you're well, you won't need insurance to pay for expensive autoimmune medications, because you've already healed yourself.

Another option is to start a health savings account (HSA) and then use that money to pay for a functional medicine doctor. A health savings account is money set aside to pay for medical expenses when you have a high-deductible insurance plan. You get a tax break for the money you put away, although there are penalties for taking out the money before retirement age if you use it for anything other than qualified medical expenses. If this approach appeals to you, talk to an accountant to find out more.

You might also ask if there's someone else in the office you can see for less, such as a registered dietitian (R.D.) or nurse-practitioner (N.P.). There are many ways in which a dietitian or nurse-practitioner can work with you, reducing the number of more expensive hours that have to be billed to the actual physician.

Yet another possibility is to find out if conventional doctors, who are covered by insurance, can do some of the work. You can often get at least some of your labs done through your regular doctor, although functional medicine practitioners frequently ask for tests that conventional doctors do not order.

Finally, there are many laboratories across the country where you can order your own lab work. You have to pay out of pocket for these tests, of course, but it can often be significantly cheaper than what your insurance company might charge for them. (I've listed a few good labs in "Resources.")

BE HONEST WITH YOUR PHYSICIAN

Your conventional medicine physician may not agree with the approach you are taking on The Myers Way, but you need to share with him or her what you are doing and which supplements you are taking.

Be prepared for them to respond by telling you that supplements are bogus or even that studies show that "supplements are dangerous." In my opinion, those studies are flawed, because they were not conducted with high-quality products. But it's not worth your while to argue with your physician.

You have the right to make your own health decisions; in the end, you are the only person who can.

If your physician says that something recommended on The Myers Way is harmful or contraindicated for one of your own medications, ask to see the study or the documentation. I've reviewed the literature closely, and I can tell you that nothing I'm asking you to do is contraindicated.

Although it makes things nicer if you get support from your physician, you don't really need it. You just want them to agree that anything you are doing on The Myers Way will not be actively harmful or interfere with their medications, and you want them to track your labs. If you get to the place where your numbers are good enough that you might be weaned off your medications, you want your doctor to be receptive to that.

If you feel you absolutely cannot work with your doctor, or that he or she is completely opposed to even the possibility of you getting off your medications, you might need to look for another physician. This is of course a very personal decision that will be influenced by your geographic location, your finances, and your insurance, among other things.

DON'T GIVE UP

Whatever your experiences with the medical maze, don't give up. Some of my patients have seen as many as a dozen doctors before they get to me, so you just have to believe that help is out there.

Meanwhile, this book has covered all the basics of what you need to consider for an autoimmune condition. It's also a good resource to take to your conventional practitioner or to help you find a functional medicine provider. So stay committed to taking care of your own health and keep going. Good health is your birthright. You deserve every chance to enjoy it.

CHAPTER 12

A World of Hope

Success Stories

Now that you have almost finished this book, I hope you share my own sense of excitement about what The Myers Way makes possible. I often think I have the most wonderful job in the world, because I get to come to work every day and see people's lives change—often within a few weeks, sometimes within a few months. I am so thrilled to be able to share this life-changing approach with you. I know that if you follow the program faithfully, you will feel better very soon, and you can ultimately look forward to a life free of pain, medications, side effects, and symptoms—a life in which your focus is on enjoying your vibrant, radiant health instead of managing a challenging condition or fearing the potential development of another autoimmune disease.

In this chapter I'd like you to meet some of my favorite reasons for hope—a sampling of patients who have enjoyed success on The Myers Way. Before I introduce my Myers Way patients to you, though, I'd like you to hear about quite a different patient, one whose conventional medical experience was part of what inspired me to stay the course and keep looking until I could come up with a better way.

Angela was a young, very sick patient whom I met in the ER when I was a first-year resident. I was working in the intensive care unit (ICU), where the most critically ill patients are treated. Patients in the ICU are often considered "touch and go." Most can't breathe on their own, so they have to rely on ventilators. Their vital signs are so unstable, they have to be monitored by machines at all times and by nurses every hour.

Angela—who was in her midtwenties—came in because her liver had started to fail, almost overnight. If she was to survive, she needed a liver transplant. Even at her young age, she had a history of rheumatoid arthritis, and her medications—prednisone and methotrexate— had stopped being effective in treating her symptoms. So she had been put on an even stronger medication known as Remicade (infliximab), which sent her, almost overnight, into acute liver failure.

Angela's whole family was holding vigil in the waiting room. She was a twin, and her twin sister was there, looking eerily like a healthy, vibrant version of the deathly sick Angela. Angela had just gotten married, and her husband was there too. Her parents were there, and her grandparents. I remember thinking how lucky she was to have such a close, loving family—and how unlucky she was to be fighting for her life at such a young age. Working in the ICU, you mainly see very old people, many of whom have been rushed in from nursing homes after long, debilitating illnesses. To see a young woman, cut down in the prime of her life, was a painful shock. Knowing that she had an autoimmune condition, just as I did, made me feel even closer to her and even more upset at what she had to go through.

Angela basically needed a liver transplant or she was going to die—that was the conversation I had to have with her family. But livers are always very much in demand, and ironically, Angela was not yet sick enough to be pushed to the top of the transplant list. We simply had to watch and wait, I told her anxious husband and her worried family. The instant her liver got worse, I could notify the transplant team, and then she would be eligible for the procedure that we all hoped would save her life.

All that night I monitored Angela's labs, tracking exactly how high her liver enzymes had risen. I kept returning to her bedside, kept checking in on her and speaking with her silent family still sitting in the waiting room. I was torn between feeling terrifically grateful that I was able to do this work, to help these people, and so angry that the medical system I was part of had failed Angela in this way. Why hadn't we been able to find another way to treat her, other than medications that produced such dreadful side effects?

Why hadn't we been able to show this young woman, this beloved daughter, this new wife, how to support her immune system and take back her life?

The next day Angela's labs showed hepatic distress (evidence of liver failure), so she did indeed get pushed to the top of the transplant list. As we were prepping her for surgery, I gave her my little guardian angel—a small metal coin—that I always carried in my wallet as a reminder of my mother. I had given a matching one to my mother when she was sick, and it had been buried with her. Now I wanted to give mine to Angela to help her get through surgery. Angela had hepatic encephalopathy, though—the worsening of brain function that occurs when the liver can no longer filter toxins out of the blood—so she was completely out of it: foggy, disoriented, and confused. I gave the angel to Angela's twin instead and asked her to keep it for her sister.

The surgery, thank heavens, was successful, and I assumed that was the end of the story. I finished my ICU rotation and went back to working in the ER. When you work in the ER, you don't really expect to see any of your patients again; with luck, they recover and return to their regular doctors. One day, though, I heard that a patient wanted to see me. Puzzled, I went where I was directed—and there was Angela.

All during her travail, Angela had been out of her head with hallucinations caused by her toxic liver. So she didn't remember me at all, but her family had told her all about the young ER resident who had, in effect, kept vigil with them all night long.

"Thank you for saving my life," she said shyly. She showed me her angel, and I was so moved to see that she still had it with her.

"That wasn't me; it was the transplant team!" I told her. We hugged, and then I had to rush right back to attend to an emergency. I haven't seen her since—although "Angela," if you're reading this, please come find me, because I could offer you so much more help now. Now I could show you how to get off your medications once and for all, how to reverse your condition and keep yourself from developing more autoimmune disorders down the line. (Seriously, Angela, please do contact me! I think of you often.)

Meanwhile, I've never forgotten that young woman and her family. Now that I have the opportunity to practice a more effective type of medicine, I'm so grateful to be able to offer help *before* the problem gets to the level of an ICU and a transplant team. And I'm pleased to introduce you to some of the other patients whom I've been able to help.

SUSAN, AGE SIXTY-SEVEN: "I CAN FINALLY PLAY WITH MY GRANDKIDS!"

If you saw Susan today, you would not recognize her as the woman who first came into my office. You actually *can* see Susan, if you want to, or at least check out her photograph next to the name "Susan R." in the testimonials section of my website. There you'll find a vital, energetic-looking woman with an absolutely radiant smile. In the picture, it looks as though she's just gotten the most wonderful news, but I can tell you that's how Susan looked a lot of the time once we had reversed her condition and gotten her off her medication. Every time I see Susan's photo, I'm reminded of why I got into this work in the first place and why I feel lucky to keep doing it, every day.

When Susan first came into my office, she was in horrific pain pretty much all the time. A naturally upbeat, determined person, she did her best to stay calm, focused, and positive as she told me her story. In those early appointments, I saw only a faint shadow of that radiant smile; Susan was grimacing in pain even as she sat in the comfortable chair in my office, listing her medications and describing her symptoms.

Susan had a condition known as transverse myelitis in which the immune cells attack the spinal cord. In later stages of the disorder, you can get a lot of muscle weakness, but so far Susan had been spared that. She was simply in severe pain.

Susan took pills for the pain, but she also had a special pain cream that brought her the most relief she had known so far. Unfortunately, she couldn't use it all the time, or her body would develop a tolerance to it and it would lose its effectiveness. So for three weeks out of the month, Susan got some measure of pain relief, and the fourth week was simply excruciating.

"I can make it through that fourth week, though," Susan told me, "just knowing that it won't always be like this. At this point that's all that keeps me going."

Susan jumped into The Myers Way with both feet. She followed the diet to the letter and carefully undertook the 4Rs protocol to heal her gut, especially the serious case of yeast overgrowth she had developed. Since 80 percent of the immune system is in the gut, this healing was crucial to her recovery. She also took steps to detoxify her life and looked for ways to relieve stress.

"My favorite form of stress relief is playing with my grandkids," she told me ruefully, explaining that they lived with her daughter and son-in-law in Southern California, "but because of the pain, I'm not really able to be as involved with them as I would like."

About two months into The Myers Way, Susan went to visit her grandkids and gave me a call from California. We chatted about how things were going, and I noticed that she hadn't said one word about her pain. Finally, I asked her about it.

I could hear the gasp on the other end of the phone.

"Oh my God!" Susan exclaimed. "I can't even believe it. I've been out here for two weeks with the kids, and I completely forgot to bring my cream with me. But *I didn't even notice*, because I haven't felt any pain!"

A few months later, Susan's daughter and husband went on vacation, and Susan was able to invite her grandchildren to spend a couple of weeks with her. She sent me a delighted e-mail. "I couldn't even play with them before," she wrote. "And now I'm taking care of them full-time for two weeks." Then she added the sentence she would later put on my website: "For the first time in my life, I feel as though my body is in 'sync' with itself, and I could not be happier."

JENNIFER, AGE THIRTY-SIX: "NOW I'M TRAINING FOR A 5K!"

Jennifer was an attractive woman in her midthirties whose dark, wavy hair fell to her shoulders. She still had a kind of athletic look about her, even though by the time I met her, she hadn't been physically active for some time, thanks to the almost constant pain and muscle weakness from her polymyositis, an autoimmune condition in which your antibodies trigger an attack on your own muscles. My dad has the same condition, so I had seen firsthand over the years just how debilitating this disorder could be. Jennifer was a high school volleyball coach whose idea of a good time was to go out and train for a race, so this disease hit her even harder than most. She missed being in peak physical condition, she couldn't run up and down the court to properly coach her team, and she knew that if we couldn't do a better job of reversing her disorder than her current doctor had done, she was in danger of losing her job.

Jennifer lived in a small Texas town where she had managed to find the one specialist within miles, a rheumatologist who had put her on prednisone. The side effects were fairly hard to take—in her case, they included weight gain, fatigue, and digestive issues—so Jennifer was not always the most compliant of patients, sometimes skipping a few days just to give herself a break. She was doing her best, though, and she told me that she would follow The Myers Way to the letter if it would help her reverse her disease.

While she continued to see her other doctor, Jennifer and I worked together for a few months. Following The Myers Way diet and our 4Rs protocol for a healthy gut, Jennifer gave up gluten and other inflammatory foods, healed her gut, and treated the SIBO and yeast overgrowth she had been struggling with. She was doing so much better, in fact, that her doctor had actually decreased her medications.

Then Jennifer asked if she could get off medication entirely, and her doctor hit the ceiling. "I decide when we're ready to do that, not you," he told her. "If you're not going to listen to me, you can't be my patient anymore."

Jennifer was devastated. Even though she was working with me, being fired by her doctor was very upsetting. She knew he was the only rheumatologist for miles around—she had to drive quite a few hours to get to me—and not having medical care nearby really scared her.

Although she was getting better slowly, neither she nor I was completely satisfied with her progress. Jennifer had had some initial success in healing her yeast overgrowth, but the yeast kept coming back, despite her strictly following our gut-healthy diet. Whenever a patient has persistent yeast overgrowth, I think about the possibility that either heavy metals or toxic mold caused it, and I assess the patient's risk factors for both.

So I asked Jennifer if there were any water leaks at her house or school. She told me that she and her husband were in the middle of an ongoing house renovation, which her husband was doing himself. In fact, he remembered seeing some mold in the kitchen. At the same time, Jennifer had noticed that several of the ceiling tiles in her school gym had water stains.

I tested Jennifer, and sure enough, her urine test came back high for levels of toxic molds. Okay, so toxic mold was the issue, but where was she being exposed? I decided to test her husband because if he too had a positive urine test, we would know that her house—and not her school—was the problem. As you read in chapter 6, only one-quarter of the population have the genes that respond to mycotoxins—the volatile compounds released by certain molds—so I knew Jennifer's husband could be exposed and display no symptoms.

And sure enough, he was. He had mistakenly thought a little bleach was enough to clear the mold he had noticed in the kitchen, but although the outward signs of the mold disappeared, the mold still lurked beneath the surface.

So Jennifer's husband set to work eliminating the mold problem (for more on coping with toxic mold, see appendix C), and Jennifer, at my urging, went to stay with relatives while I treated her with antifungal medications and cholestyramine, a binding agent that draws out the mycotoxins. I also had her take plenty of glutathione to help her detox.

The change was swift and dramatic. Within a week Jennifer felt better, and within a month her symptoms had markedly improved. We were able to get Jennifer completely off her medications, while an inflammatory marker called CPK (creatine phosphokinase, an enzyme involved in muscle damage), which had never been at a normal level even when she *was* being medicated, dropped to a completely normal level. Problem solved.

A few months later, Jennifer moved back into her mold-free house. Her physical strength returned, her symptoms stayed away, her lab values remained completely normal—and her job was safe. The last I heard, she was training for a 5K, thrilled and relieved to reclaim her health.

PETER, AGE TEN:
"I DON'T HAVE TO TAKE MY MEDICINE ANYMORE!"

Peter was a lively little boy whose parents brought him into my office with juvenile rheumatoid arthritis. I always have such mixed feelings whenever a child comes to see me. On the one hand, it's heartbreaking to see someone so young struggling with autoimmune symptoms, particularly the disabling pain of rheumatoid arthritis. On the other hand, because the stakes are so high, I'm so glad to be able to intervene and really make a difference. After all, autoimmune diseases are incurable, so if a ten-year-old child walks in with an autoimmune condition, they are going to have this disease for decades to come. I know that if I don't succeed in turning things around, there are years ahead when the disease can get worse and worse and worse. I need to make sure that we reverse the condition, support the child's immune system, and hold off the possibility of additional autoimmune disorders. Otherwise, that kid is facing a very difficult road.

Despite his young age, Peter's journey had already been fairly rocky. He had been born by C-section and bottle-fed, which, as you saw in chapter 4, are two risk factors that can set you up for leaky gut and immune problems later on. Indeed, even as a baby Peter had lots of ear infections and had tubes in his ears twice. As you also saw in chapter 4, ear infections are often an indication of dairy sensitivity, and they are usually treated with antibiotics, which destroy friendly bacteria, set you up for leaky gut, and ultimately stress your immune system.

At eighteen months, Peter had hernia surgery—more stress and more antibiotics. And at age five, he had an emergency appendectomy—still more stress and more antibiotics. So after just five years on this planet, Peter's immune system had already taken several hits.

To the great relief of his parents, Peter went on to have four relatively peaceful years. Peter's father was a high-ranking executive in a health food chain, while Peter's mother was a physician. Between the two of them, you would think they would have a healthy diet covered, and Peter probably did eat in a healthier way than most U.S. children—no sugary cereals, sodas laden with high-fructose corn syrup, or even much fast food.

But like most well-meaning parents, Peter's mother and father gave their son sandwiches made with whole-grain bread, spaghetti and meatballs, mac and cheese, tall glasses of milk, and, at least a few times a week, cookies, pudding, or ice cream. The gluten- and dairy-laden diet was slowly but surely triggering attacks on Peter's immune system, exacerbated by the occasional sugar. Eventually these attacks would create clusters of inflammatory chemicals known as "immune complexes," which would float through Peter's body and settle in his joints.

There were a few more warning signs, if only his parents had known how to read them. The fall that Peter turned eight, he got strep throat, followed soon after by the flu—indicators of a vulnerable immune system. The following spring, he woke up with a bad case of hives—another sign of immune stress and probably also indicating some problems with gluten.

Well, that's what I would have thought if I'd seen Peter at that point, but I wasn't yet Peter's physician. The doctor he did have thought the hives were an allergic reaction to a neighborhood cat and prescribed Benadryl. That helped for a few days, but then the hives came back. In the way of conventional medicine, the doctor's next response was to up the medications, so for the next several months Peter was given steroids.

All this while, Peter's immune system was getting more and more stressed—picture those guys in the Command Central being fired at for hours without a break until finally they crack under the strain. Peter's immune system went rogue, and Peter woke up with joint pain so bad that he could not walk.

Juvenile rheumatoid arthritis is relatively rare (though sadly it's becoming more common), so it took a while for Peter to be diagnosed. The little boy went through a battery of x-rays—first his elbow, then his wrist—and meanwhile, he just kept getting both hives and joint pain every afternoon. Finally, he ended up at Dell Children's Medical Center, where he got his diagnosis.

This whole time Peter's mother was convinced that her colleagues in conventional medicine were going to find a way to relieve her son of his pain. And at first Peter's father agreed. He went along with conventional treatments when his son was given prednisone. After all, the doctors told him, this was standard of care. And when the prednisone wasn't enough, he deferred to the doctors—and to his wife—when they gave his son methotrexate, a harsh immunosuppressant.

Initially, the methotrexate seemed to be working. Peter's rash and joint pain went away that August, and the whole family excitedly began to prepare Peter for the new school year. Then, in November, the joint pain and the rash came back, along with an itchiness so intense that Peter could not sleep at night. Peter's doctor put him on an even harsher drug known as Kineret, which costs something like a thousand dollars per injection and produces numerous side effects—and Peter's father put his foot down.

"This has got to stop!" he told his wife. "Our son is only ten years old and already he's on three major medications? What can his future possibly be like?"

Somehow Peter's father convinced his wife to give me a try. It certainly helped that I had an M.D. behind my name and could speak her language. I was relieved that she was willing to give my approach a try. You need 100 percent compliance for the first few months of The Myers Way, and that is such a difficult situation when one parent isn't on board. The worst is when the parents are divorced and only one is supportive. The poor kid stays gluten-free and dairy-free at one parent's house but eats all sorts of unhealthy food at the other's. Luckily, Peter's parents agreed to maintain a united front, and I was able to treat him with their full support.

So Peter began The Myers Way, and, in solidarity, his parents went on it with him. Both of them soon noticed that they were losing weight without making any special effort other than to maintain the eating plan. Peter's mother's migraines vanished. Peter's father had struggled with mild depression, but after switching to The Myers Way, he noticed a real lift in mood.

Meanwhile, Peter was improving by leaps and bounds. His tests confirmed that he was indeed sensitive to gluten and dairy. Cutting out those foods really agreed with this little boy, who had probably been suffering from sensitivities since infancy. I had also suspected a yeast infection, which a stool test further confirmed, and we found out that he had a parasite as well—probably something he picked up on a family camping trip. Once he was treated for these common gut infections, his hives cleared up and his itching completely disappeared.

So, one by one, Peter began to let go of his medications. First, he got off prednisone. A few months later, his conventional medicine doctor agreed that he no longer needed the methotrexate. And last but certainly not least, Peter was able to give up the Kineret injections.

Peter's parents had first brought him to see me in March. By the beginning of the next school year, Peter was like a new boy, growing stronger and more energetic by the day. Best of all, no more medication.

"I don't have to take my medicine anymore!" Peter informed me triumphantly on his last visit. "I'll miss you, Dr. Myers. My parents say I'm not coming back here."

"I'll miss you too, Peter," I told him. I watched him bounding out of the office, finally able to skip and run the way any ten-year-old should be able to do. I didn't know who Peter would grow up to be, but I was so happy to think that whatever future he created, it would be free of symptoms, medications, and side effects. The Myers Way had given him the tools to live a long and healthy life.

JIM MYERS, AGE SEVENTY-SEVEN: "I'M SO GLAD MY DAUGHTER'S A DOCTOR!"

Yep, this one's about my dad, which makes it maybe my favorite success story of all time. The success was all the sweeter because it came after what seemed like several years of failure.

If anyone out there has ever tried to get a family member to do something that you believed was good for their health—quit smoking, lose weight, exercise more, maybe even go gluten-free—you know how hard that is. *You* know that if your mom, dad, sister, brother, or whoever would just listen to you, their lives would get much, much better. *They* remember when you were just a baby in diapers or a passionate teenager with a million theories, and to your frustration, they treat you like you're still that kid, instead of the mature, sensible, and very well-informed adult who is now giving them this good advice.

Now, if you are thinking, "But it must be different for Amy. She's a *doctor*," well, think again. You know that saying a prophet gets no honor in his own country? That's what it was like being a functional medicine physician in my own family. I'd spend my days helping people like Susan, Jennifer, Peter, or the thousands of other patients who thanked me for giving them their lives back. Then I'd go spend the holidays with my family, and despite my excellent advice, my dad just kept on eating gluten!

As it happens, my dad has a condition called polymyositis—the same disorder that Jennifer had, the one that attacks your muscles and brings on the pain. He ended up with very weak muscles, several surgeries, and three powerful medications: prednisone, methotrexate, and CellCept. Those were also the same medications that Jennifer had been on—they're standard treatment for advanced polymyositis. These drugs are often sadly ineffective against weakness and pain. Plus they bring with them a whole slew of side effects, including, in my dad's case, weight gain and depression.

However, the biggest concern was the fact that these drugs work by suppressing the immune system—and that made Dad way too vulnerable to infection. A couple of years ago he ended up with a bad case of pneumonia that turned into a significant lung infection, requiring a long stay in the hospital and a big ol' chest tube to drain the infection. "This is it," my siblings and I all thought, and we all went home to see Dad before the end that we all thought was coming.

Well, my dad's pretty tough, so he pulled through. But at age seventy-seven, he was still practically wheelchair-bound. He could manage to get around a little bit with the help of a walker, but he spent most of his waking hours stuck in his chair. "So, Amy, what do you think about this?" my dad would ask every time I went home for the holidays.

"Dad, I told you last time you asked *and* the time before. It's your diet!" I would say, trying to sound calm and reasonable and not like an angry teenager. I just hated seeing my father in such bad shape, helping himself to a glass of wine or a piece of coffee cake, when I knew that the sugar, yeast, and gluten in those foods were literally making the problem worse, even while we sat there talking about it.

Finally I decided enough was enough. I didn't want every holiday to be spent in fruitless arguments, which I found both frustrating and, if the truth be known, heartbreaking. Worse, I was starting to feel like my proselytizing was making Dad more stubborn, not less. If he was ever going to change his diet, he would have to do it for his own reasons, in his own time.

"I'm not having any more conversations about this," I told him. "I don't want this to be what my holidays are about. You engage with me because you're curious, but then you challenge everything I say. That's fine, but now that you know what I think, we don't have to keep doing it. When you are ready to *really* hear what I have to say, let me know."

Now, to be fair to my dad, he has always been super proud of me, and it wasn't like he didn't believe in my abilities as a physician. The problem was more that he was in his seventies, and by that time, it's hard to change. He did give up gluten for a while, but he didn't really notice any difference. I believe that's because he had to let go of some other foods too; plus, at his age and after all those decades of autoimmunity, it was just going to take a while longer for him to improve. But I get it. When you don't see immediate results, it's hard to keep going.

Not only did my dad have this debilitating disease, on top of it, his joints were really bad. He was going to need a hip replacement, and the surgery was scheduled for January 2014. When I went home for Thanksgiving, he looked at me with his usual loving pride and said, "Oh, Amy, you look so great! What is going on with you?"

"Dad, it's just my diet," I told him. And then I realized that maybe here was the opening I had been waiting for. I knew my father was really scared about his upcoming surgery, and I was scared for him. A hip replacement for a healthy individual is not such a frightening procedure. But for a man in his late seventies on all these immunosuppressants, that's a whole other ball game.

"Um, Dad," I said, "you have thirty days before the operation. Maybe you want to try my diet and just see how you do? You know, just to give yourself the best shot?"

And for some reason, at that moment, something just clicked. "Okay," my dad said, just as though he hadn't been fighting me on this for the past five years. "I guess I could give it a try."

So my dad began to follow The Myers Way. As I told you in chapter 10, he lost fifteen pounds, which was a huge improvement, since he had been about forty-five pounds overweight at the time. He felt better and he could move more easily, even with the hip pain—maybe because he was carrying less weight, maybe because The Myers Way was calming his immune system and dialing back the attacks on his muscles.

I went home for Christmas, just before the surgery, and we had the Myers family Christmas I told you about in chapter 10. Finally all of us were preparing and enjoying the same food, a family united around the dinner table. For me, it was my own private Christmas miracle.

Meanwhile, thirty days before the surgery, my dad's doctor had taken him off the CellCept so as not to suppress his immune system during a long and stressful operation. Thankfully, the surgery went very well, and my father recovered more quickly than he had from his other surgeries. I was sure that the immune support he had gotten from The Myers Way was already helping him heal.

"Dad," I said to him after the surgery, "why don't we check your CPK?" Because of the polymyositis, my dad's CPK levels had been very high for a long time—in fact, the CellCept he had been on was supposed to help lower the levels. After the stress of muscle-damaging surgery and after thirty days without CellCept, my father and his doctors expected his CPK levels to be through the roof. Nobody wanted to check the levels; they didn't think my dad needed any more bad news.

Well, I got them to do the test, and lo and behold, my father's CPK levels were lower than they had ever been. Here was medical proof that The Myers Way had made a measurable difference.

Dad went home, but his surgical wound wasn't healing properly—doubtless because his other immunosuppressants were keeping his immune system from doing its job. I told him to get off those medications, and for once, his other doctors agreed. He was readmitted to the hospital and treated for infections.

Now, in theory, without the medications to keep them down, Dad's CPK levels should have been going up. But guess what. When they tested his CPK levels again, they were now *completely normal*—without any medications at all!

My dad doesn't call me very often. But he called me that day. "Amy," he said, grinning so broadly I could hear it all the way over the phone lines back in Austin, "you'll never believe it. My CPK is perfect!"

I almost couldn't answer him, I was so close to tears. I thought once more of that holiday dinner, everybody sharing the same meal—a dream I had given up on years ago. And now here we were, my father doing better than he had in years, my stepmother blooming on The Myers Way, and me so happy that I could finally share everything I had learned with the people who mattered most.

YOUR OWN WORLD OF HOPE

Now that you've finished this book, I hope you're ready to start your journey—or maybe you've even already begun. Whether you've already been diagnosed with an autoimmune condition or are simply somewhere on the spectrum, I know The Myers Way will help you feel better and look better, opening the door to a whole new world of energy, well-being, and radiant good health. This book will continue to be your resource, and I'm always here for you at AmyMyersMD .com, along with the rest of The Myers Way family. I wish you all the best on your life's journey.

Acknowledgments

Writing this book was a team effort, and I had the most amazing team possible, who made this daunting task seem almost effortless.

Yes, it was hard work and long hours, but it was possible because of the efficient, brilliantly talented Rachel Kranz, who was able to give wings to my words and tell them in a way I never could have done without her.

Enormous thanks to Gideon Weil, my editor, who believed in me from very early on. This book would not have been written had Gideon not seen something in me and encouraged me to tell my story and share what I knew about autoimmune conditions. From the first, he coached me on how to think about this project and was there for me from beginning to end.

My agent, Stephanie Tade, you've looked out for my best interests every step of the way. Your dedication to me and to this project means so much to me. You could not have helped me pick a better team.

Thanks to Brianne Williams, R.D., L.D., who helped to create each of the delicious, nutrient-dense, and healing recipes in this book. You are such a bright star, and I am so grateful to have you working with me and our patients every day.

As you have read, I have had many amazing experiences in life as well as many setbacks. I am who I am because of those experiences and because of the friends and family who have been on this journey with me from the beginning. I am unable to personally thank you all, so please know that I appreciate each of you and that you are part of making this dream a reality.

A few outstanding supporters I would like to thank by name:

Dr. Mark Hyman, I absolutely would not be here today without you and your support. You are one of the greatest blessings in my life.

My Austin UltraHealth team: It is because of you that I am able to do all the things outside of the clinic that I do. Julie Swan, R.N., your care and devotion to our patients is incredible. Thanks to Ali Fine for overseeing the store and social media, as well as creating the amazing illustrations in this book. Caroline Haltom for your never-ending kind, upbeat, and can-do attitude. Jen Cannon, you are the mother hen and the glue that keeps it all together. Thank you for hanging in there with me through thick and thin; I absolutely could not do it without you.

Dhru Purohit, you are one of the most selfless and generous people I have ever met. You are solely responsible for so many introductions, and for so much of the advice and support that have helped to get me here. I appreciate you and everything that you and the entire CLEAN team have done for me.

Dr. Katie Hendricks, you changed my life!

Thanks to those who have blazed the trail before me and opened many doors for me: Drs. Jeffrey Bland, Alejandro Junger, David Perlmutter, Frank Lipman, and Susan Blum. My IFM tribe and journal club, Drs. Kara Fitzgerald, David Brady, David Hasse, Patrick Hanaway, and Bethany Hays: You all inspire me with your brilliance and dedication to the field. Thanks to Dr. Todd Lepine for being my "go-to guy" for the latest research articles and for helping to ensure that this book was scientifically sound.

Shout-outs to the Paleo community for embracing my message, Paleo (f)x for giving me a platform to get it out, and Robb Wolf for your support and advice along the way.

Thanks to the team at MindBodyGreen, who gave me a platform early on to spread my message; to my AmyMyersMD.com community, who continue to support and spread that message every day; to the producers at *The Dr. Oz Show*, who helped me spread that message even further; and to HarperOne and your entire team for ensuring that this message will be heard around the world.

Deep, heartfelt thanks to my patients for placing your faith and trust in me. And for your dedication to The Myers Way program and reclaiming your health. You are what gets me up in the morning. I am so blessed to be able to work with each of you.

Xavier, you are all that I need. You complete me. I love you.

Most important, I'd like to thank my guardian angel, my mother. She taught me to never accept status quo, to be curious and to question, to take the road less traveled, to be authentic, and to not ever be afraid to be different or stand up for what I believe. I am the woman and the doctor I am today because of my mother.

Genetically Modified Organisms (GMOs)

Genetically modified organisms (GMOs) are potentially one of the greatest health concerns of our time—and yet many people are not even aware of their existence. In chapter 5, I explain what GMOs are and how they affect your gut and immune system. I encourage you to inform yourself about this major new threat to our food supply and to take action as a consumer and a citizen to protect yourself against it. Here's just a short introduction, with some resources for learning more.

Although GMOs now dominate many foods available in the United States, their long-term effects have barely been studied. One of the first significant long-term studies was recently completed in France. Over the course of two years, rats were given a diet of which 30 percent was GMO corn. I realize that two years doesn't sound that long, but for a rat, that's just about an entire lifetime, since the average rat rarely makes it past age three. In this study, some 70 percent of the GMO-eating female rats died prematurely of cancer, as compared to only 20 percent of the non-GMO control group.

First of all, that's a scary statistic. I wish there were more studies to compare it to, but so far, we don't have them. Which brings up the question, why not?

You're not going to like the answer. I certainly don't. Basically, whenever a company seeks FDA approval for a new product, it's required to do the research to prove that product's safety. That company-funded research is what the FDA uses to determine safety, especially if no other research has been done. And who is likely to fund research on an untested product, other than the manufacturer? After a product hits the market, who wants to go up against such corporate giants as Monsanto? As a result, many genetically modified foods have only been studied for three months or less.

Europe is much stricter in their regulations than we are, which brings up another question: Why aren't we as concerned as they are?

Again, you won't like the answer, and neither do I, but I can give it to you in one word: money! Our government is far more influenced by the wealth and power of corporations than most European governments, and as a result, corporations like Monsanto have a lot more leeway to bring GMOs to market. Consequently, we here in the United States don't even realize how many genetically modified foods we are consuming. So far, there are no federal regulations saying that GMOs have to be labeled, despite numerous polls showing that some 90 percent of the public would prefer that.

It's not like no one has tried. In 2012, the first bill to require labeling of genetically modified foods was voted on in California and defeated by a narrow margin—about 52 percent to 48 percent. Significantly, the opponents of that bill outspent the supporters by a factor of about five to one: $46 million to defeat the bill versus only $9.2 million to support it. A very tiny piece of that $9.2 million came from me and my clinic, Austin UltraHealth, and I also did a podcast at the time, urging my listeners to send in their contributions. So you can see that I put my money where my mouth is!

The top opponents of the GMO labeling bill reads like a Who's Who in the U.S. food industry: Monsanto, DuPont, PepsiCo, the Grocery Manufacturers Association, Kraft Foods, and Coca-Cola. These companies rely on GMOs at this point, and they don't want people to stop buying their GMO-laden products.

Even though we don't have all the research we need, we have a lot of evidence to suggest that genetically modified foods are associated with allergies, autism, ADD/ADHD, leaky gut, and digestive illnesses. You also saw in chapter 5 how GMOs are likely to be denser in the very elements that provoke inflammation and overburden your immune system.

Now, you might be wondering just where GMOs show up in our food supply. It would be faster to tell you where they *don't* show up:

- In any food labeled "non-GMO."

- In any food labeled "100 percent organic"—but it has to be 100 percent. A food labeled "organic" can be 30 percent GMO and still get the "organic" label. (Tell that to the rats in the French study!)

- In beef that is labeled "100 percent grass-fed" or "grass-fed, grass-finished." A lot of cattle are grass-fed but then "finished" with grain feeding. And in those grains are GMOs.

- In foods that your local farmers' market supplier tells you are 100 percent okay. Make sure to ask them the right questions, though, because often, even if they are raising free-range animals, they are giving them corn-, soy-, or alfalfa-based feed. And guess what. Virtually all the corn, soy, and alfalfa grown in the United States are genetically modified. So when you consume nonorganic meats and poultry, you're consuming GMOs.

- In any food you grow yourself—as long as you buy non-GMO seeds.

Now that you know where GMOs are *not*, I'll share with you a brief and definitely not complete list of some of the top places where they *are*. I say "not complete" because the use of GMOs keeps expanding, and so does our knowledge about where they are being used. So by the time this book comes out, we might want to put some more items on the list. Check out the always valuable resources from the Environmental Working Group to find out the latest, including their shopper's guide: www.ewg.org/research/shoppers-guide-to-avoiding -ge-food. And while you're at it, make a donation. They do amazing work that helps to protect us all.

You won't be eating rice, tomatoes, or wheat during your first thirty days on The Myers Way, but you might be adding in some tomatoes later on. Play it safe: Buy organic!

Here are your takeaways to protect you from eating GMOs:

- Read the labels.

- Avoid packaged foods.

- Be aware that even establishments like Whole Foods and other "organic" grocery stores are often full of genetically modified products—although Whole Foods did make a commitment to label all GMO products by 2018, and they have a section on their website intended to help you figure out how to avoid GMOs.

GMO FOODS IN THE USA

- **Corn,** including all products made with high-fructose corn syrup. (Now you know why Coca-Cola and PepsiCo spent so much to oppose California's labeling bill, since high-fructose corn syrup is the main sweetener used in sodas.) Many animal feeds include corn, so eating nonorganic meats probably means you're consuming GMO corn.

- **Soy,** including soy lecithin, which is used in a lot of packaged food, including "organic" dark chocolate bars! You won't be eating chocolate bars during your first thirty days on The Myers Way, but many of you will be adding them in later on. They are one of my personal favorite treats, but I have to either go for "100 percent organic" or else read that fine print on the label very carefully to avoid soy lecithin. Again, many animal feeds include soy, so eating nonorganic meats probably means you're consuming GMO soy.

- **Alfalfa.** Of course you won't be eating it, but the animals *you* eat may well have been fed GMO alfalfa.

- **Cotton and cottonseed oil.** You don't eat cotton, obviously, and as far as I know there's no reason not to *wear* GMO cotton. However, cottonseed oil is used in a lot of packaged products, so either avoid all packaged foods (not a bad rule!) or read the label carefully.

- **Canola or rapeseed oils.** These are oils made from genetically modified seeds; there is by definition no non-GMO version of them.

- **Sugar.** Some 55 percent of U.S. sugar is made from sugar beets—and about 95 percent of them have been genetically modified. Of course you are already avoiding sugar on The Myers Way.

- **Papaya.** More than 75 percent of the papaya grown in Hawaii has been genetically modified.

- **Zucchini and yellow summer squash.** Some varieties are genetically engineered, so buy organic, just to be safe.

- Other potential genetically modified foods, either approved by the FDA or being considered for approval:

Flax	**Radicchio**	**Salmon**	**Wheat**
Plums	**Rice**	**Tomatoes**	

TO LEARN MORE . . .

I encourage you to visit the website (www.responsibletechnology.org) of the Institute for Responsible Technology (IRT), the true pioneers in alerting us all to the dangers of GMOs. If you can, make a donation to support their valuable work. When I interviewed the IRT's founder, Jeffrey Smith, he told me that the most effective way to get rid of GMOs is to vote with our dollars (www.autoimmunesummit .com). If we stop buying GMO-laden products and focus on natural foods and those specifically labeled as "not containing any GMOs," the companies that make GMOs will be motivated to start providing us with non-GMO alternatives.

Also, check out the Environmental Working Group's shopper's guide, updated regularly, and update your overall knowledge by periodically visiting the site (www.ewg.org).

Finally, if you have the opportunity to vote for a GMO labeling bill or to donate to an effort to label, regulate, or restrict GMOs, take action. Your family's health is too important to be left to giant corporations like Monsanto. Your bottom line is your family; their bottom line is, well, the bottom line!

Heavy Metals

If you have followed The Myers Way for three months and haven't seen the improvement you would like, you might consider whether heavy metals are part of the problem, particularly if you have one or more of the following risk factors. You

- have amalgam fillings, either currently or in the past;
- live near a coal-burning plant (check out this link to find out whether one is near you: www.epa.gov/mats/where.html);
- have spent time in China, which is a heavy coal-burning country;
- eat tuna more than once a month;
- have recurrent yeast overgrowth (sometimes the yeast is there to protect you from the mercury);
- have one or more genetic mutations in the *MTHFR* gene (pages 145–46); or
- regularly drink or shower in unfiltered water.

If you want to find out more about whether heavy metals are a concern for you, take these next two steps:

GET A FUNCTIONAL MEDICINE PHYSICIAN TO TEST YOU

There are two tests I rely on. One is a red blood cell (RBC) test, which looks at your exposure to heavy metals over the previous three months (since that is the life of a red blood cell). The results of your RBC test will let me know how much heavy metal you have been consuming through the food you eat, via your fillings, or through the air you breathe.

If I want to know more about your long-term exposure to heavy metals and their possible accumulation in your body, I do a "challenge" test. First I take a urine sample to give me a baseline (how much heavy metal is in your urine, reflecting again current exposure). Then I have you swallow a solution of 2,3-dimercapto-1-propanesulfonic acid (DMPS), which will help your body "chelate," or filter out, the heavy metals from where they have been stored, primarily in your bones. Over the next six hours, I collect urine so that the lab can measure how much heavy metal is released or has been stored in your system.

IF NECESSARY, GET CHELATED

Based on what the challenge test reveals about the level of heavy metals stored in your bones, I might decide to chelate you—to have you undergo a process that draws out the heavy metals. If your level of heavy metals is significant but low, I might use natural chelators like cilantro. If it's higher, I'll use dimercaptosuccinic acid (DMSA), the FDA-approved substance for chelation for lead toxicity, although it's used to chelate other heavy metals as well.

I have my patients take DMSA three times a day for three days, then take eleven days off. The process can take anywhere from three to twelve months. I do a follow-up test three months later. Throughout the entire process, I make sure to support the detox pathways with lots of glutathione and minerals. Your own functional medicine physician will likely follow a similar process, though some people use slightly different protocols.

A WORD OF WARNING

Be very careful if a doctor is suggesting chelation or even a chelation test as your first step in healing. You must heal your gut, open your detox pathways, and provide them with plenty of support *before* you do either of these procedures; otherwise, you could be doing much more damage than good. Chelation is a process that pulls toxins from your bones into your system so that you can then excrete them through your urine. If your gut is leaky and your detox pathways are not working properly, you are in serious danger of reabsorbing all those toxins into your system—only instead of absorbing them little by little, you will get them in much larger quantities. *Run*, do not walk, from any physician who wants to chelate you before making absolutely sure that your gut has been healed.

Toxic Mold

I ask about mold exposure both on my intake form and during my patient's first appointment. If I hear anything that makes me think there's an obvious source of mold, I tell my patient that it might be a contributing factor to their autoimmune condition and I try to find out more.

If the patient has addressed the four pillars of The Myers Way and has still not improved sufficiently or if the person has recurrent yeast overgrowth, then I dig much deeper into toxic mold. So let's look a bit more closely right now.

WHERE ARE THE TOXINS COMING FROM?

Certain types of mold give off gases known as volatile organic compounds (VOCs). Not all molds produce these toxins, but the ones that do are obviously a huge concern. The most common culprits are

- *Aspergillus*
- *Fusarium*
- *Paecilomyces*
- *Penicillium*
- *Stachybotrys*
- *Trichoderma*

We believe that only 25 percent of the population has the genes that make them vulnerable to the deleterious effects of these molds, but for anyone who is vulnerable, the symptoms can be intense. I have seen people suffer from a number of mold-related symptoms, including the following:

- ADD/ADHD
- allergies, asthma, chronic sinus infections
- anxiety
- autoimmunity
- chronic fatigue syndrome
- depression
- fibromyalgia
- headaches
- insomnia

- neurologic issues
- recurrent yeast overgrowth
- skin rashes of all types, including eczema

However, because three-quarters of the population are not vulnerable to mycotoxins, it's not unusual for only one person in a household to show symptoms, making the cause extremely difficult to diagnose, especially for practitioners who aren't well educated about this problem.

Risk factors that cause me to suspect mold include the following:

- older homes
- homes with known leaks
- homes with basements
- homes built into hillsides
- homes with flat roofs
- humid climates

Notoriously moldy environments include the following:

- larger apartment complexes
- large office buildings
- hotels
- schools

Another factor to consider is if you live or work in a place that has a shared HVAC (heating, ventilation, and air-conditioning) system, which can carry mycotoxins from a leaky, moldy area into spaces where there is no leak—making the problem even harder to detect.

HOW TO TEST FOR TOXIC MOLD

The typical mold test is unlikely to help you, frankly, because it focuses on air quality and the level of mold spores, not on volatile organic compounds. So you have two choices:

- Cut off a piece of your air filter and send it in to RealTime Laboratories (see "Resources"); or
- check "Resources" for a company that can do what is called an ERMI (environmental relative moldiness index) test, which specifically seeks the type of mold that releases mycotoxins. However, once you run a test like this, you have to disclose it to anyone who might want to buy the house, which means that if you don't easily find the mold, you might end up ripping out walls or going

to other drastic lengths to ensure that you have indeed found and removed the mold.

All of which is to say I'm not a big fan of testing homes. I'd rather test you. But that can get tricky. The standard test is a urine test, but that only detects levels of three main mycotoxins. If you're reacting to less common mycotoxins, that won't necessarily show up. Also, the level that shows up on the test doesn't necessarily correlate with a person's symptoms: You can be very sick with low levels on the test or not so sick but test with high levels. Plus, the test is expensive. However, it's the best we have, so I do rely on it quite a bit.

If you can afford it, what I prefer to suggest is that you find somewhere else to stay for a couple of weeks—a hotel, a friend's house, a rental vacation home, an airy bed-and-breakfast—anywhere you can manage that you are reasonably certain is mold-free. Take with you as little as possible—your favorite pillow or your child's beloved stuffed animal might be mold-infested—and see if you feel better after ten days or so out of your home. After all, your body knows better than any test. If you feel better away from home, and if you feel worse when you return home, you very well might be reacting to mycotoxins.

We also have to figure out whether you seem to be reacting to mycotoxins in your home or somewhere else. If you work only at home or if your child is homeschooled, then we have only your house to worry about; but if a workplace or school is involved, then we have another problem to solve.

In that case, I'll often test someone else who is living in the home. If that person tests positive for mycotoxins—even if they aren't experiencing any symptoms—we can assume the mold is in the home. If they test negative, we can assume the mold is coming from the workplace or school.

I know this is a challenging problem. No one wants to hear that their house might be infested with mold and that it might cost a significant amount of money to clean it up. But there are some solutions:

- If you can identify a leak, then hire a certified mold remediator to remove the mold. Be careful, though, because the chemicals used to clean up mold can also cause problems to a fragile immune system.

- Take the glutathione I suggest in chapter 9, along with the rest of your supplements on The Myers Way.

- Go to a functional medicine physician for more targeted help, including prescription medications that can help you clear up your own fungi and infections as well as resist the mold attacks. The most common prescription for this condition is cholestyramine, which binds the toxins so that they can be safely eliminated from your system.

Solving a toxic mold problem can be challenging, but it is *so* worth it. See page 141 in chapter 6 as well as chapter 12 for some truly inspiring success stories that demonstrate just what extraordinary healing is possible once this problem is solved.

Biological Dentistry

In chapter 6 you learned that what's in your mouth can be a significant source of inflammation. Root canals, extracted wisdom teeth, braces, retainers, fillings, crowns, posts—your mouth is full of potential bio-hazards, and yet conventional dentists are barely aware of the problem.

Luckily, just as we have functional medical physicians to counter-act the shortcomings of conventional medicine, we have biological dentists to counter the failings of conventional dentistry. A biological dentist is concerned with more than just your teeth. He or she wants to make sure that only safe, biocompatible materials are used in your mouth and only safe procedures are performed there.

Your first takeaway is to remember that everything in your mouth affects your entire immune system. After all, you are one system—there is no "Chinese wall" separating your mouth from the rest of your anatomy. So if you have a piece of dental equipment that remains permanently in your mouth—crown, filling, wire, whatever—your immune system might be continuously exposed to it. If something in that equipment is challenging to your immune system, you are being challenged 24/7.

The solution? A biological dentist might take a sample of your blood and have a lab run tests (www.ccrlab.com) on it to discover which dental materials you might react to. If your dentist doesn't fol-low that protocol, products made by VOCO, a German company, are almost always biocompatible, so see if you can have dental materials made only by them.

THE MERCURY PROBLEM

Your next takeaway concerns the mercury that has traditionally been used in silver fillings. When I speak with biological dentists, we are all simply baffled as to why this second-most toxic substance on earth is routinely used as an element to remain permanently in people's mouths. Research shows that the mercury emitted by amalgam fillings does have an impact on our health and does indeed challenge our immune systems. Obviously, we all have a wide range of ability to tolerate toxins, just as some people can smoke heavily and never get lung cancer. But if you have an autoimmune condition or are on the spectrum, your immune system is already challenged, so you should not stress it any more. Find a biological dentist who can safely remove your silver fillings along with the mercury they contain.

Still not 100 percent convinced? Take a look at the video prepared by the International Academy of Oral Medicine and Toxicology (IAOMT), a respected organization of dentists, physicians, and researchers focused on oral and dental health. In the video, you'll see a "smoking tooth": plumes of mercury vapors rising off a tooth with a mercury-laden filling (www.youtube.com/watch?v=9ylnQ-T7oiA). If you have a conventional silver filling, that's what's happening right now in your mouth. Conventional dentists may tell you that mercury-laden fillings are safe. Don't believe them.

By the way, in the 1970s, conventional dentists also started using tin and copper in those silver fillings. Tin is toxic too, but the real danger was the copper, which raised the level of mercury exposure by a factor of fifty.

In some cases, if you've had a crown put in, your conventional dentist may have used the preexisting filling as a base. The crown on top exacerbates the effect of mercury, not least because it can create a galvanic current—literally, an electric current that competes with the natural electric currents running through your body. I've had patients report strange buzzing in their mouths from the three or four different types of metals they were carrying. I referred them to a biological dentist to have the mercury removed and heard back within a day or so that they could already feel the difference.

When you do go to replace your silver fillings, make sure you see a biological dentist. Conventional dentists simply won't know enough about how to do the procedure safely, without exposing you or themselves to the vapors.

ROOT CANALS

Your next concern should be root canals. A root canal is a procedure whereby a tooth's nerve is killed but the tooth itself remains in your mouth. Leaving a dead portion of the anatomy inside the body is done nowhere else in medicine, and in my opinion, it shouldn't be done in dentistry either. Toxic bacteria breed freely inside the dead tooth, and without the blood supply that a living tooth would receive, there are no immune factors or killer chemicals to stop them. Nor can they be effectively reached with antibiotics.

The solution is either to give the dead tooth an ozone treatment or to have it extracted. Extraction is a challenging solution in some cases, although it's obviously easier with back teeth. But remember, root canals are a breeding ground for toxic bacteria and a likely source of significant inflammation. Particularly if you have an autoimmune condition or are high on the spectrum, you don't need an additional risk factor or an added burden on your immune system. Let a biological dentist help you solve this problem.

And if a conventional dentist offers you a root canal, run, don't walk, to a biological dentist and see if there is any other option.

CAVITATIONS

A cavitation is an area of dead bone inside a bone, most commonly in the jaw. If you've had a trauma, such as the extraction of a wisdom tooth, bacteria flow into the open area. Then gum tissue grows over the hollow, and bone grows over that. Meanwhile, highly toxic bacteria remain inside the hollow area, presenting your immune system with a daily challenge.

A biological dentist can clean the area by making a small surgical incision, irrigating the area, and using ozone to attack the bacteria. Then he or she can get the area to heal properly as your immune system breathes a huge heartfelt sigh of relief.

Cavitations can be difficult to detect on an x-ray or even a CAT scan. That's why you need an experienced biological dentist, who knows what to look for.

BRACES AND RETAINERS

This equipment frequently contains stainless steel, which sounds safe.
Think again. Stainless steel contains nickel, a carcinogen. Most braces
are made from "NiTi wire," which is nickel and titanium—amazing
at helping to straighten teeth quickly but not so good for your health.
A biological dentist can work with you to reduce the exposure to
nickel and go with a safer material.

FINDING A BIOLOGICAL DENTIST

To my great joy, this branch of dentistry seems to be growing by leaps
and bounds, just as functional medicine is growing. So you have a
few options for finding someone:

- Search online for "biological dentist" or "holistic dentist" and
  see who comes up.
- Go to www.iaomt.org, the website of the IAOMT, and search for
  their members in your area.
- Ask your functional medicine physician for a referral.

If you're checking out a new dentist, here are three questions you
can ask to help you decide whether they might be a good choice:

❶ **Do you use a rubber dam?** A rubber dam should be used to protect the patient when mercury fillings are being removed. If your
dentist answers yes, he or she is far more likely to know how to
remove fillings safely.

❷ **What do you do to protect yourself and your staff?** If a dentist
is taking mercury out of your mouth, that dentist and their staff
are being exposed to it too. A dentist who doesn't protect him- or
herself or the office's staff might not be truly aware of the health
hazards involved—and therefore won't be fully aware of how to
protect you.

❸ **Do you have an amalgam separator?** When mercury is removed
normally, it goes right into the local wastewater supply, a thought
that just makes me shudder. An amalgam separator will separate
out the mercury so it can be disposed of safely.

TO LEARN MORE . . .

Check out this terrific book with a spot-on title: *Uninformed Consent: The Hidden Dangers in Dental Care* (Newburyport, Mass.: Hampton Roads Publishing, 1999), by Hal A. Huggins and Thomas E. Levy. Other good resources are *It's All in Your Head: The Link Between Mercury Amalgams and Illness* (Garden City Park, N.Y.: Avery Publishing, 1993), by Hal A. Huggins, or my interview with biological dentist Stuart Nunnally, DDS (www.autoimmunesummit.com).

Detoxifying Your Home

With so many toxins out there, you can easily start to feel overwhelmed by the task of protecting yourself and your immune system from their ill effects. However, as I always say, knowledge is power! Now that you know about the toxins, you *can* take steps to keep them out of your personal environment. I encourage everybody to do this, especially if you have an autoimmune condition or are on the spectrum. Your immune system doesn't need any more challenges to deal with!

You've already seen my top detox suggestions in chapter 6. Here are some additional ways to detox your home, listed in order of importance:

CONVENTIONAL MATTRESSES

Where you sleep and what you sleep on are two of the most important decisions you can make—I can't stress this enough! We spend nearly half our lives asleep, and most of our detox and body repair occurs while we sleep. Conventional mattresses contain harsh chemicals and fire retardants, which can emit gases for years.

Better Choices
- One hundred percent natural latex mattresses and organic wool mattress toppers

COMMERCIAL BEDDING

Most commercial bedding manufacturers use fire retardants, pesticides, bleaches, and dyes.

Better Choices
- Organic, untreated sheets, blankets, and pillows

CLEANING PRODUCTS

The American Society for the Prevention of Cruelty to Animals (ASPCA) listed household cleaners as one of the top ten pet poisons in 2009. Levels of brominated flame retardants in cats are up to twenty-three times higher than those found in human beings, and dogs have on average 2.4 times more perfluorinated chemicals in their bodies than people. These are chemicals that are already found in products you buy, such as fire-resistant fabrics and stain-proof rugs, so just imagine how susceptible your dog or cat is to the chemicals you spray and pour in your home.

Better Choices

- Luckily, there are several, which you can find in the "Resources" section.

DRY CLEANING

Dry cleaners are some of the most chemical-laden establishments around.

Better Choices

- Look for a clean and green eco dry cleaner.

- If you must use a traditional dry cleaner, remove your garments from the plastic bag and air them outside for several hours before hanging them in your closet.

VINYL SHOWER CURTAINS

These release more than a hundred VOCs, which can hang around in the air for more than a month. They also contain phthalates, which are hormone and endocrine disrupters.

Better Choices

- Organic cotton and linen shower curtains

CONVENTIONAL CARPETS

Conventional carpeting is made from synthetic, petroleum-based fibers, which can emit up to 120 hazardous chemicals that have been shown to contribute to asthma, allergies, neurological problems, and cancer. The toxins are found primarily in the rubber padding and adhesive glues, which might emit chemical-laden gases for years.

Better Choices

- Cotton or wool rugs
- Recycled carpet tiles, which do not require adhesive glues
- Stained concrete
- Renewable wood, such as bamboo or cork

VOLATILE ORGANIC COMPOUND (VOC) PAINTS

These are just what they sound like: paints that include toxic compounds. If you use them, you are literally surrounding yourself with potentially hazardous fumes.

Better Choices

- No-VOC paints. But make sure that's really what they are. Many companies advertise their products as "no-VOC," but that's the base white paint only. Once color is added, the paint is no longer no-VOC.

UPHOLSTERED FURNITURE

Upholstered furniture can be filled with polyurethane foams, which are petroleum-based and overflowing with chemicals and fire retardants. Any particleboard that is part of the furniture emits formaldehyde.

Better Choices

- Furniture made with solid wood, natural latex foam, wool cushions, and organic fabrics

CURTAINS AND WINDOW TREATMENTS

Most curtains contain fire retardants, pesticides, bleaches, and dyes.

Better Choices

- Organic, untreated cotton or linen curtains and valences
- Bamboo shades

TO LEARN MORE . . .

Watch my video interview with the executive director of the Environmental Working Group (EWG), Heather White (www.auto immunesummit.com).

APPENDIX F

Improving Your Sleep

Sleep disturbance and fatigue are two of the most common complaints I hear in my practice. Getting the right amount of deep, refreshing sleep is one of the best ways you can support your immune system, so here are my top ten tips for improving your sleep:

❶ Go to www.dansplan.com and download "Dan's Plan," a free online plan to optimize health and sleep created by sleep expert Dan Pardi. If you'd like to learn more about Dan's approach to sleep, you can check out the interview I did with him on my podcast: www.dramymyers.com/tag/sleep/.

❷ Buy amber lightbulbs and install them in lamps throughout your house. Use them once the sun begins to go down.

One of the main causes of sleep disturbances is exposure to the wrong spectrum of light once the sun has gone down. Your body has evolved to sleep when the sky is dark and be awake when the sky is light. This natural sleep-wake cycle can be disrupted by our twenty-four-hour electric world, in which your body is continuously exposed to bright "sun-like" light, including that given off by incandescent and fluorescent lightbulbs. Your body recognizes these electric devices as "sunlight" and cues you to stay awake. Using amber light after sundown will help sync up your body with the rhythms of the earth and cue your system for sleep rather than wakefulness.

❸ Download the free f.lux app at www.justgetflux.com if you work on your computer or read on your iPad at night. The flickering blue light of electronic devices also cues you to wakefulness—but the f.lux app will saturate your screen with an amber hue once the sun has gone down. You can set the app to give you the nighttime shade of amber that you prefer; reset it to accommodate watching a movie or TV show; and disable it short- or long-term if you'd actually like your device to help you stay awake. Ideally, though, you will use the device to follow a healthy sleep-wake cycle of becoming drowsy after sunset and going to bed relatively early.

❹ Determine your ideal number of hours of sleep. Try this one on the weekends! Go to sleep at night and see how long it takes you to wake up. Repeat this experiment a few times to determine your ideal number of sleeping hours. We are all different, and each of our sleep needs can change, also, depending on how much stress we are under or what demands we have placed on our bodies. Sleep is when your body heals, so if you are using The Myers Way to reverse your autoimmune condition, you might need more sleep than usual. You might also generally need more sleep than you assume. Find out your body's ideal sleep time so you can make sure to always get that amount of sleep.

❺ Set the intention of going to bed at the same time each night as determined by your ideal number of hours of sleep. In other words, if you need to get up at seven A.M. to be on time for work, and if you've discovered that your ideal amount of sleep is nine hours, set the intention of going to bed at ten P.M. each night. Ideally, you will go to bed at this time on weekends also, because you get better sleep when you maintain a consistent rhythm.

❻ Get blackout curtains for your bedroom. Even tiny amounts of light are perceived through your eyelids and can disrupt the depth and quality of your sleep. Your body was designed to respond to the earth's natural rhythms of sunset and sunrise, so if light from streetlamps or neighboring buildings is filtering into your bedroom, your body will perceive that it's supposed to be awake and your sleep will be affected.

❼ Before bed, take a hot bath with Epsom salts. The hot water and downtime are relaxing, and the Epsom salts contain magnesium to relax your muscles.

❽ Get outside and expose yourself to natural light at least three times a day for a minimum of thirty minutes. If your body has access to natural light to cue the "wake" cycle, it will be more ready to respond to darkness as the "sleep" cycle.

⑨ Skip the nightcap! Alcohol affects your sleep cycle. Of course you won't be drinking alcohol for the first thirty days of The Myers Way and maybe for several months thereafter. If you decide to add an occasional alcoholic beverage back into your diet, make sure you have it at least a couple of hours before bedtime so that when you sleep, you sleep deeply and can recover from the stress alcohol places on your immune system.

⑩ If you want a temporary sleep aid, go natural. Consider 5-HTP (5-hydroxytryptophan), a natural precursor to serotonin, the neurotransmitter that helps regulate sleep cycles as well as creates a natural "antidepressant" effect of optimism and calm. Another option is melatonin, a brain chemical that specifically cues your body for sleep. Magnesium is a mineral that helps to relax your muscles and is therefore helpful for the relaxation that precedes deep and restful sleep. Recommendations for high-quality versions of these supplements are in the "Resources" section.

TO LEARN MORE . . .

Watch my video interview with sleep expert Dan Pardi (www.auto immunesummit.com).

The Myers Way Symptom Tracker

Rate the following symptoms over the past seven days on a scale of 0 to 4 based on severity. 0 = None, 1 = Some, 2 = Mild, 3 = Moderate, 4 = Severe

HEAD

____headaches

____migraines

____faintness

____trouble sleeping

Total ____

MIND

____brain fog

____poor memory

____impaired coordination

____difficulty deciding

____slurred/stuttered
   speech

____learning/attention
   deficit

Total ____

EYES

____swollen, red eyelids

____dark circles

____puffy eyes

____poor vision

____watery, itchy eyes

Total ____

NOSE

____nasal congestion

____excessive mucus

____stuffy/runny nose

____sinus problems

____frequent sneezing

Total ____

EARS

____itchy ears

____earaches, infections

____drainage from ear

____ringing ears, hearing loss

Total ____

MOUTH, THROAT

____chronic cough

____frequent throat clearing

____sore throat

____swollen lips

____canker sores

Total ____

HEART

____irregular heartbeat

____rapid heartbeat

____chest pain

Total ____

LUNGS

____chest congestion
____asthma, bronchitis
____shortness of breath
____difficulty breathing
Total ____

SKIN

____acne
____hives, eczema, dry skin
____hair loss
____hot flashes
____excessive sweating
Total ____

WEIGHT

____inability to lose weight
____food cravings
____excess weight
____insufficient weight
____compulsive eating
____water retention, swelling
Total ____

DIGESTION

____nausea, vomiting
____diarrhea
____constipation
____bloating
____belching, passing gas
____heartburn, indigestion
____intestinal/stomach pain
    or cramps
Total ____

EMOTIONS

____anxiety
____depression
____mood swings
____nervousness
____irritability
Total ____

ENERGY, ACTIVITY

____fatigue
____lethargy
____hyperactivity
____restlessness
Total ____

JOINTS, MUSCLES

____joint pain/aches
____arthritis
____muscle stiffness
____muscle pain/aches
____weakness, tiredness
Total ____

OTHER

____frequent illness/
    infections
____frequent/urgent urination
____genital itch, discharge
____anal itch
Total ____

Preliminary total _____

Resources

BIOLOGICAL DENTISTRY

- "Biological Dentistry with Stuart Nunnally, DDS" (podcast): *www.dramymyers.com/2013/07/08/tmw-episode-12-biological-dentistry-with-stuart-nunnally-dds/*
- International Academy of Biological Dentistry and Medicine: *http://iabdm.org/*
- International Academy of Oral Medicine and Toxicology (IAOMT): *http://iaomt.org/*
- *It's All in Your Head: The Link Between Mercury Amalgams and Illness,* book by Hal A. Huggins (New York: Penguin, 1993)
- My Magic Mud: *www.mymagicmud.com/my-magic-mud-natural-teeth-whitening-remedy/*
- "Smoking Teeth = Poison Gas" (video by the International Academy of Oral Medicine and Toxicology): *www.youtube.com/watch?v=9ylnQ-T7oiA*
- *Uninformed Consent: The Hidden Dangers in Dental Care,* book by Hal A. Huggins and Thomas E. Levy (Newburyport, Mass.: Hampton Roads Publishing, 1999)

BODY CARE

- Babo Botanicals: *www.babobotanicals.com/*
- "Chemical-Free Gluten-Free Skin Care with Bob Root" (podcast): *www.dramymyers.com/2013/07/01/tmw-episode-11-chemical-free-gluten-free-skin-care-with-bob-root/*
- Environmental Working Group: *www.ewg.org/*
- "Green Beauty with W3LL PEOPLE" (podcast): *www.dramymyers.com/2013/08/12/tmw-episode-17-green-beauty-with-w3ll-people/*
- Keys body care products: *http://store.amymyersmd.com/page/1/?s=KEYS&post_type=product*

- Thorne shampoo: *http://store.amymyersmd.com/?s=thorne&post_type=product*
- W3LL PEOPLE makeup and beauty products: *http://w3llpeople.com*

COMMUNITY

- Amy Myers, MD: *www.amymyersmd.com*
- Facebook: *www.facebook.com/AmyMyersMD*
- Meetup: *www.meetup.com/*

DETOXIFYING YOUR HOME AND BODY

- "Detoxification with Dr. Myers" (podcast): *www.dramymyers.com/2013/12/30/the-myers-way-episode-29-detoxification-with-dr-myers/*

Air Filters

- IQAir GC MultiGas air purifier: *http://store.amymyersmd.com/shop/air-purifier/*
- IQAir HealthPro Plus air filter: *http://store.amymyersmd.com/shop/iqair-health-pro-plus-air-filter/*

Bath Accessories

- Organic cotton shower curtains: *www.westelm.com/search/results.html?words=organic+cotton+shower+curtain*
- Showerhead water filters: *www.aquasana.com/shower-head-water-filters*

Bedding

- Eco-Wise organic bedding: *www.ecowise.com/category_s/1860.htm*
- West Elm organic bedding: *www.westelm.com/shop/bedding/organic-bedding-style/?cm_type=gnav*

Cleaning Products

- CleanWell hand-sanitizing wipes: *http://store.amymyersmd.com/shop/cleanwell-hand-sanitizing-wipes/*
- Dr. Bronner's pure castile soap: *http://store.amymyersmd.com/shop/dr-bronners-pure-castile-soap/*

- Ecover automatic dishwasher tablets: *http://store.amymyersmd.com /shop/ecover-dishwashing-tablets/*
- Ecover bathroom cleaner: *http://store.amymyersmd.com/shop/ecover -bathroom-cleaner/*
- Ecover laundry liquid: *http://store.amymyersmd.com/shop/ecover -laundry-liquid/*
- Ecover toilet bowl cleaner: *http://store.amymyersmd.com/shop/ecover -toilet-bowl-cleaner/*
- Miele HEPA vacuum cleaner: *http://store.amymyersmd.com/shop /miele-hepa-vacuum-cleaner/*

Flooring

- Eco-Wise flooring: *www.ecowise.com/flooring_and_countertops _s/1857.htm*
- Green Building Supply: *www.greenbuildingsupply.com/All-Products /Flooring*
- West Elm wool rugs: *www.westelm.com/shop/rugs-windows/rugs-by -material/wool-rugs/?cm_type=lnav*

Furniture

- West Elm furniture: *www.westelm.com/shop/furniture/?cm_type =gnav*

Mattresses

- Urban Mattress: *www.urbanmattress.com/*

Paint

- Eco-Wise zero VOC paint: *www.ecowise.com/category_s/1817.htm*
- Home Depot low and zero VOC paint: *www.ecooptions.homedepot .com/clean-air/low-zero-voc-paint/*

Saunas

- Sunlighten saunas: *http://store.amymyersmd.com/shop/sunlighten -saunas/*

Water Filters

- Aquasana water filters: *www.aquasana.com/?discountcode=drmyers &utm_medium=referral&utm_source=drmyers&utm_campaign=_*

Window Treatments

- West Elm curtains: *www.westelm.com/shop/rugs-windows/window-panels-curtains-shades/*

FOOD AND DINING

Grocery Stores

- Natural Grocers: *www.naturalgrocers.com/*
- Sprouts Farmers Market: *www.sprouts.com/*
- Trader Joe's: *www.traderjoes.com/*
- Whole Foods Market: *www.wholefoodsmarket.com/*

Organic Meat and Fish

- US Wellness Meats: *www.grasslandbeef.com/StoreFront.bok?affId=168453*
- Vital Choice: *www.vitalchoice.com/shop/pc/home.asp?idaffiliate=3198*

Shopping Guides

- Environmental Working Group's Dirty Dozen Plus and Clean Fifteen: *www.ewg.org/foodnews/*
- Environmental Working Group's Fish List: *http://static.ewg.org/files/fishguide.pdf*
- Environmental Working Group's Shopper's Guide to Avoiding GE Food: *www.ewg.org/research/shoppers-guide-to-avoiding-ge-food*
- Mercury levels in fish: *www.nrdc.org/health/effects/mercury/guide.asp*

Special Diet Apps

- Locate Special Diet: *http://locatespecialdiet.com/*
- Urbanspoon: *www.urbanspoon.com/*

GENETICALLY MODIFIED ORGANISMS

- Environmental Working Group's Shopper's Guide to Avoiding GE Food: *www.ewg.org/research/shoppers-guide-to-avoiding-ge-food*
- Food Democracy Now!: *www.fooddemocracynow.org*

- *Genetic Roulette*, film by Jeffrey M. Smith and the Institute for Responsible Technology: *www.geneticroulettemovie.com*
- The Institute for Responsible Technology: *www.responsible technology.org*
- *Seeds of Deception: Exposing Industry and Government Lies About the Safety of the Genetically Engineered Foods You're Eating*, book by Jeffrey M. Smith (Portland, Me.: Yes! Books, 2003)

KITCHEN PRODUCTS

Beverage Storage

- Aquasana glass bottles: *http://store.amymyersmd.com/shop/aquasana -glass-bottles-6-pack/*
- Kleen Kanteen (20 ounce size): *http://store.amymyersmd.com/shop /klean-kanteen-20oz/*
- Kleen Kanteen (27 ounce size): *http://store.amymyersmd.com/shop /klean-kanteen-27oz/*

Food Storage

- Ball Mason jars: *http://store.amymyersmd.com/shop/ball-mason-jars/*
- BPA-free Ziploc bag information: *www.ziploc.com/Sustainability/ Pages/Safety-and-Plastics.aspx*
- Pyrex glass storage containers: *http://store.amymyersmd.com/shop /pyrex-glass-storage-10-piece-set/*
- up & up BPA-free freezer bags: *www.target.com/p/up-up-trade- double-zipper-quart-size-freezer-bags-50-ct/-/A-14730774#prodSlot =medium_1_3*

Cooking Equipment

- All-Clad stainless steel saucepan: *http://store.amymyersmd.com/shop /all-clad-stainless-steel-sauce-pan/*
- Crock-Pot slow cooker: *http://store.amymyersmd.com/shop/crock-pot -5-qt-slow-cooker/*
- KitchenAid Artisan stand mixer: *http://store.amymyersmd.com/shop /kitchenaid-artisan-5-qt-stand-mixer/*
- Lodge enameled cast-iron Dutch oven: *http://store.amymyersmd .com/shop/lodge-enameled-cast-iron-dutch-oven/*

- Lodge enameled cast-iron skillet: *http://store.amymyersmd.com/shop/lodge-enameled-cast-iron-skillet/*
- Lodge preseasoned cast-iron skillet: *http://store.amymyersmd.com/shop/lodge-preseasoned-cast-iron-skillet/*
- Oceanstar bamboo kitchen utensils: *http://store.amymyersmd.com/shop/oceanstar-bamboo-kitchen-utensils-7-piece-set/*

Juicers and Blenders

- Breville juicer: *http://store.amymyersmd.com/shop/breville-juicer/*
- Vitamix 5200 blender: *http://store.amymyersmd.com/shop/vitamix-5200-blender/*

LABORATORIES

- 23andMe: *www.23andme.com*
- Clifford Consulting and Research: *www.ccrlab.com*
- Commonwealth Laboratories: *www.hydrogenbreathtesting.com*
- Cyrex Laboratories: *www.cyrexlabs.com*
- DiagnosTechs: *www.diagnostechs.com/*
- Doctor's Data: *www.doctorsdata.com*
- Dunwoody Labs: *www.dunwoodylabs.com*
- Fertility and Cryogenics Lab: *www.fclab.us*
- Genova Diagnostics: *www.gdx.net*
- IGeneX: *www.igenex.com/Website/*
- Immuno Laboratories: *www.immunolabs.com/patients/*
- Immunosciences Lab: *www.immunoscienceslab.com*
- iSpot Lyme: *http://ispotlyme.com/*
- Laboratory Corporation of America: *www.labcorp.com/wps/portal/*
- Pharmasan Labs: *www.pharmasanlabs.com*
- Quest Diagnostics: *www.questdiagnostics.com/home.html*
- RealTime Laboratories: *www.realtimelab.com*

RELAXATION AND STRESS REDUCTION

- Acupuncture information and resources: *www.nccaom.org/*

- HeartMath emWave2 personal stress reliever: *http://store.amymyers md.com/shop/heartmath-emwave-2-personal-stress-reliever/*
- HeartMath Inner Balance sensor for iOS: *http://store.amymyersmd .com/shop/heartmath-inner-balance-sensor-for-ios/*
- HeartMath Inner Balance sensor for iPhone5 and iPad Air: *http:// store.amymyersmd.com/shop/heartmath-inner-balance-sensor-for -iphone5-and-ipad-air/*
- Lavender oil: *http://store.amymyersmd.com/shop/now-foods-organic -lavender-oil/*
- Relaxation and meditation CDs: *www.healthjourneys.com*

RESEARCH AND TREATMENT

- American Academy of Environmental Medicine: *www.aaemonline .org/*
- American Board of Integrative and Holistic Medicine: *www.holistic board.org/*
- American Botanical Council: *www.abc.herbalgram.org*
- American College for Advancement in Medicine: *www.acamnet.org/*
- American College of Nutrition: *www.americancollegeofnutrition.org*
- Cancer Treatment Centers of America: *www.cancercenter.com*
- Center for Integrative Medicine, University of Maryland School of Medicine: *www.compmed.umm.edu*
- Clinton Foundation: *www.clintonfoundation.org*
- The Institute for Functional Medicine: *www.functionalmedicine.org/*
- The Institute for Molecular Medicine: *www.immed.org*
- The Institutes for the Achievement of Human Potential: *www .iahp.org*
- Linus Pauling Institute, Oregon State University: *http://lpi.oregon state.edu*
- National Center for Complementary and Alternative Medicine: *www.nccam.nih.gov*
- National Institutes of Health: *www.nih.gov*
- Personalized Lifestyle Medicine Institute: *http://plminstitute.org/*
- Personalized Medicine Coalition: *www.personalizedmedicine coalition.org*
- Preventive Medicine Research Institute: *www.pmri.org*

- Slow Food USA: *www.slowfoodusa.org*
- United Natural Products Alliance: *www.unpa.com*

Autoimmune Disease Research and Support

- American Autoimmune Related Diseases Association: *www.aarda.org/*
- Autism Research Institute: *www.autism.com*
- Autoimmune Summit: *www.autoimmunesummit.com*
- Crohn's & Colitis Foundation of America: *www.ccfa.org/*
- Graves' Disease & Thyroid Foundation: *www.gdatf.org/*
- Lupus Foundation of America: *www.lupus.org/*
- Multiple Sclerosis Association of America: *www.mymsaa.org/*
- National Psoriasis Foundation: *www.psoriasis.org/*
- Scleroderma Foundation: *www.scleroderma.org/*

Gluten Intolerance and Celiac Disease Research and Support

- Celiac Disease Foundation: *http://celiac.org/*
- Celiac Support Association: *www.csaceliacs.info/*
- Center for Celiac Research and Treatment, Massachusetts General Hospital for Children: *www.celiaccenter.org*
- Gluten Intolerance Group: *www.gluten.net/*
- National Foundation for Celiac Awareness: *www.celiaccentral.org/support-groups/*

Stress Research and Support

- The Center for Mind-Body Medicine: *www.cmbm.org*
- The Hendricks Institute: *www.hendricks.com/*

SLEEP AIDS

- Bucky Luggage 40 Blinks ultralight sleep mask: *http://store.amymyersmd.com/shop/bucky-luggage-40-blinks-ultralight-sleep-mask/*
- Bulbrite amber lightbulbs: *http://store.amymyersmd.com/shop/bulbrite-amber-light-bulbs/*
- Dan's Plan: *www.dansplan.com*
- Feit amber lightbulbs: *http://store.amymyersmd.com/shop/feit-amber-light-bulbs/*

- Free f.lux app: *www.justgetflux.com*
- Simply Right Epsom salts: *http://store.amymyersmd.com/shop/simply-right-epsom-salts/*
- "Sleep Expert Dan Pardi" (podcast): *www.dramymyers.com/2013/06/24/tmw-episode-10-sleep-expert-dan-pardi/*

SUPPLEMENTS

- Allergy Research Group: *www.allergyresearchgroup.com*
- Bairn Biologics: *www.bairnbiologics.com*
- Biotics Research: *www.bioticsresearch.com*
- CitriSafe: *www.citrisafecertified.com*
- Designs for Health: *www.designsforhealth.com*
- Douglas Laboratories: *www.douglaslabs.com*
- Great Lakes Gelatin: *www.greatlakesgelatin.com*
- Lauricidin: *www.lauricidin.com*
- Metabolic Maintenance: *www.metabolicmaintenance.com*
- Metagenics: *www.metagenics.com*
- NeuroScience: *www.neurorelief.com*
- Prescript-Assist: *www.prescript-assist.com*
- ProThera/Klaire Labs: *www.protherainc.com*
- Pure Encapsulations: *www.pureencapsulations.com*
- Thorne Research: *www.thorne.com*
- Xymogen: *www.xymogen.com*

TOXIC MOLDS/MYCOTOXINS

- Environmental Relative Moldiness Index and ERMI testing services: *www.emlab.com/s/services/ERMI_testing.html*
- The Myers Way Podcast: *www.amymyersmd.com/2013/05/19/TMW-episode-5-mycotoxins*
- Real Time Laboratories: *www.realtimelab.com/*
- Surviving Mold: *www.survivingmold.com/*

Selected Bibliography

Chapter 1: My Autoimmune Journey—and Yours

Boelaert, K., P. R. Newby, M. J. Simmonds, R. L. Holder, J. D. Carr-Smith, J. M. Heward, N. Manji, et al. "Prevalence and Relative Risk of Other Autoimmune Diseases in Subjects with Autoimmune Thyroid Disease." *American Journal of Medicine* 123, no. 2 (February 2010): 183.

Ch'ng, C. L., M. Keston Jones, and Jeremy G. C. Kingham. "Celiac Disease and Autoimmune Thyroid Disease." *Clinical Medicine and Research* 5, no. 3 (October 2007): 184–92.

Harel, M., and Y. Shoenfeld. "Predicting and Preventing Autoimmunity, Myth or Reality?" *Annals of the New York Academy of Sciences* 1069 (June 2006): 322–45.

Hewagama, A., and B. Richardson. "The Genetics and Epigenetics of Autoimmune Diseases." *Journal of Autoimmunity* 33, no. 1 (August 2009): 3.

Okada, H., C. Kuhn, H. Feillet, and J.-F. Bach. "The 'Hygiene Hypothesis' for Autoimmune and Allergic Diseases: An Update." *Clinical and Experimental Immunology* 160, no. 1 (April 2010): 1–9.

Rook, G. A., C. A. Lowry, and C. L. Raison. "Hygiene and Other Early Childhood Influences on the Subsequent Function of the Immune System." *Brain Research* (April 13, 2014).

Selgrade, M. K., G. S. Cooper, D. R. Germolec, and J. J. Heindel. "Linking Environmental Agents and Autoimmune Disease: An Agenda for Future Research." *Environmental Health Perspectives* 107, suppl. 5 (October 1999): 811–13.

Shoenfeld, Y., B. Gilburd, M. Abu-Shakra, H. Amital, O. Barzilai, Y. Berkun, M. Blank, et al. "The Mosaic of Autoimmunity: Genetic Factors Involved in Autoimmune Diseases: 2008." *Israel Medical Association Journal* 10, no. 1 (January 2008): 3–7.

Smyk, D., E. Rigopoulou, H. Baum, A. K. Burroughs, D. Vergani, and D. P. Bogdanos. "Autoimmunity and Environment: Am I at Risk?" *Clinical Reviews in Allergy and Immunology* 42, no. 2 (April 2012): 199–212.

University of Michigan Health System. "The Hygiene Hypothesis: Are Cleanlier Lifestyles Causing More Allergies for Kids?" *ScienceDaily.* September 9, 2007.

Weight-Control Information Network. "Overweight and Obesity Statistics." http://win.niddk.nih.gov/statistics/.

Willett, W. C. "Balancing Life-Style and Genomics Research for Disease Prevention." *Science* 296, no. 5568 (April 2002): 695–98.

Autoimmune and Inflammation Symptoms

Adams, J. B., L. J. Johansen, L. D. Powell, D. Quig, and R. A. Rubin. "Gastrointestinal Flora and Gastrointestinal Status in Children with Autism: Comparisons to Typical Children and Correlation with Autism Severity." *BMC Gastroenterology* 11 (March 2011): 22.

Doe, W. F. "The Intestinal Immune System." *Gut* 30 (1989): 1679–85.

Ginsberg, J. "Diagnosis and Management of Graves' Disease." *Canadian Medical Association Journal* 168, no. 5 (March 2003): 575–85.

Herbert, M. R. "Autism: A Brain Disorder, or a Disorder That Affects the Brain?" *Clinical Neuropsychiatry* 2, no. 6 (2005): 354–79.

Holmdahl, R., V. Malmström, and H. Burkhardt. "Autoimmune Priming, Tissue Attack, and Chronic Inflammation: The Three Stages of Rheumatoid Arthritis." *European Journal of Immunology* 44, no. 6 (June 2014): 1593–99.

The Institute for Functional Medicine. "21st Century Medicine: A New Model for Medical Education and Practice." www.functionalmedicine.org/functional medicine-in-practice/deeper/.

MedlinePlus. "Propylthiouracil." www.nlm.nih.gov/medlineplus/druginfo/meds /a682465.html.

National Institute of Arthritis and Musculoskeletal and Skin Diseases website. www .niams.nih.gov.

Office on Women's Health, U.S. Department of Health and Human Services. "Autoimmune Diseases Fact Sheet." www.womenshealth.gov/publications/our -publications/fact-sheet/autoimmune-diseases.html.

Vojdani, A., E. Mumper, D. Granpeesheh, L. Mielke, D. Traver, K. Bock, K. Hirani, et al. "Low Natural Killer Cell Cytotoxic Activity in Autism: The Role of Glutathione, IL-2, and IL-15." *Journal of Neuroimmunology* 205, nos. 1–2 (December 2008): 148–54.

Vojdani, A., T. O'Bryan, J. A. Green, J. McCandless, K. N. Woeller, E. Vojdani, A. A. Nourian, and E. L. Cooper. "Immune Response to Dietary Proteins, Gliadin, and Cerebellar Peptides in Children with Autism." *Nutritional Neuroscience* 7, no. 3 (June 2004): 151–61.

"Autoimmunity in America" Statistics

American Autoimmune Related Diseases Association. "Autoimmune Statistics." www.aarda.org/autoimmune-information/autoimmune-statistics/.

American Autoimmune Related Diseases Association and National Coalition of Autoimmune Patient Groups. "The Cost Burden of Autoimmune Disease: The Latest Front in the War on Healthcare Spending." 2011. www.diabetesed.net /page/_files/autoimmune-diseases.pdf.

National Institutes of Health. "Autoimmune Diseases Coordinating Committee: Autoimmune Diseases Research Plan." 2002. www.niaid.nih.gov/topics/auto immune/Documents/adccreport.pdf.

"Inflammatory Conditions Along the Autoimmune Spectrum"

American Academy of Allergy Asthma and Immunology. "Asthma Statistics." www .aaaai.org/about-the-aaaai/newsroom/allergy-statistics.aspx.

Arthritis Foundation website. www.arthritis.org.

Centers for Disease Control and Prevention website. www.cdc.gov.

Chapter 2: Myths and Facts About Autoimmunity

Cooper, G. S., M. L. K. Bynum, and E. C. Somers. "Recent Insights in the Epidemiology of Autoimmune Diseases: Improved Prevalence Estimates and Understanding of Clustering of Diseases." *Journal of Autoimmunity* 33, nos. 3–4 (November–December 2009): 197–207.

Cooper, G. S., F. W. Miller, and J. P. Pandey. "The Role of Genetic Factors in Autoimmune Disease: Implications for Environmental Research." *Environmental Health Perspectives* 107, suppl. 5 (October 1999): 693–700.

Dooley, M. A., and S. L. Hogan. "Environmental Epidemiology and Risk Factors for Autoimmune Disease." *Current Opinion in Rheumatology* 15, no. 2 (March 2003): 99–103.

Fasano, A. *Gluten Freedom*. Hoboken, N.J.: John Wiley & Sons, 2014.

Fasano, A. "Systemic Autoimmune Disorders in Celiac Disease." *Current Opinion in Gastroenterology* 22, no. 6 (November 2006): 674–79.

Hewagama, A., and B. Richardson. "The Genetics and Epigenetics of Autoimmune Diseases." *Journal of Autoimmunity* 33, no. 1 (August 2009): 3.

Invernizzi, P., and M. E. Gershwin. "The Genetics of Human Autoimmune Disease." *Journal of Autoimmunity* 33, nos. 3–4 (November–December 2009): 290–99.

Kussmann, M., and P. J. van Bladeren. "The Extended Nutrigenomics—Understanding the Interplay Between the Genomes of Food, Gut Microbes, and Human Host." *Frontiers in Genetics* 2 (May 2011): 21.

Lu, Q. "The Critical Importance of Epigenetics in Autoimmunity." *Journal of Autoimmunity* 41 (March 2013): 1–5.

Powell, J. J., J. van de Water, and M. E. Gershwin. "Evidence for the Role of Environmental Agents in the Initiation or Progression of Autoimmune Conditions." *Environmental Health Perspectives* 107, suppl. 5 (October 1999): 667–72.

Radbruch, A., and P. E. Lipsky, eds. *Current Concepts in Autoimmunity and Chronic Inflammation*. Vol. 305 of *Current Topics in Microbiology and Immunology*. Berlin: Springer Verlag, 2006.

Walsh, S. J., and L. M. Rau. "Autoimmune Diseases: A Leading Cause of Death Among Young and Middle-Aged Women in the United States." *American Journal of Public Health* 90, no. 9 (September 2000): 1463–66.

CellCept (Mycophenolic Acid)

American College of Rheumatology. "Mycophenolate Mofetil (CellCept) and Mycophenolate Sodium (Myfortic)." www.rheumatology.org/Practice/Clinical/Patients/Medications/Mycophenolate_Mofetil_(CellCept)_and_Mycophenolate_Sodium_(Myfortic)/.

Genentech USA. "Frequently Asked Questions About CellCept." www.cellcept.com/cellcept/about.htm.

MedicineNet.com. "Mycophenolate Mofetil—Oral, CellCept." Last modified April 16, 2014. www.medicinenet.com/mycophenolate_mofetil-oral/article.htm.

Enbrel (Etanercept)

Immunex Corporation. "Safety Information and Side Effects of ENBREL." www.enbrel.com/possible-side-effects.jspx.

Humira (Adalimumab)

AbbVie. "Humira (Adalimumab)." www.humira.com.

Imuran (Azathioprine)

American College of Rheumatology. "Azathioprine (Imuran)." www.rheumatology.org/Practice/Clinical/Patients/Medications/Azathioprine_(Imuran)/.

Kineret (Anakinra)

MedicineNet.com. "Anakinra—Injection, Kineret." Last modified April 16, 2014. www.medicinenet.com/anakinra-injectable/article.htm.

Swedish Orphan Biovitrum. "Kineret (Anakinra)." www.kineretrx.com/patient /about-kineretr/side-effects/.

NSAIDs, Prednisone

Berner, J., and C. Gabay. "Best Practice Use of Corticosteroids in Rheumatoid Arthritis." [In French.] *Revue Médicale Suisse* 10, no. 421 (March 2014): 603–6, 608.

MedicineNet.com. "What Are the Side Effects of NSAIDS?" Last modified October 22, 2013. www.medicinenet.com/nonsteroidal_antiinflammatory_drugs/page2.htm #what_are_the_side_effects_of_nsaids.

MedlinePlus. "Ibuprofen." www.nlm.nih.gov/medlineplus/druginfo/meds/a682159.html.

MedlinePlus. "Prednisone." www.nlm.nih.gov/medlineplus/druginfo/meds/a601102 .html.

Plaquenil (Hydroxychloroquine)

American College of Rheumatology. "Hydroxychloroquine (Plaquenil)." www .rheumatology.org/Practice/Clinical/Patients/Medications/Hydroxychloroquine _(Plaquenil)/.

MedlinePlus. "Hydroxychloroquine." www.nlm.nih.gov/medlineplus/druginfo /meds/a601240.html.

Semmelweis, Ignaz Philipp

The Complete Dictionary of Scientific Biography. New York: Charles Scribner's Sons, 2008. www.encyclopedia.com/topic/Ignaz_Philipp_Semmelweis.aspx.

Trexall (Methotrexate)

American College of Rheumatology. "Methotrexate (Rheumatrex, Trexall)." www .rheumatology.org/Practice/Clinical/Patients/Medications/Methotrexate _(Rheumatrex,_Trexall)/.

Chan, E. S., and B. N. Cronstein. "Methotrexate—How Does It Really Work?" *Nature Reviews: Rheumatology* 6, no. 3 (March 2010): 175–78.

MedlinePlus. "Methotrexate." www.nlm.nih.gov/medlineplus/druginfo/meds /a682019.html.

Chapter 3: Your Enemy, Yourself

American Association of Physicians of Indian Origin. *AAPI's Nutrition Guide to Optimal Health: Using Principles of Functional Medicine and Nutritional Genomics.* 2012. http://aapiusa.org/uploads/files/docs/AAPI%20E%20book-%20Entire%20 E%20Book%202-2-2012.pdf.

Arizona Center for Advanced Medicine. "Inflammation." June 26, 2013. http:// arizonaadvancedmedicine.com/inflammation/.

Avena, N. M., P. Rada, and B. G. Hoebel. "Evidence for Sugar Addiction: Behavioral and Neurochemical Effects of Intermittent, Excessive Sugar Intake." *Neuroscience and Biobehavioral Reviews* 32, no. 1 (2008): 20–39.

Backes, C., N. Ludwig, P. Leidinger, C. Harz, J. Hoffmann, A. Keller, E. Meese, et al. "Immunogenicity of Autoantigens." *BMC Genomics* 12 (July 2011): 340.

Bosma-den Boer, M. M., M.-L. van Wetten, and L. Pruimboom. "Chronic Inflammatory Diseases Are Stimulated by Current Lifestyle: How Diet, Stress Levels, and Medication Prevent Our Body from Recovering." *Nutrition and Metabolism* 9, no. 1 (April 2012): 32.

Eisenmann, A., C. Murr, D. Fuchs, and M. Ledochowski. "Gliadin IgG Antibodies and Circulating Immune Complexes." *Scandinavian Journal of Gastroenterology* 44, no. 2 (2009): 168–71.

The Institute for Functional Medicine. "A New Era in Preventing, Managing, and Reversing Cardiovascular and Metabolic Dysfunction." Annual International Conference, Scottsdale, Ariz., May 31–June 3, 2012.

The Institute for Functional Medicine. "Immune Advanced Practice Module." www.functionalmedicine.org/listing.aspx?cid=35.

Isasi, C., I. Colmenero, F. Casco, E. Tejerina, N. Fernandez, J. I. Serrano-Vela, M. J. Castro, et al. "Fibromyalgia and Non-Celiac Gluten Sensitivity: A Description with Remission of Fibromyalgia." *Rheumatology International* (April 12, 2014).

Kantamala, D., M. Vongsakul, and J. Satayavivad. "The In Vivo and In Vitro Effects of Caffeine on Rat Immune Cells Activities: B, T, and NK Cells." *Asian Pacific Journal of Allergy and Immunology* 8, no. 2 (December 1990): 77–82.

Kovarik, J. "From Immunosuppression to Immunomodulation: Current Principles and Future Strategies." *Pathobiology* 80, no. 6 (2013): 275–81.

LeBert, D. C., and A. Huttenlocher. "Inflammation and Wound Repair." *Seminars in Immunology* (May 19, 2014).

Mannik, M., F. A. Nardella, and E. H. Sasso. "Rheumatoid Factors in Immune Complexes of Patients with Rheumatoid Arthritis." *Springer Seminars in Immunopathology* 10, nos. 2–3 (1988): 215–30.

Massachusetts General Hospital. "Inflammation 101: Your Immune System." www.gluegrant.org/immunesystem.htm.

Mathsson, L., J. Lampa, M. Mullazehi, and J. Rönnelid. "Immune Complexes from Rheumatoid Arthritis Synovial Fluid Induce FcγRIIa Dependent and Rheumatoid Factor Correlated Production of Tumour Necrosis Factor-α by Peripheral Blood Mononuclear Cells." *Arthritis Research and Therapy* 8 (2006): R64.

Morris, G., M. Berk, P. Galecki, and M. Maes. "The Emerging Role of Autoimmunity in Myalgic Encephalomyelitis/Chronic Fatigue Syndrome (ME/cfs)." *Molecular Neurobiology* 49, no. 2 (April 2014): 741–56.

Muñoz, L. E., C. Janko, C. Schulze, C. Schorn, K. Sarter, G. Schett, and M. Herrmann. "Autoimmunity and Chronic Inflammation—Two Clearance-Related Steps in the Etiopathogenesis of SLE." *Autoimmunity Reviews* 10, no. 1 (November 2010): 38–42.

Pawelec, G., D. Goldeck, and E. Derhovanessian. "Inflammation, Ageing, and Chronic Disease." *Current Opinion in Immunology* 29C (April 2014): 23–28.

Pollard, K. M., ed. *Autoantibodies and Autoimmunity: Molecular Mechanisms in Health and Disease.* Hoboken, N.J.: John Wiley & Sons, 2006.

Pomorska-Mól, M., I. Markowska-Daniel, K. Kwit, E. Czyżewska, A. Dors, J. Rachubik, and Z. Pejsak. "Immune and Inflammatory Response in Pigs During Acute Influenza Caused by H1N1 Swine Influenza Virus." *Archives of Virology* (May 21, 2014).

Radbruch, A., and P. E. Lipsky, eds. *Current Concepts in Autoimmunity and Chronic Inflammation.* Vol. 305 of *Current Topics in Microbiology and Immunology.* Berlin: Springer Verlag, 2006.

Rescigno, M. "Intestinal Microbiota and Its Effects on the Immune System." *Cellular Microbiology* (May 1, 2014).

Sompayrac, L. M. *How the Immune System Works.* 4th ed. New York: John Wiley & Sons, 2012.

Vojdani, A., and I. Tarash. "Cross-Reaction Between Gliadin and Different Food and Tissue Antigens." *Food and Nutrition Sciences* 4, no. 1 (January 2013): 20–32.

Wang, J., and H. Arase. "Regulation of Immune Responses by Neutrophils." *Annals of the New York Academy of Sciences* (May 21, 2014).

Chapter 4: Heal Your Gut

Adebamowo, C. A., D. Spiegelman, C. S. Berkey, F. W. Danby, H. H. Rockett, G. A. Colditz, W. C. Willett, et al. "Milk Consumption and Acne in Adolescent Girls." *Dermatology Online Journal* 12, no. 4 (May 2006): 1.

Adebamowo, C. A., D. Spiegelman, C. S. Berkey, F. W. Danby, H. H. Rockett, G. A. Colditz, W. C. Willett, et al. "Milk Consumption and Acne in Teenaged Boys." *Journal of the American Academy of Dermatology* 58, no. 5 (May 2008): 787–93.

Ashraf, R., and N. P. Shah. "Immune System Stimulation by Probiotic Microorganisms." *Critical Reviews in Food Science and Nutrition* 54, no. 7 (2014): 938–56.

Aydoğan, B., M. Kiroğlu, D. Altintas, M. Yilmaz, E. Yorgancilar, and Ü. Tuncer. "The Role of Food Allergy in Otitis Media with Effusion." *Otolaryngology: Head and Neck Surgery* 130, no. 6 (June 2004): 747–50.

Biasucci, G., B. Benenati, L. Morelli, E. Bessi, and G. Boehm. "Cesarean Delivery May Affect the Early Biodiversity of Intestinal Bacteria." *Journal of Nutrition* 138, no. 9 (September 2008): 1796S–1800S.

Blum, K., and J. Payne. *Alcohol and the Addictive Brain*, 99–216. New York: Free Press, 1991.

Brandtzaeg, P. "Gatekeeper Function of the Intestinal Epithelium." *Beneficial Microbes* 4, no. 1 (March 2013): 67–82.

Brown, K., D. DeCoffe, E. Molcan, and D. L. Gibson. "Corrections to Article: Diet-Induced Dysbiosis of the Intestinal Microbiota and the Effects on Immunity and Disease. *Nutrients* 4, no. 8 (2012): 1095–119." *Nutrients* 4, no. 11 (2012): 1552–53.

Brown, K., D. DeCoffe, E. Molcan, and D. L. Gibson. "Diet-Induced Dysbiosis of the Intestinal Microbiota and the Effects on Immunity and Disease." *Nutrients* 4, no. 8 (2012): 1095–119.

Buendgens, L., J. Bruensing, M. Matthes, H. Dückers, T. Luedde, C. Trautwein, F. Tacke, et al. "Administration of Proton Pump Inhibitors in Critically Ill Medical Patients Is Associated with Increased Risk of Developing Clostridium Difficile-Associated Diarrhea." *Journal of Critical Care* 29, no. 4 (August 2014): 696.e11–15.

Charalampopoulos, D., and R. A. Rastall, eds. *Prebiotics and Probiotics Science and Technology*. Vols. 1–2. New York: Springer, 2009.

Chen, J., X. He, and J. Huang. "Diet Effects in Gut Microbiome and Obesity." *Journal of Food Science* 79, no. 4 (April 2014): R442–51.

Corleto, V. D., S. Festa, E. Di Giulio, and B. Annibale. "Proton Pump Inhibitor Therapy and Potential Long-Term Harm." *Current Opinion in Endocrinology, Diabetes, and Obesity* 21, no. 1 (February 2014): 3–8.

Crook, W. G. *The Yeast Connection: A Medical Breakthrough*. New York: Vintage, 1986.

Danby, F. W. "Acne, Dairy, and Cancer." *Dermato-Endocrinology* 1, no. 1 (January–February 2009): 12–16.

Danby, F. W. "Nutrition and Acne." *Clinics in Dermatology* 28, no. 6 (November–December 2010): 598–604.

Decker, E., G. Engelmann, A. Findeisen, P. Gerner, M. Laaβ, D. Ney, C. Posovszky, et al. "Cesarean Delivery Is Associated with Celiac Disease but Not Inflammatory Bowel Disease in Children." *Pediatrics* 125, no. 6 (June 2010): e1433–40.

Doe, W. F. "The Intestinal Immune System." *Gut* 30 (1989): 1679–85.

Dominguez-Bello, M. G., E. K. Costello, M. Contreras, M. Magris, G. Hidalgo, N. Fierer, and R. Knight. "Delivery Mode Shapes the Acquisition and Structure of the Initial Microbiota Across Multiple Body Habitats in Newborns." *Proceedings of the National Academy of Sciences of the United States of America* 107, no. 26 (June 2010): 11971–75.

Eberl, G. "A New Vision of Immunity: Homeostasis of the Superorganism." *Mucosal Immunology* 3, no. 5 (September 2010): 450–60.

Fasano, A. "Celiac Disease Insights: Clues to Solving Autoimmunity." *Scientific American*, August 2009.

Fasano, A. "Leaky Gut and Autoimmune Diseases." *Clinical Reviews in Allergy and Immunology* 42, no. 1 (February 2012): 71–78.

Fasano, A. "Zonulin and Its Regulation of Intestinal Barrier Function: The Biological Door to Inflammation, Autoimmunity, and Cancer." *Physiological Reviews* 91, no. 1 (January 2011): 151–75.

Fasano, A., and T. Shea-Donohue. "Mechanisms of Disease: The Role of Intestinal Barrier Function in the Pathogenesis of Gastrointestinal Autoimmune Diseases." *Nature Clinical Practice: Gastroenterology and Hepatology* 2, no. 9 (September 2005): 416–22.

Hamad, M., K. H. Abu-Elteen, and M. Ghaleb. "Estrogen-Dependent Induction of Persistent Vaginal Candidosis in Naïve Mice." *Mycoses* 47, no. 7 (August 2004): 304–9.

Hardy, H., J. Harris, E. Lyon, J. Beal, and A. D. Foey. "Probiotics, Prebiotics, and Immunomodulation of Gut Mucosal Defences: Homeostasis and Immunopathology." *Nutrients* 5, no. 6 (June 2013): 1869–1912.

Hawrelak, J. A., and S. P. Myers. "The Causes of Intestinal Dysbiosis: A Review." *Alternative Medicine Review* 9, no. 2 (June 2004): 180–97.

Hering, N. A., and J. D. Schulzke. "Therapeutic Options to Modulate Barrier Defects in Inflammatory Bowel Disease." *Digestive Diseases* 27, no. 4 (2009): 450–54.

Huebner, F. R., K. W. Lieberman, R. P. Rubino, and J. S. Wall. "Demonstration of High Opioid-Like Activity in Isolated Peptides from Wheat Gluten Hydrolysates." *Peptides* 5, no. 6 (November–December 1984): 1139–47.

Huurre, A., M. Kalliomäki, S. Rautava, M. Rinne, S. Salminen, and E. Isolauri. "Mode of Delivery—Effects on Gut Microbiota and Humoral Immunity." *Neonatology* 93, no. 4 (2008): 236–40.

The Institute for Functional Medicine. "Advanced Practice GI Module." www.functionalmedicine.org/conference.aspx?id=2744&cid=35&section=t324.

The Institute for Functional Medicine. *Textbook of Functional Medicine.* September 2010. www.functionalmedicine.org/listing_detail.aspx?id=2415&cid=34.

Juntti, H., S. Tikkanen, J. Kokkonen, O. P. Alho, and A. Niinimäki. "Cow's Milk Allergy Is Associated with Recurrent Otitis Media During Childhood." *Acta Oto-Laryngologica* 119, no. 8 (1999): 867–73.

Kazi, Y. F., S. Saleem, and N. Kazi. "Investigation of Vaginal Microbiota in Sexually Active Women Using Hormonal Contraceptives in Pakistan." *BMC Urology* 18, no. 12 (August 2012): 22.

Kitano, H., and K. Oda. "Robustness Trade-Offs and Host–Microbial Symbiosis in the Immune System." *Molecular Systems Biology* 2 (2006): 2006.0022.

Krause, R., E. Schwab, D. Bachhiesl, F. Daxböck, C. Wenisch, G. J. Krejs, and E. C. Reisinger. "Role of Candida in Antibiotic-Associated Diarrhea." *Journal of Infectious Diseases* 184, no. 8 (October 2001): 1065–69.

Kumar, V., M. Jarzabek-Chorzelska, J. Sulej, K. Karnewska, T. Farrell, and S. Jablonska. "Celiac Disease and Immunoglobulin A Deficiency: How Effective Are the Serological Methods of Diagnosis?" *Clinical and Vaccine Immunology* 9, no. 6 (November 2002): 1295–1300.

Lam, J. R., J. L. Schneider, W. Zhao, and D. A. Corley. "Proton Pump Inhibitor and Histamine 2 Receptor Antagonist Use and Vitamin B12 Deficiency." *Journal of the American Medical Association* 310, no. 22 (December 2013): 2435–42.

Lammers, K. M., R. Lu, J. Brownley, B. Lu, C. Gerard, K. Thomas, P. Rallabhandi, et al. "Gliadin Induces an Increase in Intestinal Permeability and Zonulin Release by Binding to the Chemokine Receptor CXCR3." *Gastroenterology* 135, no. 1 (July 2008): 194–204, e3.

Lankelma, J. M., M. Nieuwdorp, W. M. de Vos, and W. J. Wiersinga. "The Gut Microbiota in Sickness and Health." [In Dutch.] *Nederlands Tijdschrift voor Geneeskunde* 157 (2014): A5901.

Ludvigsson, J. F., M. Neovius, and L. Hammarström. "Association Between IgA Deficiency and Other Autoimmune Conditions: A Population-Based Matched Cohort Study." *Journal of Clinical Immunology* 34, no. 4 (May 2014): 444–51.

Man, A. L., N. Gicheva, and C. Nicoletti. "The Impact of Ageing on the Intestinal Epithelial Barrier and Immune System." *Cellular Immunology* 289, nos. 1–2 (May–June 2014): 112–18.

McDermott, A. J., and G. B. Huffnagle. "The Microbiome and Regulation of Mucosal Immunity." *Immunology* 142, no. 1 (May 2014): 24–31.

Melnik, B. C. "Evidence for Acne-Promoting Effects of Milk and Other Insulinotropic Dairy Products." *Nestlé Nutrition Institute Workshop Series: Pediatric Program* 67 (2011): 131–45.

Naglik, J. R., D. L. Moyes, B. Wächtler, and B. Hube. "*Candida albicans* Interactions with Epithelial Cells and Mucosal Immunity." *Microbes and Infection* 13, nos. 12–13 (November 2011): 963–76.

National Digestive Diseases Information Clearinghouse (NDDIC), U.S. Department of Health and Human Services. "The Digestive System and How It Works." Last modified September 18, 2013. http://digestive.niddk.nih.gov/ddiseases/pubs/yrdd/.

Nicholson, J. K., E. Holmes, J. Kinross, R. Burcelin, G. Gibson, W. Jia, and S. Pettersson. "Host-Gut Microbiota Metabolic Interactions." *Science* 336, no. 6086 (June 2012): 1262–67.

Pizzorno, J. E., and M. T. Murray. *Textbook of Natural Medicine.* 4th ed. London: Churchill Livingstone, 2012.

Proal, A. D., P. J. Albert, and T. G. Marshall. "The Human Microbiome and Autoimmunity." *Current Opinion in Rheumatology* 25, no. 2 (March 2013): 234–40.

Rescigno, M. "Intestinal Microbiota and Its Effects on the Immune System." *Cellular Microbiology* (May 1, 2014).

Rigon, G., C. Vallone, V. Lucantoni, and F. Signore. "Maternal Factors Pre- and During Delivery Contribute to Gut Microbiota Shaping in Newborns." *Frontiers in Cellular and Infection Microbiology* (July 4, 2012).

Roberfroid, M., G. R. Gibson, L. Hoyles, A. L. McCartney, R. Rastall, I. Rowland, D. Wolvers, et al. "Prebiotic Effects: Metabolic and Health Benefits." *British Journal of Nutrition* 104, suppl. 2 (August 2010): S1–S63.

Rogier, E. W., A. L. Frantz, M. E. Bruno, L. Wedlund, D. A. Cohen, A. J. Stromberg, and C. S. Kaetzel. "Secretory Antibodies in Breast Milk Promote Long-Term Intestinal Homeostasis by Regulating the Gut Microbiota and Host Gene Expression." *Proceedings of the National Academy of Sciences of the United States of America* 111, no. 8 (February 2014): 3074–79.

Ruscin, J. M., R. L. Page II, and R. J. Valuck. "Vitamin B(12) Deficiency Associated with Histamine(2)-Receptor Antagonists and a Proton-Pump Inhibitor." *Annals of Pharmacotherapy* 36, no. 5 (May 2002): 812–16.

Sapone, A., K. M. Lammers, V. Casolaro, M. Cammarota, M. T. Giuliano, M. de Rosa, R. Stefanile, et al. "Divergence of Gut Permeability and Mucosal Immune Gene Expression in Two Gluten-Associated Conditions: Celiac Disease and Gluten Sensitivity." *BMC Medicine* 9 (March 2011): 23.

Sathyabama, S., N. Khan, and J. N. Agrewala. "Friendly Pathogens: Prevent or Provoke Autoimmunity." *Critical Reviews in Microbiology* 40, no. 3 (August 2014): 273–80.

Scrimgeour, A. G., and M. L. Condlin. "Zinc and Micronutrient Combinations to Combat Gastrointestinal Inflammation." *Current Opinion in Clinical Nutrition and Metabolic Care* 12, no. 6 (November 2009): 653–60.

Shoaie, S., and J. Nielsen. "Elucidating the Interactions Between the Human Gut Microbiota and Its Host Through Metabolic Modeling." *Frontiers in Genetics* 5 (April 2014): 86.

Simonart, T. "Acne and Whey Protein Supplementation Among Bodybuilders." *Dermatology* 225, no. 3 (2012): 256–58.

Spampinato, C., and D. Leonardi. "Candida Infections, Causes, Targets, and Resistance Mechanisms: Traditional and Alternative Antifungal Agents." *BioMed Research International* 2013 (2013), Article ID 204237.

Taibi, A., and E. M. Comelli. "Practical Approaches to Probiotics Use." *Applied Physiology, Nutrition, and Metabolism* 39, no. 8 (August 2014): 980–86.

Teschemacher, H. "Opioid Receptor Ligands Derived from Food Proteins." *Current Pharmaceutical Design* 9, no. 16 (2003): 1331–44.

Teschemacher, H., and G. Koch. "Opioids in the Milk." *Endocrine Regulations* 25, no. 3 (September 1991): 147–50.

Teschemacher, H., G. Koch, and V. Brantl. "Milk Protein–Derived Opioid Receptor Ligands." *Biopolymers* 43, no. 2 (1997): 99–117.

Togami, K., Y. Hayashi, S. Chono, and K. Morimoto. "Involvement of Intestinal Permeability in the Oral Absorption of Clarithromycin and Telithromycin." *Biopharmaceutics and Drug Disposition* (May 6, 2014).

Truss, C. O. "Metabolic Abnormalities in Patients with Chronic Candidiasis: The Acetaldehyde Hypothesis." *Journal of Orthomolecular Psychiatry* 13, no. 2 (1984): 66–93.

Ul Haq, M. R., R. Kapila, R. Sharma, V. Saliganti, and S. Kapila. "Comparative Evaluation of Cow β-Casein Variants (A1/A2) Consumption on Th2-Mediated Inflammatory Response in Mouse Gut." *European Journal of Nutrition* 53, no. 4 (June 2014): 1039–49.

Van de Wijgert, J. H., M. C. Verwijs, A. N. Turner, and C. S. Morrison. "Hormonal Contraception Decreases Bacterial Vaginosis but Oral Contraception May Increase

Candidiasis: Implications for HIV Transmission." *AIDS* 27, no. 13 (August 2013): 2141–53.

Vieira, S., O. Pagovich, and M. Kriegel. "Diet, Microbiota, and Autoimmune Diseases." *Lupus* 23, no. 6 (2014): 518–26.

Vojdani, A., P. Rahimian, H. Kalhor, and E. Mordechai. "Immunological Cross-Reactivity Between Candida albicans and Human Tissue." *Journal of Clinical and Laboratory Immunology* 48, no. 1 (1996): 1–15.

West, C. E., M. C. Jenmalm, and S. L. Prescott. "The Gut Microbiota and Its Role in the Development of Allergic Disease: A Wider Perspective." *Clinical and Experimental Allergy* (April 29, 2014).

Wilhelm, S. M., R. G. Rjater, and P. B. Kale-Pradhan. "Perils and Pitfalls of Long-Term Effects of Proton Pump Inhibitors." *Expert Review of Clinical Pharmacology* 6, no. 4 (July 2013): 443–51.

Wright, J., and L. Lenard. *Why Stomach Acid Is Good for You: Natural Relief from Heartburn, Indigestion, Reflux, and GERD.* New York: M. Evans, 2001.

Yu, L. C., J. T. Wang, S. C. Wei, and Y. H. Ni. "Host-Microbial Interactions and Regulation of Intestinal Epithelial Barrier Function: From Physiology to Pathology." *World Journal of Gastrointestinal Pathophysiology* 3, no. 1 (February 2012): 27–43.

Zakout, Y. M., M. M. Salih, and H. G. Ahmed. "Frequency of Candida Species in Papanicolaou Smears Taken from Sudanese Oral Hormonal Contraceptives Users." *Biotech and Histochemistry* 87, no. 2 (February 2012): 95–97.

Chapter 5: Get Rid of Gluten, Grains, and Legumes

Antoniou, M., C. Robinson, and J. Fagan. "GMO Myths and Truths: An Evidence-Based Examination of the Claims Made for the Safety and Efficacy of Genetically Modified Crops and Foods." Earth Open Source. June 2012. http://earthopensource.org/files/pdfs/GMO_Myths_and_Truths/GMO_Myths_and_Truths_1.3.pdf.

Ballantyne, S. *The Paleo Approach: Reverse Autoimmune Disease and Heal Your Body.* Las Vegas: Victory Belt, 2013.

Bergmans, H., C. Logie, K. van Maanen, H. Hermsen, M. Meredyth, and C. van der Vlugt. "Identification of Potentially Hazardous Human Gene Products in GMO Risk Assessment." *Environmental Biosafety Research* 7, no. 1 (January–March 2008): 1–9.

Bjarnason, I., P. Williams, A. So, G. D. Zanelli, A. J. Levi, J. M. Gumpel, T. J. Peters, et al. "Intestinal Permeability and Inflammation in Rheumatoid Arthritis: Effects of Non-Steroidal Anti-Inflammatory Drugs." *Lancet* 2, no. 8413 (November 1984): 1171–74.

Bonds, R. S., T. Midoro-Horiuti, and R. Goldblum. "A Structural Basis for Food Allergy: The Role of Cross-Reactivity." *Current Opinion in Allergy and Clinical Immunology* 8, no. 1 (February 2008): 82–86.

Catassi, C., J. C. Bai, B. Bonaz, G. Bouma, A. Calabrò, A. Carroccio, G. Castillejo, et al. "Non-Celiac Gluten Sensitivity: The New Frontier of Gluten Related Disorders." *Nutrients* 5, no. 10 (October 2013): 3839–53.

Cordain, L., L. Toohey, M. J. Smith, and M. S. Hickey. "Modulation of Immune Function by Dietary Lectins in Rheumatoid Arthritis." *British Journal of Nutrition* 83 (2000): 207–17.

David, W. *Wheat Belly.* Emmaus, PA: Rodale, 2011.

Dieterich, W., B. Esslinger, D. Trapp, E. Hahn, T. Huff, W. Seilmeier, H. Wieser, et al. "Cross Linking to Tissue Transglutaminase and Collagen Favours Gliadin Toxicity in Coeliac Disease." *Gut* 55, no. 4 (April 2006): 478–84.

Drago, S., R. el Asmar, M. di Pierro, M. Grazia Clemente, A. Tripathi, A. Sapone, M. Thakar, et al. "Gliadin, Zonulin, and Gut Permeability: Effects on Celiac and Non-Celiac Intestinal Mucosa and Intestinal Cell Lines." *Scandinavian Journal of Gastroenterology* 41, no. 4 (April 2006): 408–19.

Eswaran, S., J. Tack, and W. D. Chey. "Food: The Forgotten Factor in the Irritable Bowel Syndrome." *Gastroenterological Clinics of North America* 40, no. 1 (March 2011): 141–62.

Farrell, R. J., and C. P. Kelly. "Celiac Sprue." *New England Journal of Medicine* 346, no. 3 (January 2002): 180–88.

Fasano, A. "Physiological, Pathological, and Therapeutic Implications of Zonulin-Mediated Intestinal Barrier Modulation: Living Life on the Edge of the Wall." *American Journal of Pathology* 173, no. 5 (November 2008): 1243–52.

Fasano, A. "Zonulin, Regulation of Tight Junctions, and Autoimmune Diseases." *Annals of the New York Academy of Sciences* 1258, no. 1 (July 2012): 25–33.

Freed, D. L. J. "Do Dietary Lectins Cause Disease?" *British Medical Journal* 318 (April 17, 1999): 1023.

Gasnier, C., C. Dumont, N. Benachour, E. Clair, M. C. Chagnon, and G. E. Séralini. "Glyphosate-Based Herbicides Are Toxic and Endocrine Disruptors in Human Cell Lines." *Toxicology* 262, no. 3 (August 2009): 184–91.

Hadjivassiliou, M., R. A. Grünewald, M. Lawden, G. A. Davies-Jones, T. Powell, and C. M. Smith. "Headache and CNS White Matter Abnormalities Associated with Gluten Sensitivity." *Neurology* 56, no. 3 (February 2001): 385–88.

Hadjivassiliou, M., D. S. Sanders, R. A. Grünewald, N. Woodroofe, S. Boscolo, and D. Aeschlimann. "Gluten Sensitivity: From Gut to Brain." *Lancet Neurology* 9 (2010).

Hansen, C. H., L. Krych, K. Buschard, S. B. Metzdorff, C. Nellemann, L. H. Hansen, D. S. Nielsen, et al. "A Maternal Gluten-Free Diet Reduces Inflammation and Diabetes Incidence in the Offspring of NOD Mice." *Diabetes* (April 2, 2014).

Hausch, F., L. Shan, N. A. Santiago, G. M. Gray, and C. Khosla. "Intestinal Digestive Resistance of Immunodominant Gliadin Peptides." *American Journal of Physiology: Gastrointestinal and Liver Physiology* 283, no. 4 (October 2002): G996–G1003.

Humbert, P., F. Pelletier, B. Dreno, E. Puzenat, and F. Aubin. "Gluten Intolerance and Skin Diseases." *European Journal of Dermatology* 16, no. 1 (January–February 2006): 4–11.

Ingenbleek, Y., and K. S. McCully. "Vegetarianism Produces Subclinical Malnutrition, Hyperhomocysteinemia, and Atherogenesis." *Nutrition* 28, no. 2 (February 2012): 148–53.

The Institute for Responsible Technology. "Health Risks." www.responsible tecnology.org/health-risks.

The Institute for Responsible Technology website. www.responsibletechnology.org.

Jackson, J. R., W. W. Eaton, N. G. Cascella, A. Fasano, and D. L. Kelly. "Neurologic and Psychiatric Manifestations of Celiac Disease and Gluten Sensitivity." *Psychiatric Quarterly* 83, no. 1 (March 2012): 91–102.

Ji, S. *The Dark Side of Wheat: A Critical Appraisal of the Role of Wheat in Human Disease.* http://curezone.com/upload/PDF/Articles/jurplesman/DarkSideWheat _GreenMedInfo.pdf.

Jönsson, T., S. Olsson, B. Ahrén, T. C. Bøg-Hansen, A. Dole, and S. Lindeberg. "Agrarian Diet and Diseases of Affluence—Do Evolutionary Novel Dietary Lectins Cause Leptin Resistance?" *BMC Endocrine Disorders* 5 (December 2005): 10.

Junker, Y., S. Zeissig, S. J. Kim, D. Barisani, H. Wieser, D. A. Leffler, V. Zevallos, et al. "Wheat Amylase Trypsin Inhibitors Drive Intestinal Inflammation via Activation of Toll-Like Receptor 4." *Journal of Experimental Medicine* 209, no. 13 (December 2012): 2395–408.

Kagnoff, M. F. "Celiac Disease: Pathogenesis of a Model Immunogenetic Disease." *Journal of Clinical Investigation* 117, no. 1 (January 2007): 41–49.

Kharrazian, D. "The Gluten, Leaky Gut, Autoimmune Connection™ Seminar." Apex Seminars, 2013.

Koerner, T. B., C. Cléroux, C. Poirier, I. Cantin, A. Alimkulov, and H. Elamparo. "Gluten Contamination in the Canadian Commercial Oat Supply." *Food Additives and Contaminants: Part A; Chemistry, Analysis, Control, Exposure, and Risk Assessment* 28, no. 6 (June 2011): 705–10.

Kornbluth, A., D. B. Sachar, and the Practice Parameters Committee of the American College of Gastroenterology. "Ulcerative Colitis Practice Guidelines in Adults: American College of Gastroenterology, Practice Parameters Committee." *American Journal of Gastroenterology* 105, no. 3 (March 2010): 501–23.

Ludvigsson, J. F., and A. Fasano. "Timing of Introduction of Gluten and Celiac Disease Risk." *Annals of Nutrition and Metabolism* 60, suppl. 2 (2012): 22–29.

Mesnage, R., S. Gress, N. Defarge, and G.-E. Séralini. "Human Cell Toxicity of Pesticides Associated to Wide Scale Agricultural GMOs." *Theorie in der Ökologie* 17 (2013): 118–20.

Nachbar, M. S., and J. D. Oppenheim. "Lectins in the United States Diet: A Survey of Lectins in Commonly Consumed Foods and a Review of the Literature." *American Journal of Clinical Nutrition* 33, no. 11 (November 1980): 2338–45.

Pascual, V., R. Dieli-Crimi, N. López-Palacios, A. Bodas, L. M. Medrano, and C. Núñez. "Inflammatory Bowel Disease and Celiac Disease: Overlaps and Differences." *World Journal of Gastroenterology* 20, no. 17 (May 2014): 4846–56.

Pellegrina, D., O. Perbellini, M. T. Scupoli, C. Tomelleri, C. Zanetti, G. Zoccatelli, M. Fusi, et al. "Effects of Wheat Germ Agglutinin on Human Gastrointestinal Epithelium: Insights from an Experimental Model of Immune/Epithelial Cell Interaction." *Toxicology and Applied Pharmacology* 237, no. 2 (June 2009): 146–53.

Perlmutter, D. *Grain Brain*. New York: Little Brown, 2013.

Richard, S., S. Moslemi, H. Sipahutar, N. Benachour, and G. E. Seralini. "Differential Effects of Glyphosate and Roundup on Human Placental Cells and Aromatase." *Environmental Health Perspectives* 113, no. 6 (2005): 716–20.

Rubio-Tapia, A., R. A. Kyle, E. L. Kaplan, D. R. Johnson, W. Page, F. Erdtmann, T. L. Brantner, et al. "Increased Prevalence and Mortality in Undiagnosed Celiac Disease." *Gastroenterology* 137, no. 1 (July 2009): 88–93.

Samsel, A., and S. Seneff. "Glyphosate, Pathways to Modern Diseases II: Celiac Sprue and Gluten Intolerance." *Interdisciplinary Toxicology* 6, no. 4 (2013): 159–84.

Samsel, A., and S. Seneff. "Glyphosate's Suppression of Cytochrome P450 Enzymes and Amino Acid Biosynthesis by the Gut Microbiome: Pathways to Modern Diseases." *Entropy* 15 (2013): 1416–63.

Sapone, A., L. de Magistris, M. Pietzak, M. G. Clemente, A. Tripathi, F. Cucca, R. Lampis, et al. "Zonulin Upregulation Is Associated with Increased Gut Permeability in Subjects with Type 1 Diabetes and Their Relatives." *Diabetes* 55, no. 5 (May 2006): 1443–49.

Sapone, A., K. M. Lammers, G. Mazzarella, I. Mikhailenko, M. Cartenì, V. Casolaro, and A. Fasano. "Differential Mucosal IL–17 Expression in Two Gliadin-Induced Disorders: Gluten Sensitivity and the Autoimmune Enteropathy Celiac Disease." *International Archives of Allergy and Immunology* 152, no. 1 (2010): 75–80.

Shaoul, R., and A. Lerner. "Associated Autoantibodies in Celiac Disease." *Autoimmunity Reviews* 6, no. 8 (September 2007): 559–65.

Shor, D. B. B., O. Barzilai, M. Ram, D. Izhaky, B. S. Porat-Katz, J. Chapman, M. Blank, et al. "Gluten Sensitivity in Multiple Sclerosis: Experimental Myth or Clinical Truth?" *Annals of the New York Academy of Sciences* 1173 (September 2009): 343–49.

Sjöberg, V., O. Sandström, M. Hedberg, S. Hammarström, O. Hernell, and M. L. Hammarström. "Intestinal T-Cell Responses in Celiac Disease—Impact of Celiac Disease Associated Bacteria." *PLoS ONE* 8, no. 1 (2013): e53414.

Smith, J. M. "Genetically Engineered Foods May Cause Rising Food Allergies—Genetically Engineered Corn." In the Institute for Responsible Technology newsletter *Spilling the Beans*. June 2007.

Smith, J. M., and the Institute for Responsible Technology. *Genetic Roulette*. DVD. Directed by Jeffrey M. Smith. Fairfield, Ia.: The Institute for Responsible Technology, 2012. 85 mins. http://geneticroulettemovie.com.

Sollid, L. M., and B. Jabri. "Triggers and Drivers of Autoimmunity: Lessons from Coeliac Disease." *Nature Reviews: Immunology* 13, no. 4 (April 2013): 294–302.

Thompson, T., A. R. Lee, and T. Grace. "Gluten Contamination of Grains, Seeds, and Flours in the United States: A Pilot Study." *Journal of the American Dietetic Association* 110, no. 6 (June 2010): 937–40.

Tripathi, A., K. M. Lammers, S. Goldblum, T. Shea-Donohue, S. Netzel-Arnett, M. S. Buzza, T. M. Antalis, et al. "Identification of Human Zonulin, a Physiological Modulator of Tight Junctions, as Prehaptoglobin–2." *Proceedings of the National Academy of Sciences of the United States of America* 106, no. 39 (September 2009): 16799–804.

Urbano, G., M. López-Jurado, P. Aranda, C. Vidal-Valverde, E. Tenorio, and J. Porres. "The Role of Phytic Acid in Legumes: Antinutrient or Beneficial Function?" *Journal of Physiology and Biochemistry* 56, no. 3 (September 2000): 283–94.

Verdu, E. F., D. Armstrong, and J. A. Murray. "Between Celiac Disease and Irritable Bowel Syndrome: The 'No Man's Land' of Gluten Sensitivity." *American Journal of Gastroenterology* 104 (June 2009): 1587–94.

Vojdani, A. "The Characterization of the Repertoire of Wheat Antigens and Peptides Involved in the Humoral Immune Responses in Patients with Gluten Sensitivity and Crohn's Disease" *ISRN Allergy* 2011 (2011), Article ID 950104.

Vojdani, A., and I. Tarash. "Cross-Reaction Between Gliadin and Different Food and Tissue Antigens." *Food and Nutrition Sciences* 4, no. 1 (January 2013): 20–32.

Chapter 6: Tame the Toxins

Amy Myers MD. "Biological Dentistry with Stuart Nunnally DDS." Podcast audio. www.dramymyers.com/2013/07/08/tmw-episode-12-biological-dentistry-with -stuart-nunnally-dds/.

Burazor, I., and A. Vojdani. "Chronic Exposure to Oral Pathogens and Autoimmune Reactivity in Acute Coronary Atherothrombosis." *Autoimmune Diseases* 2014 (2014), Article ID 613157.

Carvalho, A. N., J. L. Lim, P. G. Nijland, M. E. Witte, and J. van Horssen. "Glutathione in Multiple Sclerosis: More than Just an Antioxidant?" *Multiple Sclerosis* (May 19, 2014).

Centers for Disease Control and Prevention. "Fourth National Report on Human Exposure to Environmental Chemicals." 2009. www.cdc.gov/exposurereport/pdf/ FourthReport.pdf. [The Fourth Report presents data for 212 chemicals and includes the findings from nationally representative samples for 1999–2004.]

Centers for Disease Control and Prevention. "Fourth National Report on Human Exposure to Environmental Chemicals. Updated Tables, July 2014." 2014. www. cdc.gov/exposurereport/pdf/FourthReport_UpdatedTables_Jul2014.pdf.

Clauw, D. J. "Fibromyalgia: A Clinical Review." *Journal of the American Medical Association* 311, no. 15 (April 2014): 1547–55.

Crinnion, W. *Clean, Green, and Lean.* New York: John Wiley & Sons, 2010.

Darbre, P. D., and P. W. Harvey. "Paraben Esters: Review of Recent Studies of Endocrine Toxicity, Absorption, Esterase, and Human Exposure, and Discussion of Potential Human Health Risks." *Journal of Applied Toxicology* 28, no. 5 (July 2008): 561–78.

Di Pietro, A., B. Baluce, G. Visalli, S. La Maestra, R. Micale, and A. Izzotti. "Ex Vivo Study for the Assessment of Behavioral Factor and Gene Polymorphisms in Individual Susceptibility to Oxidative DNA Damage Metals-Induced." *International Journal of Hygiene and Environmental Health* 214, no. 3 (June 2011): 210–18.

Dr. Ben Lynch Network Sites. "MTHFR.Net." http://MTHFR.net.

Environmental Working Group. "EWG's 2014 Shopper's Guide to Pesticides in Produce." April 2014. www.ewg.org/foodnews/.

Environmental Working Group. "Pollution in People: Cord Blood Contaminants in Minority Newborns." 2009. http://static.ewg.org/reports/2009/minority_cord _blood/2009-Minority-Cord-Blood-Report.pdf.

Fujinami, R. S., M. G. von Herrath, U. Christen, and J. L. Whitton. "Molecular Mimicry, Bystander Activation, or Viral Persistence: Infections and Autoimmune Disease." *Clinical Microbiology Reviews* 19, no. 1 (January 2006): 80–94.

Genetics Home Reference. "What Are Single Nucleotide Polymorphisms (SNPs)?" http://ghr.nlm.nih.gov/handbook/genomicresearch/snp.

Gill, R. F., M. J. McCabe, and A. J. Rosenspire. "Elements of the B Cell Signalosome Are Differentially Affected by Mercury Intoxication." *Autoimmune Diseases* 2014 (2014), Article ID 239358.

Houlihan, J., R. Wiles, K. Thayer, and S. Gray. "Body Burden: The Pollution in People." Environmental Working Group. 2003.

Huggins, H. A. *Uninformed Consent: The Hidden Dangers in Dental Care.* Newburyport, MA: Hampton Roads Publishing, 1999.

Hybenova, M., P. Hrda, J. Procházková, V. D. Stejskal, and I. Sterzl. "The Role of Environmental Factors in Autoimmune Thyroiditis." *Neuro Endocrinology Letters* 31, no. 3 (2010): 283–89.

The Institute for Functional Medicine. "Advanced Practice Detoxification Modules." www.functionalmedicine.org/conference.aspx?id=2744&cid=35&section=t324.

The Institute for Functional Medicine. "Illuminating the Energy Spectrum: Exploring the Evidence and Emerging Clinical Solutions for Managing Pain, Fatigue, and Cognitive Dysfunction." Annual International Conference, Dallas, TX, May

30–June 1, 2013. https://www.functionalmedicine.org/conference.aspx?id=2664& cid=0&section=t241.

Johansson, O. "Disturbance of the Immune System by Electromagnetic Fields—A Potentially Underlying Cause for Cellular Damage and Tissue Repair Reduction Which Could Lead to Disease and Impairment." *Pathophysiology* 16, nos. 2–3 (August 2009): 157–77.

Kaur, S., S. White, and P. M. Bartold. "Periodontal Disease and Rheumatoid Arthritis: A Systematic Review." *Journal of Dental Research* 92, no. 5 (May 2013): 399–408.

Liang, S., Y. Zhou, H. Wang, Y. Qian, D. Ma, W. Tian, V. Persaud-Sharma, et al. "The Effect of Multiple Single Nucleotide Polymorphisms in the Folic Acid Pathway Genes on Homocysteine Metabolism." *BioMed Research International* 2014 (2014), Article ID 560183.

Motts, J. A., D. L. Shirley, E. K. Silbergeld, and J. F. Nyland. "Novel Biomarkers of Mercury-Induced Autoimmune Dysfunction: A Cross-Sectional Study in Amazonian Brazil." *Environmental Research* 132C (July 2014): 12–18.

Nakazawa, D. J. *The Autoimmune Epidemic: Bodies Gone Haywire in a World Out of Balance and the Cutting Edge Science That Promises Hope.* New York: Simon and Schuster, 2008.

Nuttall, S. L., U. Martin, A. J. Sinclair, and M. J. Kendall. "Glutathione: In Sickness and in Health." *Lancet* 351, no. 9103 (February 1998): 645–46.

Ong, J., E. Erdei, R. L. Rubin, C. Miller, C. Ducheneaux, M. O'Leary, B. Pacheco, et al. "Mercury, Autoimmunity, and Environmental Factors on Cheyenne River Sioux Tribal Lands." *Autoimmune Diseases* 2014 (2014), Article ID 325461.

Pinhel, M. A., C. L. Sado, S. Longo Gdos, M. L. Gregório, G. S. Amorim, G. M. Florim, C. M. Mazeti, et al. "Nullity of GSTT1/GSTM1 Related to Pesticides Is Associated with Parkinson's Disease." *Arquivos de Neuropsiquiatr* 71, no. 8 (August 2013): 527–32.

Procházková, J., I. Sterzl, H. Kucerova, J. Bartova, and V. D. Stejskal. "The Beneficial Effect of Amalgam Replacement on Health in Patients with Autoimmunity." *Neuro Endocrinology Letters* 25, no. 3 (June 2004): 211–18.

Salehi, I., K. G. Sani, and A. Zamani. "Exposure of Rats to Extremely Low-Frequency Electromagnetic Fields (ELF-EMF) Alters Cytokines Production." *Electromagnetic Biology and Medicine* 32, no. 1 (March 2013): 1–8.

Seymour, G. J., P. J. Ford, M. P. Cullinan, S. Leishman, and K. Yamazaki. "Relationship Between Periodontal Infections and Systemic Disease." *Clinical Microbiology and Infection* 13, suppl. 4 (October 2007): 3–10.

Sirota, M., M. A. Schaub, S. Batzoglou, W. H. Robinson, and A. J. Butte. "Autoimmune Disease Classification by Inverse Association with SNP Alleles." *PLoS Genetics* 5, no. 12 (December 2009): e1000792.

Song, G. G., S. C. Bae, and Y. H. Lee. "Association of the MTHFR C677T and A1298C Polymorphisms with Methotrexate Toxicity in Rheumatoid Arthritis: A Meta-Analysis." *Clinical Rheumatology* (May 3, 2014).

Stejskal, J., and V. D. Stejskal. "The Role of Metals in Autoimmunity and the Link to Neuroendocrinology." *Neuro Endocrinology Letters* 20, no. 6 (1999): 351–64.

Teens Turning Green. "Sustainable Food Resources: Dirty Thirty." http://www.teensturninggreen.org/wordpress/wp-content/uploads/2013/03/dirtythirty-10-11-10.pdf.

Tsai, C. P., and C. T. Lee. "Multiple Sclerosis Incidence Associated with the Soil Lead and Arsenic Concentrations in Taiwan." *PLoS ONE* 8, no. 6 (June 2013): e65911.

Yang, Q., Y. Xie, and J. W. Depierre. "Effects of Peroxisome Proliferators on the Thymus and Spleen of Mice." *Clinical and Experimental Immunology* 122, no. 2 (November 2000): 219–26.

Bisphenol A (BPA)

Alizadeh, M., F. Ota, K. Hosoi, M. Kato, T. Sakai, and M. A. Satter. "Altered Allergic Cytokine and Antibody Response in Mice Treated with Bisphenol A." *Journal of Medical Investigation* 53, nos. 1–2 (February 2006): 70–80.

Kharrazian, D. "The Potential Roles of Bisphenol A (BPA) Pathogenesis in Autoimmunity." *Autoimmune Diseases* 2014 (2014), Article ID 743616.

Rogers, J. A., L. Metz, and V. W. Yong. "Review: Endocrine Disrupting Chemicals and Immune Responses: A Focus on Bisphenol-A and Its Potential Mechanisms." *Molecular Immunology* 53, no. 4 (April 2013): 421–30.

The EPA's Statistics on Chemicals

Faber, S., and T. Cluderay. "1,000 Chemicals." *EnviroBlog* (blog). Environmental Working Group. May 15, 2014. www.ewg.org/enviroblog/2014/05/1000-chemicals.

U.S. Environmental Protection Agency. "TSCA Chemical Substance Inventory." www.epa.gov/oppt/existingchemicals/pubs/tscainventory/basic.html.

U.S. Environmental Protection Agency website. www.epa.gov.

Flame Retardants

Lunder, S. "Flame Retardants Are Everywhere in Homes, New Studies Find." *EnviroBlog* (blog). Environmental Working Group. November 28, 2012. www .ewg.org/enviroblog/2012/12/toxic-fire-retardants-are-everywhere-homes -new-studies-find.

Indoor Air Quality

American Thoracic Society. "HEPA Filters Reduce Cardiovascular Health Risks Associated with Air Pollution, Study Finds." Science Daily. January 21, 2011. www.sciencedaily.com/releases/2011/01/110121144009.htm.

Environmental Working Group. "EWG's Healthy Home Tips for Parents." 2008. http://static.ewg.org/reports/2008/EWGguide _ goinggreen.pdf.

Reisman, R. E., P. M. Mauriello, G. B. Davis, J. W. Georgitis, and J. M. DeMasi. "A Double-Blind Study of the Effectiveness of a High-Efficiency Particulate Air (HEPA) Filter in the Treatment of Patients with Perennial Allergic Rhinitis and Asthma." *Journal of Allergy and Clinical Immunology* 85, no. 6 (June 1990): 1050–57.

U.S. Environmental Protection Agency. "Indoor Air Quality (IAQ)." www.epa.gov /iaq/.

U.S. Environmental Protection Agency. "Targeting Indoor Air Pollutants: EPA's Approach and Progress." March 1993. http://nepis.epa.gov

Perfluorooctanoic Acid (PFOA)

Environmental Working Group and Commonweal. "PFOA (Perfluorooctanoic Acid)." Human Toxome Project. www.ewg.org/sites/humantoxome/chemicals /chemical.php?chemid=100307.

U.S. Environmental Protection Agency. "Perfluorooctanoic Acid (PFOA) and Fluorinated Telomers." www.epa.gov/oppt/pfoa/pubs/pfoainfo.html.

Skin Care, Cosmetics

Amy Myers MD. "Chemical-Free, Gluten-Free Skin Care with Bob Root." Podcast audio. www.dramymyers.com/2013/07/01/tmw-episode-11-chemical-free-gluten -free-skin-care-with-bob-root/.

Amy Myers MD. "Green Beauty with W3LL PEOPLE." Podcast audio. www.dramy myers.com/2013/08/12/tmw-episode-17-green-beauty-with-w3ll-people/.

Environmental Working Group. "EWG's Skin Deep Cosmetics Database." www.ewg .org/skindeep/.

Root, B. *Chemical-Free Skin Health.* N.p.: M42 Publishing, 2010.

Sigurdson, T., and S. Fellow. "Exposing the Cosmetics Cover-Up: True Horror Stories of Cosmetic Dangers." Environmental Working Group. October 29, 2013. www.ewg.org/research/exposing-cosmetics-cover/true-horror-stories -of-cosmetic-dangers.

Toxic Mold / Mycotoxins

Guilford, F. T., and J. Hope. "Deficient Glutathione in the Pathophysiology of Mycotoxin-Related Illness." *Toxins* [Basel] 6, no. 2 (February 2014): 608–23.

Schaller, J. *Mold Illness and Mold Remediation Made Simple: Removing Mold Toxins from Bodies and Sick Buildings.* Tampa, Fla.: Hope Academic Press, 2005.

Shoemaker, R. C. *Mold Warriors: Fighting America's Hidden Health Threat.* Baltimore: Gateway Press, 2005.

Shoemaker, R. C. *Surviving Mold: Life in the Era of Dangerous Buildings.* Baltimore: Otter Bay Books, 2010.

Surviving Mold website. www.survivingmold.com.

Trichloroethylene (TCE)

Gilbert, K. M., B. Przybyla, N. R. Pumford, T. Han, J. Fuscoe, L. K. Schnackenberg, R. D. Holland, et al. "Delineating Liver Events in Trichloroethylene-Induced Autoimmune Hepatitis." *Chemical Research in Toxicology* 22, no. 4 (April 2009): 626–32.

Gilbert, K. M., B. Rowley, H. Gomez-Acevedo, and S. J. Blossom. "Coexposure to Mercury Increases Immunotoxicity of Trichloroethylene." *Toxicological Sciences* 119, no. 2 (February 2011): 281–92.

Water Safety, Fluoride

Centers for Disease Control and Prevention. "Community Water Fluoridation." www.cdc.gov/fluoridation/faqs/.

Choi, A. L., G. Sun, Y. Zhang, and P. Grandjean. "Developmental Fluoride Neuro-toxicity: A Systematic Review and Meta-Analysis." *Environmental Health Perspectives* 120, no. 10 (October 2012): 1362–68.

Connett, P. "50 Reasons to Oppose Fluoridation." Fluoride Action Network. Last modified September 2012. http://fluoridealert.org/articles/50-reasons/.

Diesendorf, M., J. Colquhoun, B. J. Spittle, D. N. Everingham, and F. W. Clutter-buck. "New Evidence on Fluoridation." *Australia and New Zealand Journal of Public Health* 21, no. 2 (April 1997): 187–90.

Environmental Working Group. "Dog Food Comparison Shows High Fluoride Levels: Health Effects of Fluoride." June 26, 2009. www.ewg.org/research /dog-food-comparison-shows-high-fluoride-levels/health-effects-fluoride.

Environmental Working Group. "EPA Proposes to Phase Out Fluoride Pesticide." July 14, 2011. www.ewg.org/news/testimony-official-correspondence/epa-proposes -phase-out-fluoride-pesticide.

Environmental Working Group. "FDA Should Adopt EPA Tap Water Health Goals as Enforceable Limits for Bottled Water." November 18, 2008. www.ewg .org/news/testimony-official-correspondence/fda-should-adopt-epa-tap -water-health-goals-enforceable.

Environmental Working Group. "Is Your Bottled Water Worth It?: Bottle Vs. Tap—Double Standard." June 10, 2009. www.ewg.org/research/your-bottled -water-worth-it/bottle-vs-tap-double-standard.

Environmental Working Group. "Over 300 Pollutants in U.S. Tap Water." December 2009. www.ewg.org/tapwater/.

Null, G. "Fluoride: Killing Us Softly." Global Research. December 5, 2013. www .globalresearch.ca/fluoride-killing-us-softly/5360397.

U.S. Environmental Protection Agency. "Ground Water and Drinking Water." http://water.epa.gov/drink/.

Chapter 7: Heal Your Infections and Relieve Your Stress

Adrenal Fatigue website. www.adrenalfatigue.org.

Alam, J., Y. C. Kim, and Y. Choi. "Potential Role of Bacterial Infection in Autoimmune Diseases: A New Aspect of Molecular Mimicry." *Immune Network* 14, no. 1 (February 2014): 7–13.

Allen, K., B. E. Shykoff, J. L. Izzo Jr. "Pet Ownership, but Not ACE Inhibitor Therapy, Blunts Home Blood Pressure Responses to Mental Stress." *Hypertension* 38 (October 2001): 815–20.

American College of Rheumatology. "Study Provides Greater Understanding of Lyme Disease-Causing Bacteria." Press release. July 2009. www.rheumatology .org/about/newsroom/2009/2009_07_steere.asp.

Assaf, A. M. "Stress-Induced Immune-Related Diseases and Health Outcomes of Pharmacy Students: A Pilot Study." *Saudi Pharmaceutical Journal* 21, no. 1 (January 2013): 35–44.

Bach, J.-F. "The Effect of Infections on Susceptibility to Autoimmune and Allergic Diseases." *New England Journal of Medicine* 347 (September 2002): 911–20.

Bagi, Z., Z. Broskova, and A. Feher. "Obesity and Coronary Microvascular Disease—Implications for Adipose Tissue-Mediated Remote Inflammatory Response." *Current Vascular Pharmacology* 12, no. 3 (2014): 453–61.

Brady, D. M. "Molecular Mimicry, the Hygiene Hypothesis, Stealth Infections, and Other Examples of Disconnect Between Medical Research and the Practice of Clinical Medicine in Autoimmune Disease." *Open Journal of Rheumatology and Autoimmune Diseases* 3 (2013): 33–39.

Campos-Rodríguez, R., M. Godínez-Victoria, E. Abarca-Rojano, J. Pacheco-Yépez, H. Reyna-Garfias, R. E. Barbosa-Cabrera, and M. E. Drago-Serrano. "Stress Modulates Intestinal Secretory Immunoglobulin A." *Frontiers in Integrative Neuroscience* 7 (December 2, 2013): 86.

Casiraghi, C., and M. S. Horwitz. "Epstein-Barr Virus and Autoimmunity: The Role of a Latent Viral Infection in Multiple Sclerosis and Systemic Lupus Erythematosus Pathogenesis." *Future Virology* 8, no. 2 (2013): 173–82.

Chastain, E. M. L., and S. D. Miller. "Molecular Mimicry as an Inducing Trigger for CNS Autoimmune Demyelinating Disease." *Immunological Reviews* 245, no. 1 (January 2012): 227–38.

Collingwood, J. "The Power of Music to Reduce Stress." Psych Central. http://psychcentral.com/lib/the-power-of-music-to-reduce-stress/000930?all=1.

Cusick, M. F., J. E. Libbey, and R. S. Fujinami. "Molecular Mimicry as a Mechanism of Autoimmune Disease." *Clinical Reviews in Allergy and Immunology* 42, no. 1 (February 2012): 102–11.

Davis, S. L. "Environmental Modulation of the Immune System via the Endocrine System." *Domestic Animal Endocrinology* 15, no. 5 (September 1998): 283–89.

De Brouwer, S. J., H. van Middendorp, C. Stormink, F. W. Kraaimaat, I. Joosten, T. R. Radstake, E. M. de Jong, et al. "Immune Responses to Stress in Rheumatoid Arthritis and Psoriasis." *Rheumatology* [Oxford] (May 20, 2014).

Delogu, L. G., S. Deidda, G. Delitala, and R. Manetti. "Infectious Diseases and Autoimmunity." *Journal of Infection in Developing Countries* 5, no. 10 (October 2011): 679–87.

Draborg, A. H., K. Duus, and G. Houen. "Epstein-Barr Virus in Systemic Autoimmune Diseases." *Clinical and Developmental Immunology* 2013 (2013), Article ID 535738.

Ercolini, A. M., and S. D. Miller. "The Role of Infections in Autoimmune Disease." *Clinical and Experimental Immunology* 155, no. 1 (January 2009): 1–15.

Gądek-Michalska, A., J. Tadeusz, P. Rachwalska, and J. Bugajski. "Cytokines, Prostaglandins, and Nitric Oxide in the Regulation of Stress-Response Systems." *Pharmacological Reports* 65, no. 6 (2013): 1655–62.

Gagliani, N., B. Hu, S. Huber, E. Elinav, and R. A. Flavell. "The Fire Within: Microbes Inflame Tumors." *Cell* 157, no. 4 (May 2014): 776–83.

Getts, D. R., E. M. L. Chastain, R. L. Terry, and S. D. Miller. "Virus Infection, Antiviral Immunity, and Autoimmunity." *Immunological Reviews* 255, no. 1 (September 2013): 197–209.

Godbout, J. P., and R. Glaser. "Stress-Induced Immune Dysregulation: Implications for Wound Healing, Infectious Disease, and Cancer." *Journal of Neuroimmune Pharmacology* 1, no. 4 (December 2006): 421–27.

Gomez-Merino, D., C. Drogou, M. Chennaoui, E. Tiollier, J. Mathieu, and C. Y. Guezennec. "Effects of Combined Stress During Intense Training on Cellular Immunity, Hormones, and Respiratory Infections." *Neuroimmunomodulation* 12, no. 3 (2005): 164–72.

Grossman, P., L. Niemann, S. Schmidt, and H. Walach. "Mindfulness-Based Stress Reduction and Health Benefits: A Meta-Analysis." *Journal of Psychosomatic Research* 57, no. 1 (July 2004): 35–43.

Gupta, A., R. Rezvani, M. Lapointe, P. Poursharifi, P. Marceau, S. Tiwari, A. Tchernof, et al. "Downregulation of Complement C3 and C3aR Expression in Subcutaneous Adipose Tissue in Obese Women." *PLoS ONE* 9, no. 4 (April 2014): e95478.

The Institute for Functional Medicine. "The Challenge of Emerging Infections in the 21st Century: Terrain, Tolerance, and Susceptibility." Annual International Conference, Bellevue, Wash., April 28–30, 2011.

Irwin, M., M. Daniels, S. C. Risch, E. Bloom, and H. Weiner. "Plasma Cortisol and Natural Killer Cell Activity During Bereavement." *Biological Psychiatry* 24, no. 2 (June 1988): 173–78.

Kabat-Zinn, J., A. O. Massion, J. Kristeller, L. G. Peterson, K. E. Fletcher, L. Pbert, W. R. Lenderking, et al. "Effectiveness of a Meditation-Based Stress Reduction

Program in the Treatment of Anxiety Disorders." *American Journal of Psychiatry* 149, no. 7 (July 1992): 936–43.

Khansari, D. N., A. J. Murgo, and R. E. Faith. "Effects of Stress on the Immune System." *Immunology Today* 11 (1990): 170–75.

Labrique-Walusis, F., K. J. Keister, and A. C. Russell. "Massage Therapy for Stress Management: Implications for Nursing Practice." *Orthopedic Nursing* 29, no. 4 (July–August 2010): 254–57; quiz 258–59.

Lünemann, J. D., T. Kamradt, R. Martin, and C. Münz. "Epstein-Barr Virus: Environmental Trigger of Multiple Sclerosis?" *Journal of Virology* 81, no. 13 (July 2007): 6777–84.

Mameli, G., D. Cossu, E. Cocco, S. Masala, J. Frau, M. G. Marrosu, and L. A. Sechi. "Epstein-Barr Virus and Mycobacterium Avium Subsp. Paratuberculosis Peptides Are Cross Recognized by Anti-Myelin Basic Protein Antibodies in Multiple Sclerosis Patients." *Journal of Neuroimmunology* 270, nos. 1–2 (May 2014): 51–55.

Marshall, T. "VDR Receptor Competence Induces Recovery from Chronic Autoimmune Disease." Presented at the Sixth International Congress on Autoimmunity, Porto, Portugal, September 10–14, 2008. Directed by Autoimmunity Research Foundation. http://autoimmunityresearch.org/transcripts/ICA2008 _Transcript_TrevorMarshall.pdf.

Maru, G. B., K. Gandhi, A. Ramchandani, and G. Kumar. "The Role of Inflammation in Skin Cancer." *Advances in Experimental Medicine and Biology* 816 (2014): 437–69.

Nelson, P., P. Rylance, D. Roden, M. Trela, and N. Tugnet. "Viruses as Potential Pathogenic Agents in Systemic Lupus Erythematosus." *Lupus* 23, no. 6 (May 2014): 596–605.

Pender, M. P. "CD8+ T-Cell Deficiency, Epstein-Barr Virus Infection, Vitamin D Deficiency, and Steps to Autoimmunity: A Unifying Hypothesis." *Autoimmune Diseases* 2012 (2012), Article ID 189096.

Pohl, J., G. N. Luheshi, and B. Woodside. "Effect of Obesity on the Acute Inflammatory Response in Pregnant and Cycling Female Rats." *Journal of Neuroendocrinology* 25, no. 5 (May 2013): 433–45.

Prasad, R., J. C. Kowalczyk, E. Meimaridou, H. L. Storr, and L. A. Metherell. "Oxidative Stress and Adrenocortical Insufficiency." *Journal of Endocrinology* 221, no. 3 (June 2014): R63–R73.

Rapaport, M. H., P. Schettler, and C. Bresee. "A Preliminary Study of the Effects of Repeated Massage on Hypothalamic-Pituitary-Adrenal and Immune Function in Healthy Individuals: A Study of Mechanisms of Action and Dosage." *Journal of Alternative and Complementary Medicine* 18, no. 8 (August 2012): 789–97.

Rashid, T., and A. Ebringer. "Autoimmunity in Rheumatic Diseases Is Induced by Microbial Infections via Crossreactivity or Molecular Mimicry." *Autoimmune Diseases* 2012 (2012), Article ID 539282.

Rigante, D., M. B. Mazzoni, and S. Esposito. "The Cryptic Interplay Between Systemic Lupus Erythematosus and Infections." *Autoimmunity Reviews* 13, no. 2 (February 2014): 96–102.

Rose, N. R. "The Role of Infection in the Pathogenesis of Autoimmune Disease." *Seminars in Immunology* 10, no. 1 (February 1998): 5–13.

Sapolsky, R. *Why Zebras Don't Get Ulcers.* New York: Holt, 2004.

Segerstrom, S. C., and G. E. Miller. "Psychological Stress and the Human Immune

System: A Meta-Analytic Study of 30 Years of Inquiry." *Psychological Bulletin* 130, no. 4 (July 2004): 601–30.

Sfriso, P., A. Ghirardello, C. Botsios, M. Tonon, M. Zen, N. Bassi, F. Bassetto, et al. "Infections and Autoimmunity: The Multifaceted Relationship." *Journal of Leukocyte Biology* 87, no. 3 (March 2010): 385–95.

Shoenfeld, Y., G. Zandman-Goddard, L. Stojanovich, M. Cutolo, H. Amital, Y. Levy, M. Abu-Shakra, et al. "The Mosaic of Autoimmunity: Hormonal and Environmental Factors Involved in Autoimmune Diseases—2008." *Israel Medical Association Journal* 10, no. 1 (January 2008): 8–12.

Smolders, J. "Vitamin D and Multiple Sclerosis: Correlation, Causality, and Controversy." *Autoimmune Diseases* 2011 (2011), Article ID 629538.

Szymula, A., J. Rosenthal, B. M. Szczerba, H. Bagavant, S. M. Fu, and U. S. Deshmukh. "T Cell Epitope Mimicry Between Sjögren's Syndrome Antigen A (SSA)/Ro60 and Oral, Gut, Skin, and Vaginal Bacteria." *Clinical Immunology* 152, nos. 1–2 (May–June 2014): 1–9.

Uchakin, P. N., D. C. Parish, F. C. Dane, O. N. Uchakina, A. P. Scheetz, N. K. Agarwal, and B. E. Smith. "Fatigue in Medical Residents Leads to Reactivation of Herpes Virus Latency." *Interdisciplinary Perspectives on Infectious Diseases* 2011 (2011), Article ID 571340.

Vojdani, A. "A Potential Link Between Environmental Triggers and Autoimmunity." *Autoimmune Diseases* 2014 (2014), Article ID 437231.

Wilson, J., and J. V. Wright. *Adrenal Fatigue: The 21st Century Stress Syndrome.* Petaluma, CA: Smart Publications, 2001.

Wucherpfennig, K. W. "Mechanisms for the Induction of Autoimmunity by Infectious Agents." *Journal of Clinical Investigation* 108, no. 8 (October 2001): 1097–104.

Wucherpfennig, K. W. "Structural Basis of Molecular Mimicry." *Journal of Autoimmunity* 16, no. 3 (May 2001): 293–302.

Yang, C. Y., P. S. Leung, I. E. Adamopoulos, and M. E. Gershwin. "The Implication of Vitamin D and Autoimmunity: A Comprehensive Review." *Clinical Reviews in Allergy and Immunology* 45, no. 2 (October 2013): 217–26.

Yeung, S.-C. J. "Graves' Disease." Medscape. Last updated May 30, 2014. http://emedicine.medscape.com/article/120619-overview.

Chapter 8: Putting The Myers Way into Practice

Amy Myers MD. "Sleep Expert Dan Pardi." Podcast audio. www.dramymyers.com/2013/06/24/tmw-episode-10-sleep-expert-dan-pardi/.

Burkhart, K., and J. R. Phelps. "Amber Lenses to Block Blue Light and Improve Sleep: A Randomized Trial." *Chronobiology International* 26, no. 8 (December 2009): 1602–12.

Cordain, L., S. B. Eaton, A. Sebastian, N. Mann, S. Lindeberg, B. A. Watkins, J. H. O'Keefe, et al. "Origins and Evolution of the Western Diet: Health Implications for the 21st Century." *American Journal of Clinical Nutrition* 81, no. 2 (February 2005): 341–54.

Environmental Working Group. "Cell Phone Radiation Depends on Wireless Carrier." November 12, 2013. www.ewg.org/research/cell-phone-radiation-depends -wireless-carrier.

The Institute for Functional Medicine. *Clinical Nutrition: A Functional Approach Textbook.* 2nd ed. 2004.

The Institute for Functional Medicine. "Functional Perspectives on Food and Nutrition: The Ultimate Upstream Medicine." Annual International Conference, San Francisco, CA, May 29–31, 2014. www.functionalmedicine.org/conference .aspx?id=2711&cid=35&section=t281.

The Institute for Functional Medicine. *Textbook of Functional Medicine.* September 2010. www.functionalmedicine.org/listing _ detail.aspx?id=2415&cid=34.

Johansson, O. "Disturbance of the Immune System by Electromagnetic Fields—A Potentially Underlying Cause for Cellular Damage and Tissue Repair Reduction Which Could Lead to Disease and Impairment." *Pathophysiology* 16, nos. 2–3 (August 2009): 157–77.

Liu,Y., A. G. Wheaton, D. P. Chapman, and J. B. Croft. "Sleep Duration and Chronic Diseases Among U.S. Adults Age 45 Years and Older: Evidence from the 2010 Behavioral Risk Factor Surveillance System." *Sleep* 36, no. 10 (October 2013): 1421–27.

Wu, C., N. Yosef, T. Thalhamer, C. Zhu, S. Xiao, Y. Kishi, A. Regev, et al. "Induction of Pathogenic TH17 Cells by Inducible Salt-Sensing Kinase SGK1." *Nature* 496, no. 7446 (April 2013): 513–17.

Chapter 9: Your Thirty-Day Protocol

García-Niño, W. R., and J. Pedraza-Chaverrí. "Protective Effect of Curcumin Against Heavy Metals-Induced Liver Damage." *Food and Chemical Toxicology* 69C (July 2014): 182–201.

Gleeson, M. "Nutritional Support to Maintain Proper Immune Status During Intense Training." *Nestlé Nutrition Institute Workshop Series* 75 (2013): 85–97.

Lieberman, S., M. G. Enig, and H. G. Preuss. "A Review of Monolaurin and Lauric Acid: Natural Virucidal and Bactericidal Agents." *Alternative and Complementary Therapies* 12, no. 6 (December 2006): 310–14.

Ogbolu, D. O., A. A. Oni, O. A. Daini, and A. P. Oloko. "In Vitro Antimicrobial Properties of Coconut Oil on Candida Species in Ibadan, Nigeria." *Journal of Medicinal Food* 10, no. 2 (June 2007): 384–87.

Özdemir, Ö. "Any Role for Probiotics in the Therapy or Prevention of Autoimmune Diseases? Up-to-Date Review." *Journal of Complementary and Integrative Medicine* 10 (August 2013).

Patavino, T., and D. M. Brady. "Natural Medicine and Nutritional Therapy as an Alternative Treatment in Systemic Lupus Erythematosus." *Alternative Medicine Review* 6, no. 5 (October 2001): 460–71.

Ramadan, G., and O. El-Menshawy. "Protective Effects of Ginger-Turmeric Rhizomes Mixture on Joint Inflammation, Atherogenesis, Kidney Dysfunction, and Other Complications in a Rat Model of Human Rheumatoid Arthritis." *International Journal of Rheumatic Diseases* 16, no. 2 (April 2013): 219–29.

Wang, G., J. Wang, H. Ma, G. A. Ansari, and M. F. Khan. "N-Acetylcysteine Protects Against Trichloroethene-Mediated Autoimmunity by Attenuating Oxidative Stress." *Toxicology and Applied Pharmacology* 273, no. 1 (November 2013): 189–95.

Notes

a. Most autoimmune conditions are far more common among women. Researchers believe that this is because of women's higher estrogen levels and greater number of hormonal shifts.

b. Because this medication affects the gut lining, it is also a known risk factor for a condition known as "leaky gut." For more information on how leaky gut contributes to autoimmune disorders, see chapters 4 and 5.

c. I keep specifying "harmful" bacteria because there are actually loads of friendly bacteria that you want to welcome into your gut and into the rest of your body. We'll learn more about them in chapter 4.

d. If you have an autoimmune condition or are high on the autoimmune spectrum, you might need two or three months for full gut healing. We'll be using all-natural remedies in this book, but in some cases you might need to see a functional medicine physician to get some prescription medications. Whatever your condition, however, if you strictly follow The Myers Way, you should notice significant improvements in thirty days, and that should motivate you to keep going.

e. While scientists are not completely sure how to categorize these conditions, the latest thinking is that ulcerative colitis, Crohn's disease, and other types of irritable bowel disorder are all forms of autoimmune disorders in which the body attacks its own intestinal tissue.

Index

absorption, 76, 84, 87–88
acetyl-glutathione, 197, 198, 199
acid reflux, 7, 42, 60, 82–86
acne
  as autoimmunity indicator, 7, 21, 26
  dairy sensitivity causing, 81, 86
  and gut health, 73, 76, 77
  healing, 188, 287
  from inflammation, 58, 60
acorn squash recipe, 218
acute inflammation, 51, 59
adaptogenic herbal blend, 168, 200
Addison's disease, 166
adrenal fatigue, 166–168, 189, 200
agglutinins, 110, 112
air filters, 127, 128–129, 350
alcohol, 77, 87, 95, 182, 293–294, 346
allergies, food, 56–57, 60, 77–81, 98,
  100, 187
allergies, respiratory, 60, 73, 331, 342
aloe vera, 89, 197, 198, 259
amber lightbulbs, 344
amino acids, 82–83, 84, 89, 176
antibiotics
  pitfalls of, 28, 77, 80–82, 85, 86, 314
  repairing damage by, 88, 156, 301
antibodies
  gluten look-alikes, 99–100, 105,
    106–108
  immune system role, 53–56
  inflammatory response and, 58, 64,
    78, 79, 98
  nightshades producing, 112
  passed in birth, 177
  and TCE, 130
  types of, 56–57
  viral infection, 153, 154
antigens, 107–108
antinutrients, 111
anxiety, 7, 58, 60, 73, 76, 80–81
apple recipes, 249, 265
arsenic exposure, 139–140
arthritis, 7, 26, 37, 60, 73, 156

Artichokes with Ume Plum
  Vinaigrette, 223
Arugula, Blood Orange, and Fennel
  Salad, 233
asparagus recipes, 224, 251
asthma, 7, 60, 73, 331, 342
autism, 8, 9
autoimmune disorders
  chronic inflammation triggering,
    60–64
  conventional approaches, 3–10,
    48–49, 63 (*See also* autoimmunity
    myths)
  hygiene hypothesis, 28
  link to infections, 151–157
  medications, 36–39, 48–49
  online resources, 355–356
  prevalence of, 19, 26–27
  solutions, 18–20, 28–30, 45–47
  warning signs, 7, 20–25
  See also Myers Way Autoimmune
    Program
autoimmune spectrum, 8, 20–25, 46
Autoimmune Summit, 11–12
autoimmunity myths
  digestive issues, 40
  genetics, 34–35, 42
  gluten-free dismissal, 40–41
  irreversibility, 34–35, 46
  medication side effects, 36–39
  necessity of medication, 33–36
  overview of, 32–34
  quality of life, 42
  treating symptoms, 42–43
avocado recipes
  dressing, 237
  main dishes, 242, 243, 244, 246,
    250, 255
  salads, 230, 232, 237, 239, 241
  snacks, 236, 237, 264

bacteria
  dental work and, 337